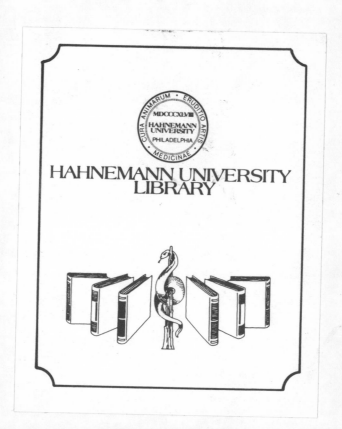

Atlas of Clinical Neuropathology

Atlas of Clinical Neuropathology

Sydney S. Schochet, Jr., M.D.
Professor of Pathology, Neurology, and Neurosurgery
Department of Pathology
West Virginia University School of Medicine
Morgantown, West Virginia

Jeannie Nelson, M.D.
Assistant Professor of Neurology
Department of Neurology
West Virginia University School of Medicine
Morgantown, West Virginia

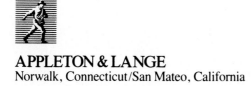

APPLETON & LANGE
Norwalk, Connecticut/San Mateo, California

0-8385-0114-1

Copyright © 1989 by Appleton & Lange
A Publishing Division of Prentice Hall

Figures 1–6D, 1–10B, 2–15D, 3–21B, 5–2D, 5–10A, 8–5C, and 8–21B are
reproduced from Schochet, SS Jr & McCormick, WF: Essentials of
Neuropathology. New York: Appleton–Century–Crofts, 1979.

89 90 91 93/ 10 9 8 7 6 5 4 3 2 1

Prentice-Hall International (UK) Limited, *London*
Prentice-Hall of Australia Pty. Limited, *Sydney*
Prentice-Hall Canada, Inc., *Toronto*
Prentice-Hall Hispanoamericana, S.A., *Mexico*
Prentice-Hall India Private Limited, *New Delhi*
Prentice-Hall of Japan, Inc., *Tokyo*
Simon & Schuster Asia Pte. Ltd., *Singapore*
Editora Prentice-Hall do Brasil Ltda., *Rio de Janeiro*
Prentice-Hall, *Englewood Cliffs, New Jersey*

Library of Congress Cataloging-in-Publication Data

Schochet, Sydney S., 1937–
      Altas of clinical neuropathology.

      1. Nervous system—Diseases—Atlases.
I. Nelson, Jeannie, 1954-   II. Title.
[DNLM: 1. Nervous System diseases—pathology
—atlases. WL 17 S363a]
RC347.S34   1989   616.8'071'0222   88–34403
ISBN 0–8385–0114–1

Production Editor: Elizabeth Ryan
Designer: Steve M. Byrum
Acquisitions Editor: William R. Schmitt

PRINTED IN THE UNITED STATES OF AMERICA

Contents

Introduction/vii

1. Congenital and Perinatal Disorders/1

2. Infections/57

3. Vascular Disease/119

4. Trauma/191

5. Intoxications and Deficiency States/225

6. Demyelinating and Metabolic Diseases/255

7. Dementias and Degenerations/283

8. Neoplasms/323

Index/383

Introduction

The authors, a neuropathologist with an interest in clinical neurology, and a clinical neurologist with an interest in neuropathology, have collaborated to prepare a book that portrays the pathology of some of the disorders that their clinical colleagues encounter in the practice of neurology and neurosurgery. Both surgical and postmortem material have been included. Postmortem gross specimens have been emphasized since the general decline in autopsies has made it more difficult for medical students and trainees in neurology, neurosurgery, and pathology to study the clinicopathological correlations provided by these specimens. Histology has been included when it facilitates further understanding of a disease process. A single volume of this nature obviously cannot present comprehensive discussions of the many topics that are presented. Therefore, numerous references are included to complement our brief text. The references have been selected from ones that the authors found especially useful in their pursuit of the various topics.

We thank our colleagues in the departments of Neurology, Neurosurgery, and Pathology for their assistance in making the clinical and pathological material available for our use. We thank Linda Kent Tomago for typing and retyping our manuscripts and Patricia Russell Turner for preparing our illustrations. Without their contributions, this book would not have been possible. We also want to thank Elizabeth Ryan of Appleton & Lange for her help with the editorial process.

1

Congenital and Perinatal Disorders

1.1   Anencephaly

Anencephaly Craniorachischisis

CLINICAL

This female infant was the second of twins delivered by cesarean section. At 36 weeks of gestation, the mother had had an ultrasound examination because of severe polyhydramnios. The study disclosed twins, one of whom was anencephalic.

PATHOLOGY

This infant displayed the typical features of anencephaly craniorachischisis (Fig. 1–1A). The calvarium was nearly absent and the base of the skull was malformed, lacking demarcation of the middle fossa. The eyes were unusually prominent due to the shallow orbits. The head was retroflexed and the neural arches were widely open with dysplastic spinal tissue exposed in the depths of the spinal canal (Fig. 1–1B). The brain was replaced by an irregular mass of reddish tissue, the area cerebrovasculosa. Microscopically, this was composed of disorganized neuroglial tissue and thin-walled blood vessels partially covered by vascularized connective tissue corresponding to the leptomeninges (Fig. 1–1C). Portions of choroid plexi and ependyma were also identified.

COMMENT

Anencephaly is the most common major malformation of the central nervous system and has a prevalence of about 1 per 1000 births. The prevalence shows considerable variation in different parts of the world. No consistent chromosomal abnormalities or maternal insults have been identified. As in the present case, twins show a low rate of concordance and there is a strong female predominance. Polyhydramnios frequently occurs during the pregnancy. The affected infants are often premature and delivered stillborn or die shortly after birth.

The eyes are usually well developed, although the optic nerves terminate blindly in the orbits. The relatively normal development of the globes suggests that the craniocerebral lesion must arise after formation of the optic vesicles. The anterior lobe of the pituitary is consistently present; however, the posterior lobe and hypothalamus are missing. The lack of normal pituitary function is responsible for the associated adrenal hypoplasia. Other visceral abnormalities may be present, including hypoplastic lungs and a relatively large thymus.

In less severe forms, so-called anencephaly acrania (Fig. 1–1D), components of the brain stem, such as the mesencephalon, pons, and medulla, may be present. Although there is no skin defect, the neural arches of the spine are generally unfused. The abnormal spinal cord is often small. Extradural spinal roots are always demonstrable.

REFERENCE

Giroud A: Anencephaly. In Vinken PJ, Bruyn GW (eds): Handbook of Clinical Neurology. Amsterdam, Elsevier, 1977, vol 30, chap 6, pp 173-208.

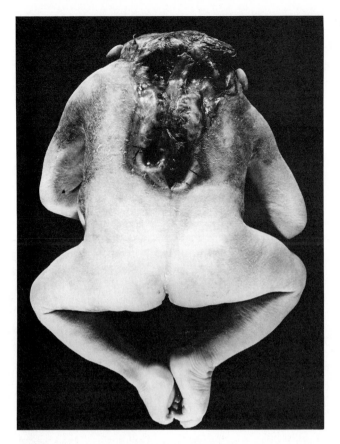

Figure 1–1A. Anencephaly craniorachischisis.

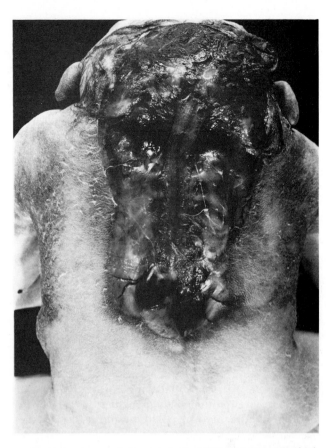

Figure 1–1B. Anencephaly craniorachischisis showing details of spinal dysraphia.

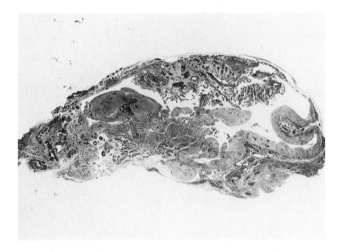

Figure 1–1C. Macrosection of a portion of the area cerebrovasculosa. Note the disorganized neural tissue and accompanying choroid plexus.

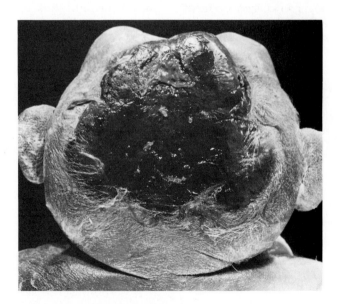

Figure 1–1D. Anencephaly acrania.

1.2   Iniencephaly

CLINICAL

This dysmorphic stillborn infant was delivered at approximately 36 weeks of gestation.

PATHOLOGY

This infant showed the characteristic external features of iniencephaly. The head was retroflexed and there was virtually no neck (Fig. 1–2A). In addition, there was a partially cystic midline mass overlying the thoracic region of the back (Fig. 1–2B).

COMMENT

Iniencephaly is a rare malformation that is encountered predominantly in female infants. The pregnancy is often complicated by polyhydramnios but the gestation usually goes to term. The infants are often stillborn or die shortly after birth. As shown in an x-ray from another case, the cervical spine and the cervical vertebrae are severely malformed (Fig. 1–2C). Portions of cerebrum, cerebellum, and malformed brain stem protrude through the enlarged foramen magnum and may be within a dorsal cyst along with dysplastic spinal cord.

The cerebrum shows a wide spectrum of anomalies including hypoplasia of various lobes, partial fusion of the hemispheres, polymicrogyria, and heterotopias. None of these abnormalities appears to be characteristic of iniencephaly and vary from case to case. We have studied one case in which the cerebrum was divided into three large masses rather than the expected two hemispheres. In this case, the ventricular system was partially obliterated and the cerebellum was hypoplastic. In other cases, the cerebellum has been described as normal, showing vermian agenesis or containing cysts.

REFERENCE

Aleksic S, Budzilovich G, Greco MA, et al: Iniencephaly: A neuropathologic study. Clin Neuropathol 1983; 2:55-61.

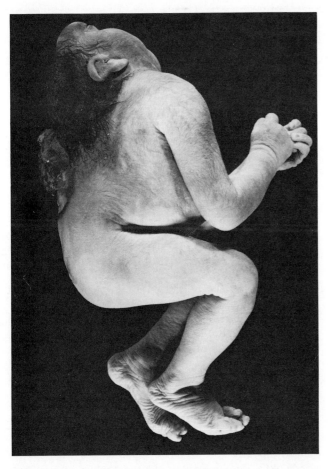

Figure 1–2A. Iniencephaly. Note the retroflexion of the head and absence of the neck.

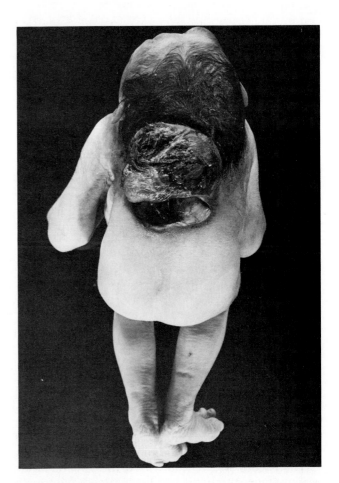

Figure 1–2B. Iniencephaly. Dorsal view showing the cystic midline mass.

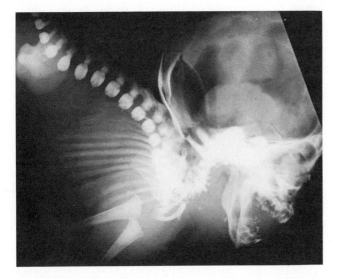

Figure 1–2C. Lateral radiograph showing the severely malformed cervical spine.

1.3 Occipital Encephalocele

CLINICAL

This female infant was born prematurely at 35 weeks of gestation. At birth she was noted to have a small head with a large occipital encephalocele. A computerized tomogram of the head demonstrated an occipital skull defect and the large encephalocele (Fig. 1–3A). At 4 months of age, the patient was attentive to her environment, able to hold her head up, and moved all four extremities spontaneously. The encephalocele was surgically removed.

PATHOLOGY

The surgical specimen consisted of a saccular dural structure covered by intact skin. Contained within the sac was a large portion of cerebral tissue (Fig. 1–3B) and a small portion of cerebellar tissue. The cortex of the cerebral tissue showed moderately complex convolutional markings. The interior of the cerebral tissue was multiloculated and had been in continuity with the occipital horn (Fig. 1–3C). The ependymal lining was partially disrupted and the periventricular white matter was reduced in volume. Gray-white and yellow foci of necrosis and mineralization were visible from the interior of the encephalocele. Grossly, the cerebellar tissue within the encephalocele was normal, but microscopically, it displayed an unusually prominent external granular cell layer (Fig. 1–3D).

COMMENT

Encephaloceles are rare lesions, with an incidence of about 1 per 10,000 births. They most commonly involve the occipital region except among orientals in whom frontal lesions are more common. Other locations are rarely affected. The head is often microcephalic and the cerebral hemispheres are of unequal size, with the encephalocele arising from the smaller hemisphere. The remainder of the cerebrum and ventricular system are often malformed. Occipital encephaloceles often contain disorganized cerebellar tissue and may contain portions of the brain stem. This obviously complicates the surgical management of these cases.

REFERENCES

Friede RL: Developmental Neuropathology. New York, Springer Verlag, 1975, pp 236-240.

Karch SB, Urich H: Occipital encephaloceles: A morphological study. J Neurol Sci 1972; 15:89-122.

Yokota A, Matsukado Y, Fuwa I, et al: Anterior basal encephalocele of the neonatal period. Neurosurgery 1986; 19:468-478.

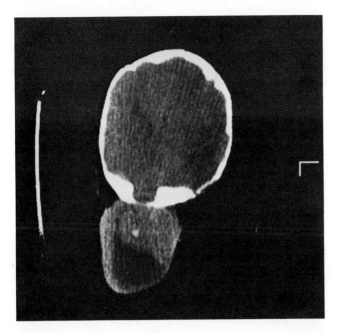

Figure 1–3A. Computerized tomogram showing partially cystic occipital encephalocele.

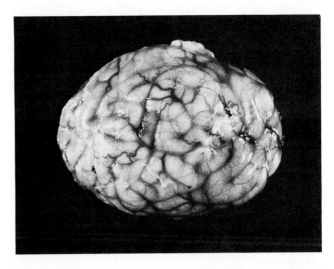

Figure 1–3B. Malformed cerebral tissue contained in the occipital encephalocele.

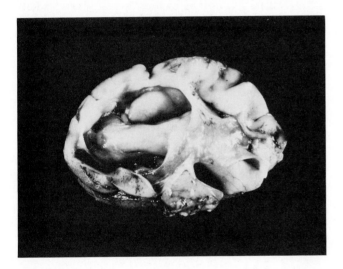

Figure 1–3C. Section of cerebral tissue from the encephalocele showing the cavity that was in communication with the occipital horn.

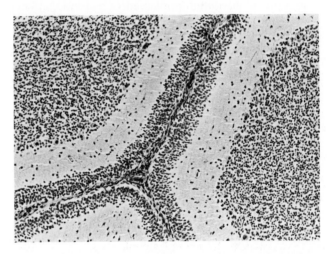

Figure 1–3D. Microscopic section of the cerebellar tissue that was contained in the encephalocele showing an unusually prominent external cerebellar granular layer.

1.4 Meningocele

Cervical Meningocele

CLINICAL

At birth, this female infant was noted to have a pedunculated mass at the base of her neck. Metrizamide myelography and computerized tomography performed at age 8 months demonstrated a dural stalk penetrating a defect in the lamina of the sixth cervical vertebra. The meningocele, stalk, and lamina were resected.

PATHOLOGY

The surgical specimen consisted of a dural sac covered by intact skin (Figs. 1–4A and 1–4B) and lined by flattened arachnoid cells (Fig. 1–4C). This was surrounded by an admixture of meningeal tissue, fibrous connective tissue, and small peripheral nerve twigs. No neuroglial tissue, nerve roots, or abnormal ectodermal structures were present.

COMMENT

Meningoceles are among the lesions included in the spectrum of malformations designated as the spinal dysraphias. In contrast to the more common meningomyelocele, meningoceles consist only of meninges herniated through a bony defect. The underlying spinal cord is intact and generally is normally located in the spinal canal.

However, nerve roots may be incorporated in the dural sac. The overlying skin may be normal or harbor a vascular malformation or a hairy nevus. Similar to meningomyeloceles, these lesions are most commonly encountered in the lumbosacral region. Some patients with high cervical meningoceles may have additional occult lesions in the lower portion of the spinal canal.

REFERENCES

Pollay M: Spinal dysraphism: Aperta and occulta. In Rosenberg RN, et al (eds): The Clinical Neurosciences. New York, Churchill Livingstone, 1983, vol 2, chap 19, pp II:1419–II:1433.

Vogter DM, Culberson JL, Schochet SS, et al: "High spinal" dysrhaphism: Case report of a complex cervical meningocele. Acta Neurochir 1987; 84:136-139.

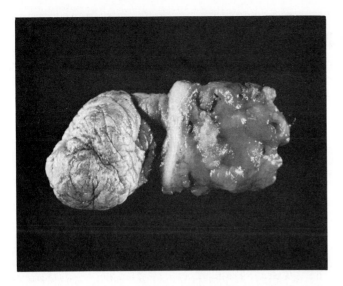

Figure 1–4A. Exterior of surgically resected cervical meningocele.

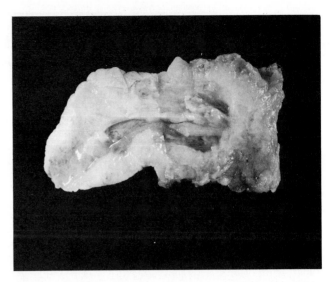

Figure 1–4B. Section of the meningocele showing the dural sac covered by skin.

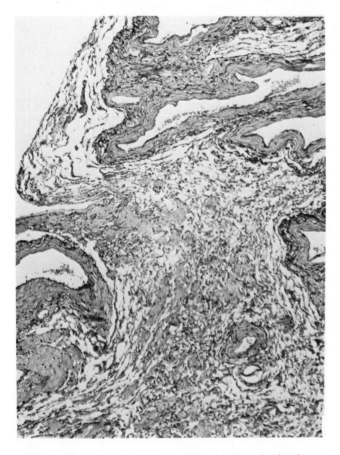

Figure 1–4C. Microscopic section of the meningocele showing an admixture of meninges, vessels, and fibrous tissue but no neuroglial tissue.

1.5   Lipomeningocele

CLINICAL

This 19-year-old man was evaluated for bowel and bladder incontinence and impotence. Sensation, motor function, and gait were normal. He had a pigmented protuberant hairy patch in his lumbosacral area. Radiological studies disclosed spina bifida, a lipomeningocele, diplomyelia, and a tethered cord. The lipomeningocele was resected and the filum released.

PATHOLOGY

The surgically resected specimen consisted of a small dural sac surrounded by a mass of adipose tissue that blended into the surrounding subcutaneous tissue (Fig. 1–5A). The interior of the sac contained dysplastic meninges (Fig. 1–5B). The overlying skin harbored a compound pigmented nevus.

COMMENT

Lipomeningoceles are meningoceles that contain and are surrounded by abnormal adipose tissue. As in this patient, the abnormal adipose tissue associated with the dural defect tends to blend into the subcutaneous tissue of the lumbosacral region. The lipomatous tissue may extend through the dura and into the spinal roots and conus of the spinal cord. The lipomeningoceles may produce symptoms by compressing the adjacent neural tissues and by tethering the spinal cord. These lesions may be designated as lipomyelomeningoceles when there is a cystic cavity within the intradural mass of adipose tissue.

REFERENCES

Hoffman HJ, Taecholarn C, Hendrick EB, Humphreys RP: Management of lipomyelomeningoceles. J Neurosurg 1985; 62:1-8.

Pollay M: Spinal dysraphism: Aperta and occulta. In Rosenberg RN el al (eds): The Clinical Neurosciences. New York, Churchill Livingstone, 1983, vol 2, chap 19, pp II:1419–II:1433.

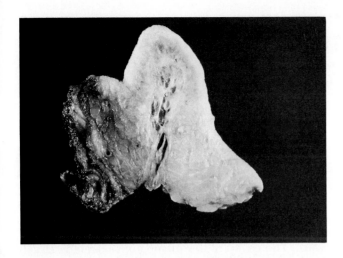

Figure 1–5A. Surgically resected lipomeningocele.

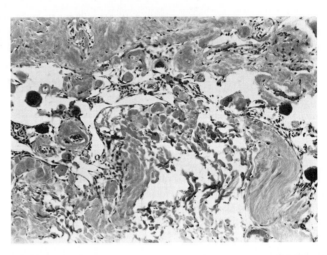

Figure 1–5B. Microscopic section showing meninges in the interior of the specimen.

1.6 Arnold–Chiari Malformation

Meningomyelocele

CLINICAL

At birth, this 42-week gestational age female was noted to have a large saccular neural tube defect covering the T8–L1 region. Her head was large, with widely separated sutures. The child died a few hours after delivery.

PATHOLOGY

The saccular neural tube defect contained dysplastic neuroglial tissue and was thus classified as a meningomyelocele. As in most, if not all cases with meningomyeloceles, the brain showed a Chiari type II or Arnold–Chiari malformation (Figs. 1–6A to 1–6D).

COMMENT

Although the major components of this malformation involve the posterior fossa structures, almost no portion of the central nervous system is unaffected. The Arnold–Chiari malformation is often complicated by hydrocephalus. This may be present at birth as in the present case but more commonly develops postnatally. The cerebrum often displays excessively complex convolutional markings. This has been variously designated as polygyria or stenogyria. The ventricular walls may contain foci of heterotopic gray matter. The mesencephalic tectum is consistently malformed and has a beaked or keel-shaped configuration (Fig. 1–6B). The aqueduct may be stenosed, forked, or merely kinked. The pons and medulla are elongated and the fourth ventricle is flattened. Since the posterior fossa is relatively small, the caudal end of the elongated medulla, the outlet foramina of the fourth ventricle, and portions of cerebellar tissue often extend into the spinal canal.

In the more severe examples, there is a Z-shaped kink at the cervicomedullary junction. This results from the dorsal components of the medulla extending further caudally than the more ventral portions of the medulla. The cerebellum is relatively small. The cerebellar hemispheres are rounded, abnormally separated from one another by a hypoplastic vermis, and

may be impacted in the foramen magnum. Tongues of dysmorphic cerebellar tissue extend caudally from the vermis over the medulla and cervical spinal cord (Fig. 1–6C).

As seen in a specimen from another case, the spinal cord is continuous with the placode of dysplastic neural tissue in the meningomyelocele (Fig. 1–6D). The cavity of the meningomyelocele is largely ventral to the neural placode and may be traversed by nerve roots. The rostral spinal cord is often abnormal and may show hydromyelia or even syringomyelia.

The pathogenesis of the Arnold–Chiari malformation is disputed. Some authors regard abnormal development of the posterior fossa as the fundamental malformation while others feel that hydrocephalus is the initial event.

The Chiari type II or Arnold–Chiari malformation must be clearly distinguished from the Chiari type I malformation. The latter lesion is often regarded as chronic cerebellar tonsillar herniation. The herniated tissue extends caudally from the cerebellar tonsils, rather than the vermis, and is not associated with the characteristic spectrum of brain stem and other cerebellar malformations. The individuals may have abnormalities such as platybasia and basilar impression but do not have meningomyeloceles. They generally do not become symptomatic until late in childhood or adult life.

REFERENCES

Gilbert JN, Jones KL, Rorke LB, et al: Central nervous system anomalies associated with meningomyelocele, hydrocephalus, and the Arnold–Chiari malformation: Reappraisal of theories regarding the pathogenesis of posterior neural tube defects. Neurosurgery 1986; 18:559-564.

Masters CL: Pathogenesis of the Arnold–Chiari malformation: The significance of hydrocephalus and aqueduct stenosis. J Neuropathol Exp Neurol 1978; 37:56-74.

McLendon RE, Crain BJ, Oakes WJ, Burger PC: Cerebral polygyria in the Chiari type II (Arnold–Chiari) malformation. Clin Neuropathol 1985; 4:200-205.

Paul KS, Lye RH, Strang FA, Dutton J: Arnold–Chiari malformation. Review of 71 cases. J Neurosurg 1983; 58:183-187.

Peach B: Arnold–Chiari malformation. Anatomic features of 20 cases. Arch Neurol 1965; 12:613-621.

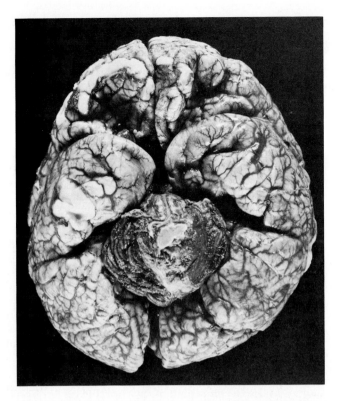

Figure 1–6A. Base of brain from a patient with the Arnold–Chiari malformation. Note the relatively small, malformed cerebellum and the enlarged cerebrum, with excessive complex gyral markings.

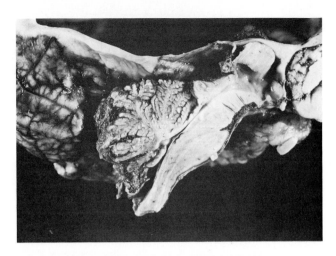

Figure 1–6B. Sagittal section of Arnold–Chiari malformation. Note the hydrocephalus, patent aqueduct, malformed quadrigeminal plate, elongated pons, flattened fourth ventricle, elongated medulla, and malformed cerebellum with a tongue of vermal tissue extending caudally over the upper cervical spinal cord.

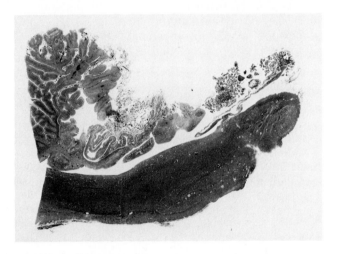

Figure 1–6C. Macrosection of the Arnold–Chiari malformation showing the caudal extension of dysplastic cerebellar vermal tissue.

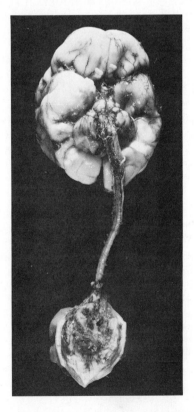

Figure 1–6D. Meningomyelocele with associated Arnold–Chiari malformation.

1.7   Dandy–Walker Malformation

CLINICAL

This newborn male infant was the product of a spontaneous vaginal delivery at 37 weeks of gestation. Multiple somatic and skeletal anomalies were noted at birth. Chromosomal analysis revealed trisomy 13. The child died on the third postnatal day.

PATHOLOGY

The brain weighed 334 grams. The cerebral hemispheres were grossly normal. There was a large posterior fossa cyst that had ruptured during removal of the brain. Sagittal section of the brain stem showed the cyst to be in continuity with the fourth ventricle (Fig. 1–7A). A malformed, hypoplastic cerebellar vermis was situated at the rostral end of the cyst. The lateral walls of the cyst were formed by the medial aspects of the cerebellar hemispheres. These surfaces had an abnormal gray white color. The membranous portion of the cyst was composed of meninges and glial tissue. Microscopically, the olivary nuclei were malformed.

COMMENT

The Dandy–Walker malformation consists of a posterior fossa cyst that is in continuity with the fourth ventricle. The cerebellar vermis may be absent or, more commonly, hypoplastic and malformed. The cerebellar hemispheres are displaced laterally by the dilated fourth ventricle. The medial walls of the displaced cerebellar hemispheres are often abnormally gliotic. The membranous portion of the cyst arises from the displaced cerebellar hemispheres and hypoplastic vermis. The expanding cyst causes enlargement of the posterior fossa, elevation of the inion, and upward displacement of the tentorium and dural sinuses. This lesion has a characteristic appearance when demonstrated by computerized tomography and can be distinguished from other forms of posterior fossa cysts (Fig. 1–7B). As seen in a surgical specimen from an older child, the cyst is lined in part by ependyma and glial tissue and covered on the exterior by fibrotic meninges (Fig. 1–7C). The lesion has also been identified in utero by ultrasonography.

The pathogenesis of the Dandy–Walker malformation is controversial. Formerly, the posterior fossa cyst was thought to result from failure of the foramina of Luschka and Magendie to develop. However, these outlet foramina are often found to be patent and hydrocephalus is not a consistent finding. The posterior fossa cyst is now thought to result from disturbances in the development of the rhombic lip and roof of the fourth ventricle. The brains from these individuals often show other malformations, including abnormal cerebral gyri, agenesis of the corpus callosum, malformations of the inferior olivary nuclei and anomalies of the cerebellar folia. Some of the patients also have skeletal abnormalities. There is no consistent association with chromosomal abnormalities, although the present case had trisomy 13.

REFERENCES

Hart MN, Malamud N, Ellis WG: The Dandy–Walker syndrome. A clinicopathological study based on 28 cases. Neurology 1972; 22:771-780.

Hirsch J-F, Pierre-Kahn A, Renier D, et al: The Dandy–Walker malformation. A review of 40 cases. J Neurosurg 1984; 61:515-522.

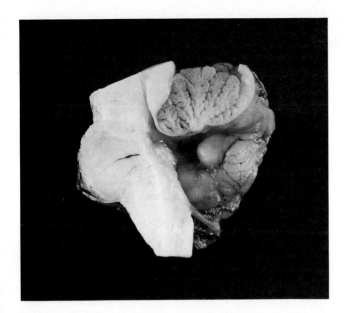

Figure 1–7A. Sagittal section of brain stem showing Dandy–Walker malformation. The cyst has been disrupted.

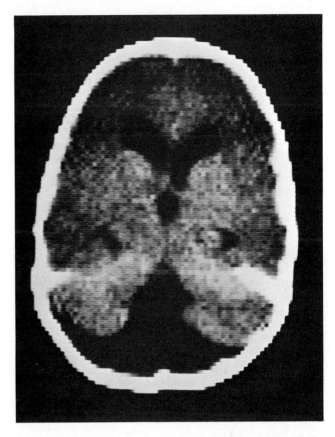

Figure 1–7B. Computerized tomogram showing a Dandy–Walker malformation.

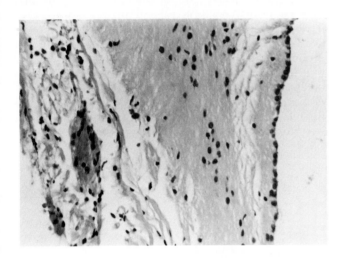

Figure 1–7C. Microscopic section from surgically resected Dandy–Walker cyst showing ependyma on interior and arachnoid on exterior.

1.8　Syringomyelia

CLINICAL

This 60-year-old man died of pneumonia. He was a nursing home resident with a history of "polio in childhood," kyphoscoliosis, hemiparesis, and arrested hydrocephalus.

PATHOLOGY

Examination of the brain demonstrated the hemispheres to be somewhat enlarged. The basilar meninges about the outlet foramina of the fourth ventricle were thickened and fibrotic (Fig. 1–8A). A horizontal section of the cerebrum disclosed massive dilatation of the lateral ventricles (Fig. 1–8B). This was accompanied by enlargement of the third ventricle, aqueduct, and fourth ventricle (Fig. 1–8C). Externally, the spinal cord was mildly flattened but appeared to have been enlarged during life. The spinal meninges were not significantly fibrotic. Transverse sections of the spinal cord revealed a syrinx (Figs. 1–8D and 1–8E).

Although the cavitation was maximal in the cervical portion of the spinal cord and approached the dilated fourth ventricle, actual communication with the ventricular system could not be identified.

COMMENT

Syringomyelia is by definition a tubular cavity in the spinal cord. Most authors separate syringomyelia, which is lined in part by astroglial tissue, from hydromyelia, which is cystic dilatation of the central canal and thus lined in part by ependyma.

Syringomyelia apparently has many causes. Much of the confusion in the older literature seems to have resulted from attempts to explain all cases by a single pathogenetic mechanism. In rare cases, syringomyelia may be a malformation related to improper fusion between the alar and basal laminae of the spinal cord. Occasionally, the lesion begins as hydromyelia that is secondary to various cerebral malformations or acquired disorders that alter the normal flow of the cerebrospinal fluid. In these cases, subsequent degeneration of the spinal cord parenchyma around the dilated central canal leads to the development of

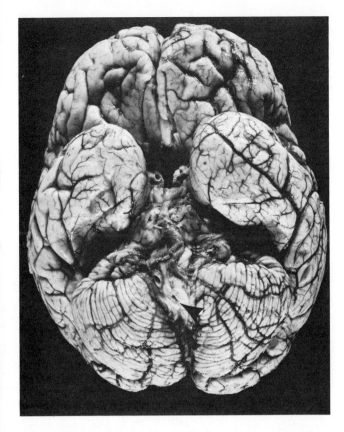

Figure 1–8A. Base of brain showing enlarged cerebral hemispheres, fibrotic basal meninges, and opening in caudal portion of brain stem (arrowhead).

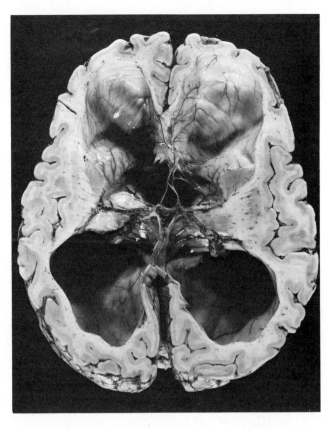

Figure 1–8B. Horizontal section showing hydrocephalus.

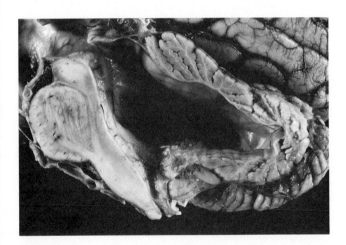

Figure 1–8C. Sagittal section of brain stem showing enlargment of fourth ventricle.

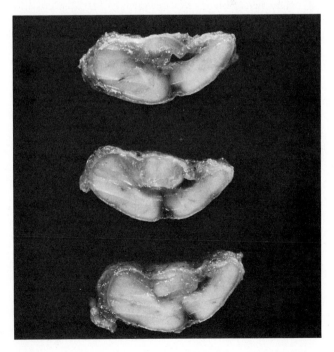

Figure 1–8D. Transverse section of spinal cord showing collapsed syrinx.

syringomyelia. In still other cases, syringomyelia arises from degeneration of the spinal cord secondary to trauma (Figs. 1–8F and 1–8G), vascular diseases, or neoplasms. Rare cases have been associated with spinal arachnoiditis. These cases may have a vascular basis mediated by impaired blood flow within the spinal cord. In still other cases, the cause is not evident despite careful study.

In the present case, the meningeal fibrosis about the outlet foramina of the fourth ventricle probably diverted cerebrospinal fluid into the central canal of the spinal cord, causing hydromyelia. Subsequent disruption of the ependyma and degeneration of the surrounding neural parenchyma could give rise to syringomyelia. Although the dilated fourth ventricle and the syrinx were separated by a thin band of tissue (Fig. 1–8C), it seems likely that these cavities were in communication earlier in the course of the disease process. As is usually the case, the cavitation was maximal in the cervical region. The cavity is usually transversely oriented, often asymmetrical, and may be duplicated at some levels. The tissue surrounding the syrinx shows demyelination and gliosis.

REFERENCES

Barnett HJM, Foster JB, Hudgson P: Syringomyelia. London, Saunders, 1973.

Larroche J-C: Malformations of the nervous system. In Adams JH, Corsellis JAN, Duchen LW (eds): Greenfield's Neuropathology, 4th ed. New York, Wiley, 1984, chap 10, pp 385-450.

McComas CF, Frost JL, Schochet SS Jr: Posttraumatic syringomyelia with paroxysmal episodes of unconsciousness. Arch Neurol 1983; 40:322-324.

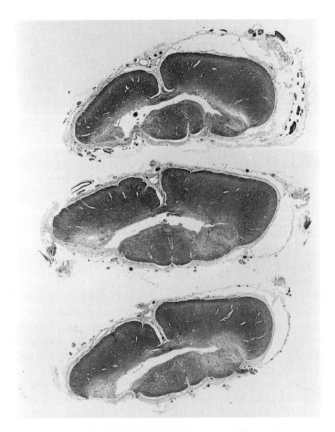

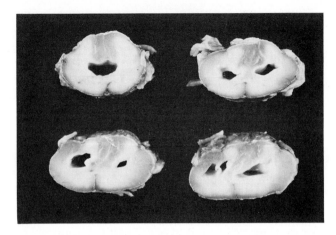

Figure 1–8F. Transverse sections of spinal cord showing post-traumatic syrinx.

Figure 1–8E. Macrosections of spinal cord showing syrinx.

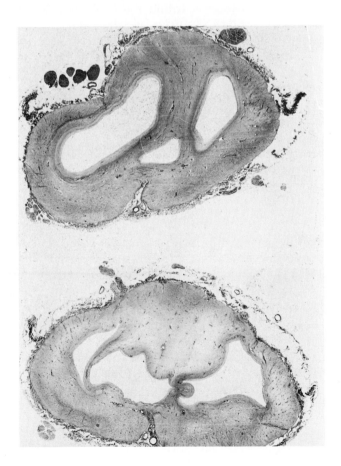

Figure 1–8G. Macrosections showing multiple lumina of post-traumatic syrinx.

1.9 Agenesis of the Corpus Callosum

CLINICAL

This 20-month-old female infant was hospitalized for evaluation of an abdominal mass. The child had multiple congenital anomalies including micrognathia, cleft palate, and hypertelorism. A computerized tomogram of the head revealed agenesis of the corpus callosum (Fig. 1–9A). Computerized tomograms of the abdomen and an intravenous pyelogram revealed a right-sided renal mass. The infant died approximately 2 weeks after resection of a nephroblastoma.

PATHOLOGY

Examination of the brain revealed nearly complete agenesis of the corpus callosum (Fig. 1–9B).

COMMENT

Agenesis of the corpus callosum is a relatively common malformation that occurs as an isolated lesion or, more commonly, in association with other abnormalities of the central nervous system. Even when other lesions are not obvious, many of the patients have seizures, mental retardation, and hydrocephalus. Most of the cases are sporadic, although some familial cases have been reported.

The corpus callosum develops in the commissural plate, a thickened portion of the lamina terminalis at the rostral end of the neural tube. The anterior commissure, fornix, and hippocampal commissure develop in the same region and may be hypoplastic or absent in patients with agenesis of the corpus callosum. The rostral portion of the corpus callosum develops first. Thus, in cases of partial agenesis, the rostrum and genu are usually intact whereas the splenium and portions of the body are missing (Fig. 1–9C).

Where the corpus callosum is absent, the medial aspects of the cerebral hemispheres are anomalous. The cingulate gyri are poorly demarcated and the remaining gyri and sulci assume an aberrant radial orientation. Fibers that would normally interconnect the hemisphere through the corpus callosum run in a rostral–caudal direction and comprise the so-called Probst's bundles. The third ventricle is covered only by ependyma and meninges. The resulting midline defect is readily visualized by computerized tomography. Occasionally, there are midline ependymal cysts or even lipomas within the interhemispheric fissure. The lateral ventricles are distorted and assume a characteristic "bat wing" configuration.

REFERENCES

Loeser JD, Alvord EC Jr: Agenesis of the corpus callosum. Brain 1968; 91:553-570.

Parrish ML, Roessmann U, Levinsohn MW: Agenesis of the corpus callosum: A study of the frequency of associated malformations. Ann Neurol 1979; 6:349-354.

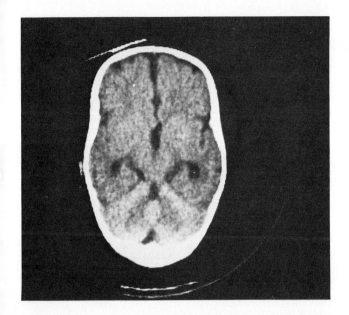

Figure 1–9A. Computerized tomogram showing agenesis of corpus callosum.

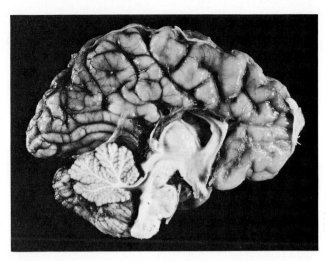

Figure 1–9B. Sagittal section showing nearly complete agenesis of corpus callosum.

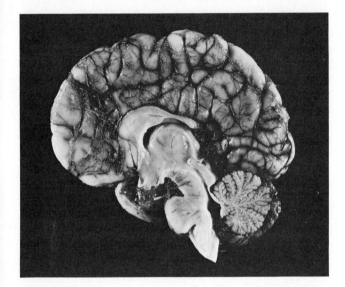

Figure 1–9C. Sagittal section of brain showing partial agenesis of corpus callosum.

1.10   Holoprosencephaly

CLINICAL

The mother of this premature male infant was a 17-year-old woman with juvenile onset diabetes mellitus. The infant was delivered by cesarean section because of maternal complications, including pyelonephritis, ketoacidosis, and polyhydramnios. The infant died shortly after delivery.

PATHOLOGY

The infant was severely malformed, with hypotelorism, microophthalmia, and a midline proboscis (cebocephaly) with atretic internal choanae (Fig. 1–10A). The thoracic and abdominal organs were normal. There were no supernumerary digits. Postmortem chromosomal studies showed a normal male karyotype.

A membranous cyst was present in the posterior half of the calvarium. The cyst was continuous with the dorsal aspect of the malformed brain (Fig. 1–10B). The cerebrum was not divided into hemispheres and contained a single large ventricle (Fig. 1–10C). There were nodular masses of heterotopic gray matter on the ventricular surface. The basal ganglia, thalamus, and hypothalamus were incompletely delineated and there was no third ventricle. The mammillary bodies were fused and formed a prominent mass on the ventral surface of the cerebrum. There were no olfactory bulbs or tracts. The optic nerves were hypoplastic. The brain stem and cerebellum were small. No medullary pyramids could be identified.

COMMENT

The term holoprosencephaly is used to designate a spectrum of cerebral malformations resulting from faulty diverticulation of the prosencephalon. The malformations involve to varying degrees derivatives of the telencephalic, optic, and olfactory vesicles. Studies by DeMyer et al have shown that cyclopia, ethmocephaly, cebocephaly, and median facial clefts with hypotelorism are consistently accompanied by some form of holoprosencephaly. In addition, individuals with bilateral lateral cleft lips, hypotelorism, and microcephaly commonly have some form of this malformation.

The most severe form of this cerebral malformation is so-called alobar holoprosencephaly. In this form there is persistence of a single prosencephalic vesicle. The holoprosencephalon is homologous to the cerebrum caudal to the gigantopyramidal cortex. The corpus callosum is unformed and the dorsal surface of the brain is a membrane derived from the tela choroidea. The corpora striate and thalamus are undivided. The pyramidal tracts are absent. Although the olfactory bulbs and tracts are absent or hypoplastic, other rhinencephalic structures, including the hippocampi, are present.

Lobar holoprosencephaly is a less severe form of this malformation in which an interhemispheric fissure divides at least the posterior portion of the cerebrum. The corpus callosum may be nearly normal, hypoplastic, or even absent. Olfactory bulbs and tracts are generally absent.

Brains with the least severe form of this malformation may have only absence of the olfactory bulbs and tracts. In these cases, the olfactory sulcus will be rudimentary.

Patients with holoprosencephaly may have normal karyotypes as in this case or show various chromosomal abnormalities. Among these, the D (13/15) trisomy is especially common. The trisomic patients with holoprosencephaly often have multiple extracephalic anomalies including polydactyly and congenital heart lesions. Figures 1–10D and 1–10E illustrate lobar holoprosencephaly with hypoplasia of the ventricular system in an infant with trisomy 13.

REFERENCES

DeMyer W: Holoprosencephaly (cyclopia–arhinencephaly). In Vinken PJ, Bruyn GW (eds): Handbook of Clinical Neurology. Amsterdam, Elsevier, 1977, vol 30, chap 18, pp 431-478.

Jellinger K, Gross H, Kaltenback E, Grisold W: Holoprosencephaly and agenesis of the corpus callosum: Frequency of associated malformations. Acta Neuropathol 1981; 55:1-10.

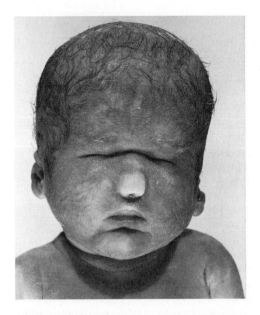

Figure 1–10A. Cebocephaly with microophthalmia.

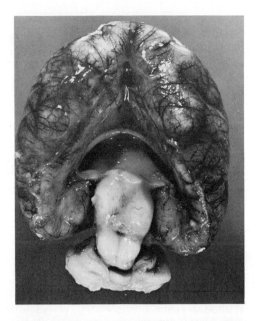

Figure 1–10B. Dorsal view of brain with holoprosencephaly.

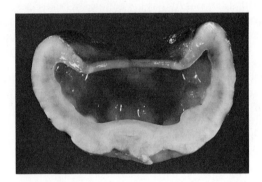

Figure 1–10C. Coronal section of brain with holoprosencephaly.

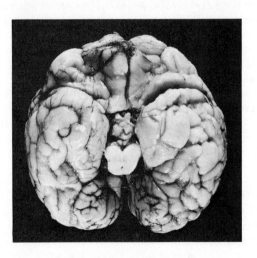

Figure 1–10D. Base of brain from infant with trisomy 13 and lobar holoprosencephaly.

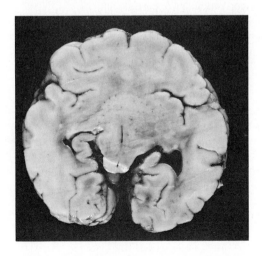

Figure 1–10E. Horizontal section of brain showing fused hemispheres and hypoplastic ventricles.

1.11 Pachygyria

CLINICAL

This young child had a history of psychomotor retardation, hypotonia, and seizures. The child had recurrent respiratory infections, developed bronchiectasis, and died of pneumonia.

PATHOLOGY

The brain was relatively small. There was a reduced number of gyri and those present were unusually broad and separated by shallow sulci (Fig 1–11A). Coronal sections accentuated these features and disclosed abnormally thick cortex overlying the white matter (Figs. 1–11B and 1–11C). This was most evident in the frontal lobes. The temporal lobe gyri and hippocampi were nearly normal. The caudate nuclei, putamena, and pallida were grossly intact. The claustra were absent. The ventricular system was only mildly enlarged.

The cerebellum was grossly normal. However, the brain stem and pyramidal tracts were small and the architecture of the inferior olivary nuclei was simplified (Fig. 1–11D).

COMMENT

The terms pachygyria, agyria, and lissencephaly refer to similar malformations. The term agyria is used to describe brains in which there is nearly complete absence of gyri, whereas pachygyria is used to describe cases in which there are a reduced number of abnormally broad gyri. The term lissencephaly refers to brains with a smooth surface.

Histological examination of the pachygyric brain reveals four layers. From the exterior inward, the first layer is a molecular layer. Next there is a relatively thin layer of cortex containing large neurons. These cells correspond to neurons that would normally be found in the deeper layers of the cortex. Beneath the external cellular layer is a band of gliotic white matter. The inner cellular layer is thicker and contains neurons that are in disarray. These cells are interpreted as heterotopic neurons derived from neuroblasts that had been arrested during their migration from the periventricular region. They correspond to the neurons that would normally be found in the second and fourth layers of the cortex.

Although pachygyria is generally regarded to arise from abnormal migration of neurons, the exact pathogenesis is unknown. Some authors have suggested that the pathological process begins as early as 8 weeks of gestation and persists throughout the stages of neuronal migration. Other authors attribute the migrational arrest to a hypoxic or ischemic injury at about the fourth month of gestation. The frequently encountered olivary abnormalities would seem to favor the first hypothesis.

REFERENCES

Friede RL: Developmental Neuropathology. New York, Springer Verlag, 1975, pp 298-300.

Larroche J-C: Malformations of the nervous system. In Adams JH, Corsellis JAN, Duchen LW (eds): Greenfield's Neuropathology, 4th ed. New York, Wiley, 1984, chap 10, pp 385-450.

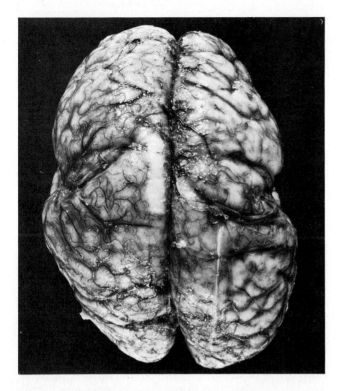

Figure 1–11A. Dorsal surface of brain with pachygyria.

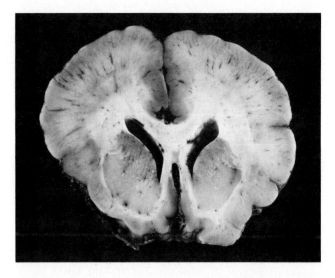

Figure 1–11B. Coronal section of brain with pachygyria.

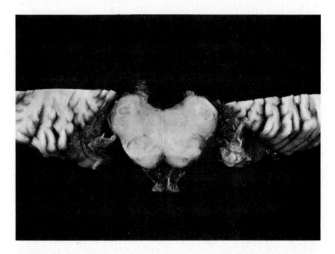

Figure 1–11D. Transverse section of brain stem showing malformed inferior olivary nuclei.

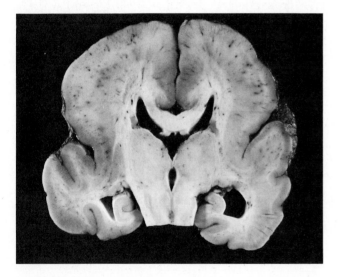

Figure 1–11C. Coronal section of brain with pachygyria showing thick frontal cortex and more nearly normal temporal lobes.

1.12 Polymicrogyria

CLINICAL

This 1495-gram male infant was delivered vaginally at 36 weeks of gestation to an 18-year-old primigravida woman. The infant was cyanotic and had multiple congenital anomalies, including a cleft palate, club foot, low set ears, and hypoplastic lungs. He died on the second postnatal day.

PATHOLOGY

The brain from this infant was small and showed features typical of polymicrogyria. On initial inspection, the gyral pattern seemed simplified. However, closer examination revealed numerous small nodular gyri covering much of the dorsal and lateral surfaces of the cerebrum (Figs. 1–12A and 1–12B). The base of the brain (Fig. 1–12C), parasagittal regions, and medial aspects of the hemispheres were less severely affected.

Horizontal sections disclosed abnormally thickened cortex (Fig. 1–12D). This appearance resulted from incomplete demarcation of the abnormal small gyri.

COMMENT

Polymicrogyria may be a focal abnormality or may affect a large portion of the brain. When extensive, the patients often have mental retardation and seizures.

The typical polymicrogyric cortex is composed of four layers. On the surface there is a sparsely cellular molecular layer. The second layer is densely cellular and irregular in arrangement. The third layer is sparsely cellular and, in older individuals, contains a horizontal plexus of myelinated fibers. The fourth layer is cellular but often discontinuous. In many cases, the four layers are not distinctly delineated.

The pathogenesis of polymicrogyria is unsettled. Some authors regard the malformation as the result of a disturbance in neuroblastic migration. Others interpret the lesion as the sequela of a hypoxic or ischemic injury early in gestation. The tendency for polymicrogyria to occur in a vascular distribution and the association with porencephaly are evidence in favor of the latter hypothesis.

Polymicrogyria must be distinguished from the excessively complex gyral markings (stenogyria) seen in some cases of the Arnold–Chiari malformation and from sclerotic ulegyria that results from hypoxic or ischemic injuries that occur later in gestation or even postnatally.

REFERENCES

Friede RL: Developmental Neuropathology. New York, Springer Verlag, 1975, pp 303-307.

Larroche J-C: Malformations of the nervous system. In Adams JH, Corsellis JAN, Duchen LW (eds): Greenfield's Neuropathology, 4th ed. New York, Wiley, 1984, chap 10, pp 385-450.

Ludwin SK, Norman MG: Congenital malformations of the nervous system. In Davis RL, Robertson DM (eds): Textbook of Neuropathology. Baltimore, Williams & Wilkins, 1985, chap 6, pp 176-242.

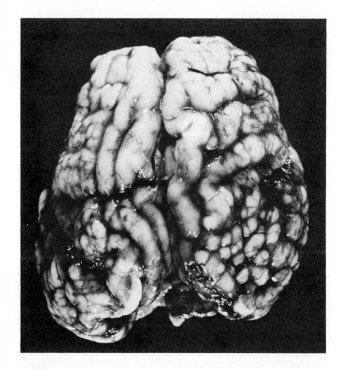

Figure 1–12A. Dorsal surface of brain with polymicrogyria.

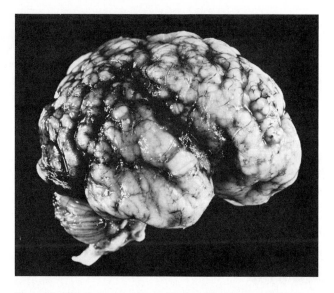

Figure 1–12B. Lateral surface of brain with polymicrogyria.

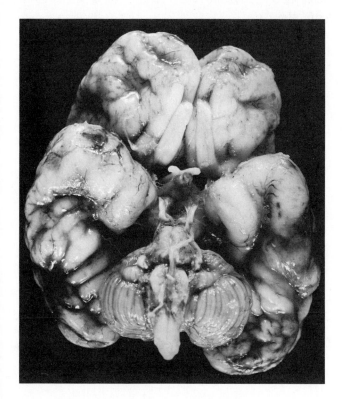

Figure 1–12C. Base of brain with polymicrogyria.

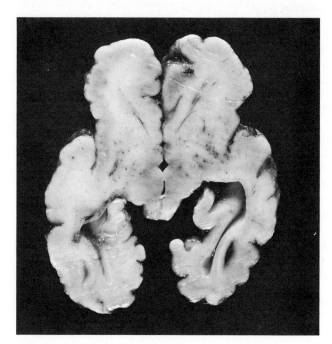

Figure 1–12D. Horizontal section of brain with polymicrogyria.

1.13 Down's Syndrome

CLINICAL

This child, who was known to have Down's syndrome, died at age 5 months from congestive heart failure due to an atrial septal defect. A pulmonary artery banding procedure had been performed at age 3 weeks. He had simian creases on both hands and syndactyly of the left foot.

PATHOLOGY

The brain weighed 612 grams and was mildly dysmorphic. The frontal and occipital poles were blunted (Fig. 1–13A). The convolutional patterns on the two hemispheres were slightly asymmetrical. The superior temporal convolutions were relatively small (Fig. 1–13B).

COMMENT

Brains from patients with Down's syndrome are generally small. In infants and young children, the cerebellum and brain stem may be especially small in proportion to the cerebrum. The cerebrum is often somewhat rounded with blunted frontal and occipital poles. This is due, in part, to hypoplasia of the frontal lobes. The convolutional markings on the two hemispheres may be quite dissimilar and asymmetrical. In some cases, the insulae are abnormally widely exposed. In about one half of the cases, the superior temporal gyri are unusually narrow. Freytag and Lindenberg emphasize the common occurrence of a square- or rectangular-shaped thalamus, even when the brains are otherwise grossly unremarkable (Fig. 1–13C).

Mild and varied histological abnormalities have been observed in the brains from children with Down's syndrome. More recently, quantitative histological studies have indicated a reduction in the neuronal population affecting especially the granular cells. By contrast, brains from patients with Down's syndrome who are over the age of 35 regularly show neurofibrillary tangles and senile plaques (Fig. 1–13D).

Down's syndrome is seen with increased frequency among children of older women. Most cases are due to trisomy 21. Occasional cases are due to translocations or mosaicisms involving this chromosome. Most of the familial cases are associated with translocations.

REFERENCES

Ball MJ, Nuttall K: Neurofibrillary tangles, granulovacuolar degeneration, and neuronal loss in Down syndrome: Quantitative comparison with Alzheimer dementia. Ann Neurol 1980; 7:462-465.

Benda CE: Mongolism. In Minckler J (ed): Pathology of the Nervous System. New York, McGraw-Hill, 1971, vol 2, chap 97, pp 1361-1371.

Freytag E, Lindenberg R: Neuropathologic findings in patients of a hospital for the mentally deficient. A survey of 359 cases. Johns Hopkins Med J 1967; 121:379-392.

Ross MH, Galaburda AM, Kemper TL: Down's syndrome: Is there a decreased population of neurons? Neurology 1984; 34:909-916.

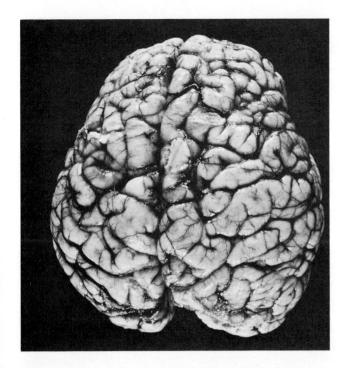

Figure 1–13A. Dorsal surface of brain from child with Down's syndrome. Note the blunted frontal and occipital poles.

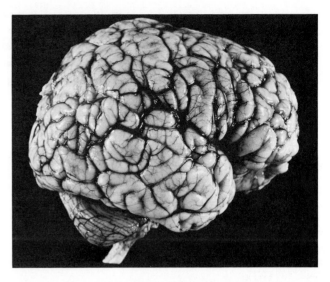

Figure 1–13B. Lateral surface of brain from child with Down's syndrome. Note the relatively small superior temporal gyrus.

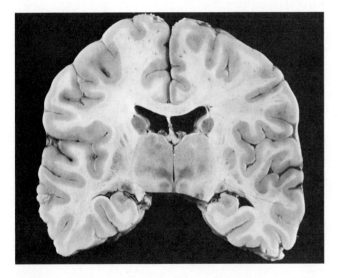

Figure 1–13C. Coronal section of brain from a patient with Down's syndrome. Note the rectangular shape of the thalamus.

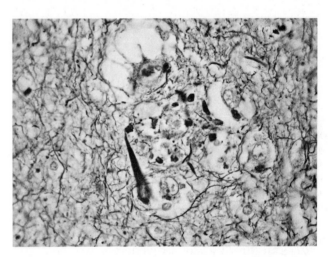

Figure 1–13D. Microscopic section showing a senile plaque and a neurofibrillary tangle in the brain of an adult with Down's syndrome.

1.14 Cerebellar Hypoplasia

Neocerebellar Hypoplasia

CLINICAL

This male infant was born at term to a primigravida woman. The infant was microcephalic with a head circumference of 31.5 cm. The infant was spastic and cried weakly. The anterior fontanelle could not be palpated. The child had cyanotic episodes and died 1 week later. Autopsy showed craniosynostosis and a patent ductus arteriosus.

PATHOLOGY

The brain weighed 211 grams and had symmetrical cerebral hemispheres with an unremarkable gyral pattern. The cerebellum and brain stem were hypoplastic (Fig. 1–14A). The cerebellar hemispheres were especially small and flattened (Fig. 1–14B). The flocculi and nodulus were relatively well developed, in comparison to the rest of the cerebellum (Fig. 1–14C). The pons was small and angular and the middle cerebellar peduncles were hypoplastic. The medulla was small and the olives could not be identified grossly.

Histologically, the nodulus and flocculi were nearly normal, with intact molecular, Purkinje, and internal granular cell layers. By contrast, the cerebellar hemispheres were severely hypoplastic, showed incomplete differentiation of the folia, and contained a reduced number of neurons. The basis pontis contained a reduced number of neurons and the inferior olivary nuclei were hypoplastic.

COMMENT

The cerebellar hypoplasias are a diverse group of entities that probably have varied etiologies. This case resembles the pontoneocerebellar hypoplasia of Brun with severe hypoplasia of neocerebellar derivatives, moderate hypoplasia of paleocerebellar structures, and relative preservation of archicerebellar components. The pontine nuclei and inferior olivary nuclei are concurrently affected.

Rare cases of cerebellar hypoplasia may show extreme hypoplasia or even aplasia of a single cerebellar hemisphere, the cerebellar vermis, or even the entire cerebellum.

REFERENCE

Friede RL: Developmental Neuropathology. New York, Springer Verlag, 1975, pp 319-324.

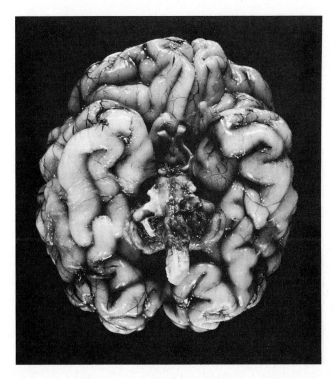

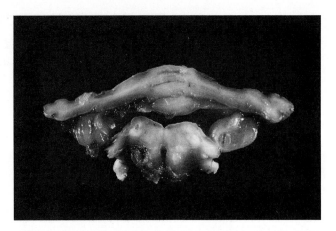

Figure 1–14B. Transverse section of cerebellum and brain stem showing neocerebellar hypoplasia.

Figure 1–14A. Base of brain showing hypoplastic cerebellum.

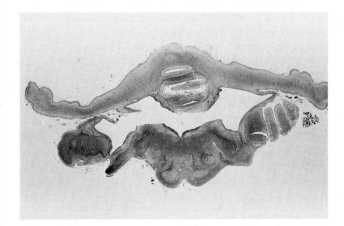

Figure 1–14C. Macrosection of brain stem and cerebellum showing neocerebellar hypoplasia.

1.15 Tuberous Sclerosis

CLINICAL

This 3460-gram male infant was born at term to a 23-year-old primigravida woman who had no known neurological disease. Her pregnancy had been complicated by polyhydramnios during the third trimester. A few hours after delivery, the infant became cyanotic and tachypneic. A chest x-ray showed a massively enlarged cardiothymic shadow. Emergency surgery was performed and disclosed an unresectable left ventricular tumor nearly twice the size of the heart. The child died on the second post-operative day.

PATHOLOGY

The brain weighed 410 grams. Abnormally firm cortical tubers were palpable on the surface of the unfixed brain even though they were not visually distinguishable from the adjacent cortex. In coronal sections of the fixed brain, the tubers appeared as abnormally widened gyri (Fig. 1–15A). Subependymal nodules or "candle gutterings" were more readily apparent since they were quite firm, partially demarcated, and tended to project into the ventricular cavities (Fig. 1–15A).

Histologically, the cortical tubers were composed predominantly of large stellate cells (Fig. 1–15B). By contrast, the subependymal nodules were composed predominantly of compact masses of spindle-shaped cells (Figs. 1–15C and 1–15D).

COMMENT

Tuberous sclerosis is an autosomal dominant disorder, although many cases result from spontaneous mutations. The prevalence is estimated to be from 1 per 50,000 to 1 per 100,000. All races are affected.

Only about one third of the cases of tuberous sclerosis display the classical triad of mental retardation, seizures, and adenoma sebacea. Some authors regard careful examination of the skin to be the most sensitive means of evaluating patients suspected of having this disease. Up to 96 percent of older children and adults with tuberous sclerosis have cutaneous lesions which are predominantly fibrovascular lesions. They include the so-called adenoma sebacea in the malar region, the sub- and periungual fibromas otherwise known as Koenen tumors, and areas of thickened skin and subcutaneous tissue on the back and thighs known as "shagreen" patches. Patients also may have hypopigmented areas known as "ash leaf macules" or hyperpigmented café-au-lait spots.

Lesions are found in many visceral organs. This case, like the neonate originally described by von Recklinghausen, had a cardiac rhabdomyoma. These tumors are found in 20 to 60 percent of the affected individuals. Another commonly encountered visceral lesion is the angiomyolipoma of the kidney. These tumors are found in about 40 percent of the cases.

The central nervous system lesions include cortical tubers, subependymal nodules ("candle gutterings"), and, rarely, subependymal giant cell astrocytomas. Cells comprising the cortical tubers have been studied extensively by electron microscopy and immunoperoxidase techniques. Although study results are somewhat conflicting, the tubers appear to be composed of aberrant multipolar neurons and astrocytes.

The cells comprising the subependymal "candle gutterings" are generally considered to be fibrillary astrocytes. These lesions are especially common along the thalamostriate sulcus. They often undergo mineralization in older patients (Figs. 1–15E and 1–15F).

The relatively uncommon subependymal giant cell tumors are composed of large bizarre glial cells with vesicular nuclei and abundant cytoplasm. They show variable immunostaining for glial fibrillary acidic protein and neuron specific enolase. The retinal hamartomas, found in about 50 percent of these patients, contain cells that are similar to these subependymal tumors.

Cranial CT has shown abnormalities, usually "candle gutterings," in about two thirds of the cases. More recently, magnetic resonance imaging (MRI) has been shown to effectively demonstrate the cortical lesions. The number of cortical lesions detected with MRI tended to correlate with the clinical severity of the disease.

REFERENCES

Bender BL, Yunis EJ: The pathology of tuberous sclerosis. In Sommers, SC, Rosen PP (eds): Pathology Annual 1982, East Norwalk, Connecticut, part 1, Appleton-Century-Crofts, 339–382.

Donegani G, Grattarola F-R, Wildi E: Tuberous sclerosis. Bourneville disease. In Vinken PJ, Bruyn GW (eds): Handbook of Clinical Neurology. Amsterdam, Elsevier, 1972, vol 14, chap 11, pp 340-389.

Huttenlocker PR, Heydemann PT: Fine structure of cortical tubers in tuberous sclerosis: A Golgi study. Ann Neurol 1984; 16:595-602.

deRecondo J, Hagueneau M: Neuropathologic survey of the phakomatoses and allied disorders. In Vinken PJ, Bruyn GW (eds). Handbook of Clinical Neurology. Amsterdam, Elsevier, 1972, vol 14, chap 3, pp 19-100.

Roach ES, Williams DP, Laster DW: Magnetic resonance imaging in tuberous sclerosis. Arch Neurol 1987; 44:301-303.

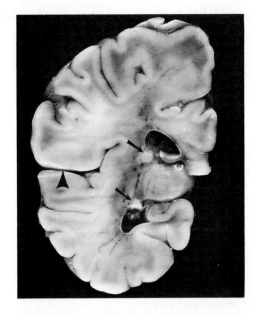

Figure 1–15A. Coronal section of brain from infant with tuberous sclerosis. Note the cortical tuber (arrowhead) and the subependymal nodules (arrows).

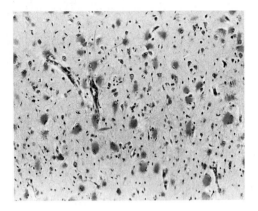

Figure 1–15B. Microscopic section of a cortical tuber.

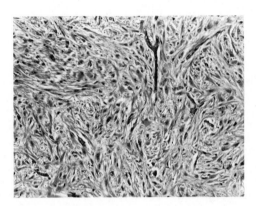

Figure 1–15D. Microscopic section showing elongated glial cells comprising a subependymal nodule.

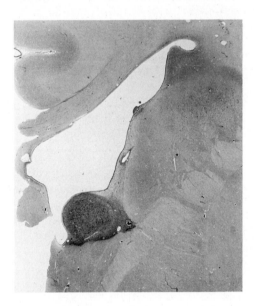

Figure 1–15C. Macrosection showing subependymal nodules.

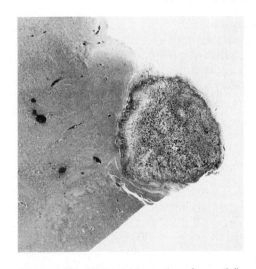

Figure 1–15F. Macroscopic section of a partially calcified subependymal nodule.

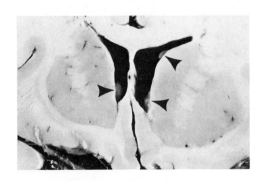

Figure 1–15E. Coronal section from older patient with calcified subependymal nodules.

1.16 Subependymal Germinal Matrix Hemorrhage

CLINICAL

This 830-gram male infant was born at approximately 28 weeks of gestation. Shortly after birth, the infant became hypotensive and bradycardic. A chest x-ray revealed changes consistent with severe respiratory distress syndrome. The infant died the following day.

PATHOLOGY

The brain was immature and weighed 100 grams. Blood was present in the subarachnoid space at the base of the brain and about the outlet foramina of the fourth ventricle (Fig. 1–16A). A sagittal section of the brain disclosed blood in all ventricular cavities (Fig. 1–16B). Coronal sections of the individual cerebral hemispheres showed the blood to be arising from the subependymal germinal matrices (Fig. 1–16C).

COMMENT

Subarachnoid and intraventricular hemorrhages are commonly encountered in the brains of neonates. In premature infants, these hemorrhages generally arise from the subependymal germinal matrix. This zone of highly cellular, incompletely differentiated tissue is maximally developed during the second trimester and subsequently involutes. Prominent masses of this tissue persist until late in the third trimester over the caudate nucleus, along the thalamostriate vein, and in the roof of the temporal horn.

The etiology and pathogenesis of the subependymal germinal matrix hemorrhages remain controversial despite extensive investigations. Most of these hemorrhages occur during the early post-natal period, although, rarely, they may occur in utero. The hemorrhages vary greatly in size and severity. Some are small and confined to the germinal matrix whereas others are massive and rupture into the ventricular system. They may be bilateral as seen in a horizontal section from another premature infant (Fig. 1–16D). Occasionally, the hemorrhages also extend into the surrounding neural parenchyma (Fig. 1–16E). Less commonly and generally in more mature infants, intraventricular hemorrhages may arise from the choroid plexi.

REFERENCES

Darrow VC, Alvord EC Jr, Mack LA, Hodson WA: Histologic evolution of the reactions to hemorrhage in the premature human infant's brain: A combined ultrasound and autopsy study and a comparison with reaction in adults. Am J Pathol 1988; 130:44-58.

Gilles FH: Perinatal neuropathology. In Davis RL, Robertson DM (eds): Textbook of Neuropathology. Baltimore, Williams & Wilkins, 1985, chap 7, pp 243-283.

Goddard-Finegold J: Periventricular, intraventricular hemorrhages in the premature newborn. Arch Neurol 1984; 41:766-771.

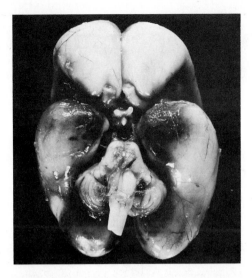

Figure 1–16A. Base of brain from premature infant with subependymal germinal matrix hemorrhage.

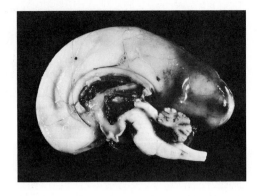

Figure 1–16B. Sagittal section of brain from premature infant with subependymal germinal matrix hemorrhage. Note the intraventricular and subarachnoid blood.

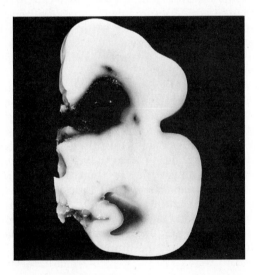

Figure 1–16C. Coronal section of cerebral hemisphere showing a subependymal germinal matrix hemorrhage with intraventricular extension.

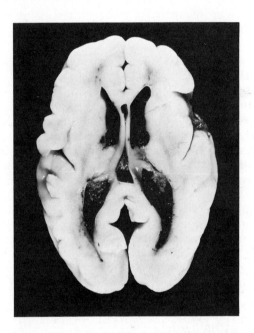

Figure 1–16D. Horizontal section of brain with bilateral germinal matrix hemorrhages.

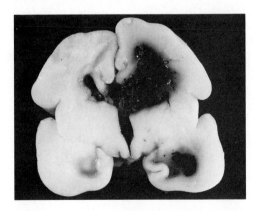

Figure 1–16E. Coronal section showing subependymal germinal matrix hemorrhage with intraventricular and intraparenchymal extensions.

35

1.17 Hydrocephalus Secondary to Remote Subependymal Germinal Matrix Hemorrhage

CLINICAL

This male infant was delivered by cesarean section at 30 weeks of gestation because of abruptio placentae. The infant's hospital course was complicated by respiratory distress syndrome, hyperbilirubinemia, intraventricular hemorrhage, and hydrocephalus. The infant died 4 months after birth.

PATHOLOGY

The brain was enlarged and moderately hydrocephalic. The convolutional markings appeared abnormally complex since the hydrocephalus effaced sulci and exposed gyri that normally would have been hidden from the surface (Fig. 1–17A). The meninges on the ventral surface of the cerebrum and inferior surfaces of the cerebellum were thickened and stained brown by hemosiderin (Fig. 1–17B). Horizontal section of the cerebrum disclosed dilatation of the ventricular system that was maximal in the occipital horns (Fig. 1–17C). The ependymal surfaces were roughened and hemosiderin stained. The choroid plexi were also brown colored.

COMMENT

Hydrocephalus is a major complication of intraventricular hemorrhage. This problem is being encountered more frequently since premature infants are now more likely to survive their initial problems. Enlargement of the entire ventricular system, including the fourth ventricle, as seen in another case (Fig. 1–17D) is evidence that the hydrocephalus results largely from obliteration of the subarachnoid space, rather than obstruction of intracerebral cerebrospinal fluid pathways.

Smaller subependymal germinal matrix hemorrhages may be completely resorbed, leaving multiloculated subependymal cysts in the regions of the germinal matrices (Fig. 1–17E). Similar lesions also may result from intrauterine viral infections and certain metabolic diseases, for example, Zellweger's syndrome.

Other cases of hydrocephalus are due to obstruction of the aqueduct in the absence of other obvious anomalies such as the Arnold–Chiari or Dandy–Walker malformation. Histological examination of the brain stem from these patients reveals narrowing of the aqueduct without gliosis or overt evidence of inflammation. The pathogenesis of this type of obstruction remains controversial. It was originally suggested that this lesion was a true developmental anomaly. Subsequently, some authors have suggested that the aqueduct is merely compressed and kinked secondary to hydrocephalus. Still others have suggested that aqueductal stenosis may be the result of inapparent intrauterine infections. This concept has received support from experimental studies. Certain intrauterine infections in laboratory animals can cause ependymitis and aqueductal stenosis without residual inflammation at the time of birth.

REFERENCES

Ahmann PA, Lazarra A, Dykes F, et al: Intraventricular hemorrhage in the high-risk preterm infant: Incidence and outcome. Ann Neurol 1980; 7:118-124.

Hill A, Volpe JJ: Seizures, hypoxic–ischemic brain injury, and intraventricular hemorrhage in the newborn. Ann Neurol 1981; 10:109-121.

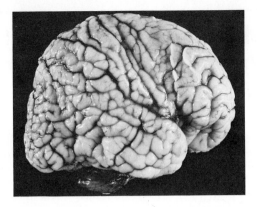

Figure 1–17A. Lateral surface of hydrocephalic brain.

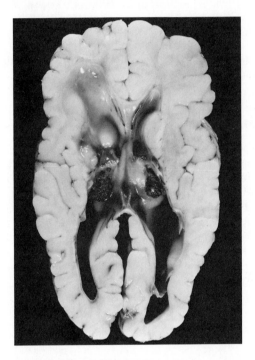

Figure 1–17C. Horizontal section of brain showing hydrocephalus and hemosiderin staining of choroid plexi.

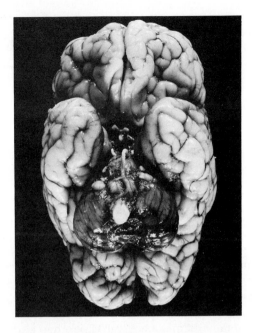

Figure 1–17B. Base of brain showing hemosiderin staining of meninges about cerebellum.

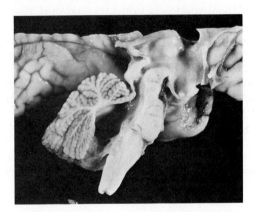

Figure 1–17D. Sagittal section of hydrocephalic brain. Note the enlarged aqueduct and fourth ventricle and the ependymal granulations.

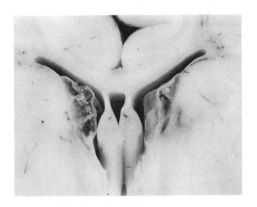

Figure 1–17E. Coronal section showing bilateral subependymal germinal matrix cysts.

1.18 Cerebellar Hemorrhage

CLINICAL

This infant was delivered by cesarean section at approximately 26 weeks of gestation because of abruptio placentae. The infant weighed only 920 grams at the time of delivery. The child had respiratory distress syndrome and died at age 4 months after a complicated hospital course.

PATHOLOGY

The brain weighed 256 grams. There was a striking discrepancy in the size of the cerebellar hemispheres (Fig. 1–18A). The leptomeninges over the lateral aspect of the smaller hemisphere were thickened and discolored yellow-brown (Fig. 1–18B). Sections of the cerebellum disclosed loss of tissue from the lateral half of the right cerebellar hemisphere (Fig. 1–18C). The surface of the lesion was yellow-brown and abnormally firm. There were lipid and pigment-laden macrophages in the area of destruction that extended medially into the lateral portion of the dentate nucleus (Fig. 1–18D). Histological examination of the medulla disclosed loss of neurons from a portion of the contralateral inferior olivary nucleus (Fig. 1–18E).

COMMENT

The tissue loss and discoloration of the right cerebellar hemisphere were the sequelae of an intracerebellar hematoma that had been resorbed by the time of the patient's demise. Cerebellar hematomas are being recognized with increased frequency in the brains of premature infants. Some authors have suggested that these lesions are caused by straps over the occiput. However, Larroche found similar hemorrhages in infants who had not been treated in this manner and correlated the increased occurrence of these lesions with more marked immaturity.

This case also displayed transsynaptic degeneration of the inferior olivary nucleus. This is seen most commonly in elderly patients with vascular lesions that interrupt the central tegmental tract. Similar changes may be seen with lesions anywhere along the so-called Guillain–Mollaret triangle.

REFERENCES

Lapresle J, Ben Hamida M: The dentato-olivary pathway. Somatotopic relationship between the dentate nucleus and the contralateral inferior olive. Arch Neurol 1970; 22:135-143.

Larroche J-C: Perinatal brain damage. In Adams JH, Corsellis JAN, Duchen LW (eds): Greenfield's Neuropathology, 4th ed. New York, Wiley, 1984, chap 11, pp 451-490.

Rorke LB: Pathology of Perinatal Brain Injury. New York, Raven Press, 1982, pp 37-44.

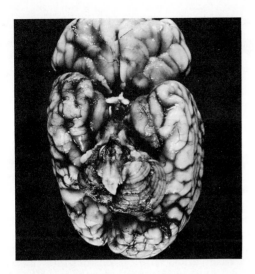

Figure 1–18A. Base of brain showing asymmetry of cerebellar hemispheres.

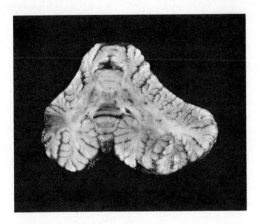

Figure 1–18C. Frontal section showing loss of tissue from right cerebellar hemisphere subsequent to previous hemorrhage.

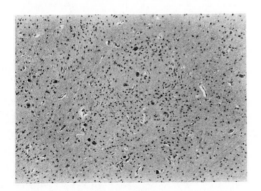

Figure 1–18E. Microscopic section showing loss of neurons and gliosis of left inferior olivary nucleus.

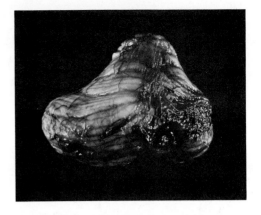

Figure 1–18B. Dorsal surface of cerebellum showing small, discolored right cerebellar hemisphere.

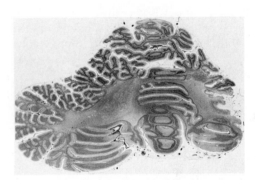

Figure 1–18D. Macrosection showing loss of tissue from lateral portion of right cerebellar hemisphere.

1.19 Periventricular Leukomalacia

CLINICAL

This 2300-gram male infant was born with an omphalocele. This was repaired surgically, but post-operatively the infant developed respiratory distress and sepsis. The infant died 10 days later.

PATHOLOGY

The brain weighed 344 grams. Externally the brain was unremarkable. On coronal sections, multiple small gray-white areas were seen in the cerebral white matter. The largest lesions were immediately rostral to the corpus callosum (Fig. 1–19A). Additional lesions were present in the white matter dorsolateral to the atria. Microscopically, the lesions appeared as sparsely cellular foci of coagulative necrosis (Fig. 1–19B).

COMMENT

Foci of white matter necrosis, otherwise known as periventricular leukomalacia, have been described in small premature infants and in larger infants with congenital heart disease, impaired cerebral perfusion, hypoxia, hypoglycemia, meningitis, or sepsis. Typically, the lesions are sparsely cellular foci of coagulative necrosis surrounded by reactive axons. Occasionally, they may be hemorrhagic. With longer survival, the lesions may become cavitated and contain varying proportions of lipid-laden macrophages and reactive astrocytes (Fig. 1–19C).

The lesions are most commonly encountered in the deep white matter near the lateral angle of the lateral ventricles, in the temporal isthmus, dorsolateral to the atrium, and in the optic radiations. Banker and Larroche interpreted these lesions as ischemic infarcts in border zones between ventriculofugal and ventriculopetal arteries. Alternatively, Gilles et al have suggested that the lesions may be caused by endotoxemia.

REFERENCES

Banker BQ, Larroche J-C: Periventricular leukomalacia of infancy: A form of neonatal anoxic encephalopathy. Arch Neurol 1962; 7:386-410.

Hill A, Volpe JJ: Seizures, hypoxic-ischemic brain injury, and intraventricular hemorrhage in the newborn. Ann Neurol 1981; 10:109-121.

Leviton A, Gilles FH: Acquired perinatal leucoencephalopathy. Ann Neurol 1984; 16:1-8.

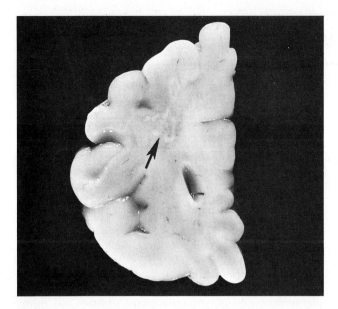

Figure 1–19A. Coronal section showing areas of periventricular leukomalacia (arrow) in the frontal white matter.

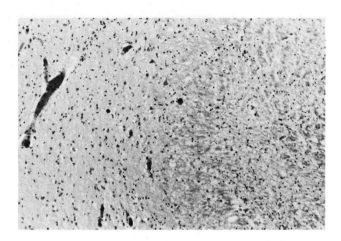

Figure 1–19B. Microscopic section showing coagulative necrosis (right) within the area of periventricular leukomalacia.

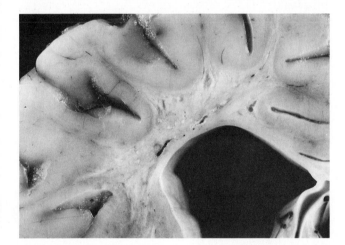

Figure 1–19C. Coronal section showing partially cavitated foci of periventricular leukomalacia in an infant with longer survival.

1.20   Multicystic Encephalopathy

CLINICAL

This 20-day-old infant was hospitalized with seizures. Although he was suspected of having encephalitis, this diagnosis was never confirmed and he was discharged 10 days later. The child was readmitted with severe lethargy at age 49 days. He did poorly and died 1 week later.

PATHOLOGY

The brain weighed 170 grams and tended to collapse, although the neural parenchyma was somewhat rubbery (Fig. 1–20A). Coronal sections revealed extensive loss of cerebral white matter, partial loss of cerebral cortex and relative preservation of the basal ganglia, thalamus, and hypothalamus (Fig. 1–20B). The cerebral hemispheres were cavitated and traversed by strands of glial tissue and blood vessels. Numerous lipid-laden macrophages were present in the margins of the white matter cysts and in the cortex. The cortex also showed severe loss of neurons and gliosis. No infectious agent could be identified and the major cerebral blood vessels were patent.

COMMENT

The pathological changes illustrated in this brain can be designated as multicystic encephalopathy. This is one of the many terms that has been used to describe this pattern of tissue destruction. The tissue loss is maximal in the cerebral white matter. The basal ganglia and thalamus are relatively well preserved. Another case, with a 4-year survival, is shown in Figure 1–20C.

Morphologically similar lesions can result from cerebral injuries sustained during the late antenatal, perinatal, or even early postnatal periods. In many cases, the lesions can be attributed to hypoxic or ischemic events associated with obstetrical complications. In other cases, an infectious etiology has been proposed.

REFERENCES

Aicardi J, Goutieres F, Hodebourg de Verbois A: Multicystic encephalomalacia of infants and its relation to abnormal gestation and hydranencephaly. J Neurol Sci 1972; 15:357-373.

Lyen KR, Lingam S, Butterfill AM, et al: Multicystic encephalomalacia due to fetal viral encephalitis. Eur J Pediatr 1981; 137:11-16.

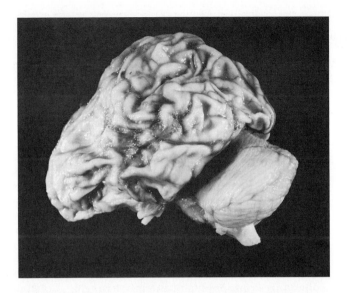

Figure 1–20A. Lateral view of brain showing partially collapsed cerebral hemispheres in an infant with multicystic encephalopathy.

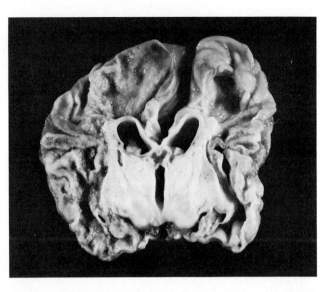

Figure 1–20B. Coronal section of brain with severe multicystic encephalopathy. Note the relative preservation of the basal ganglia and thalamus.

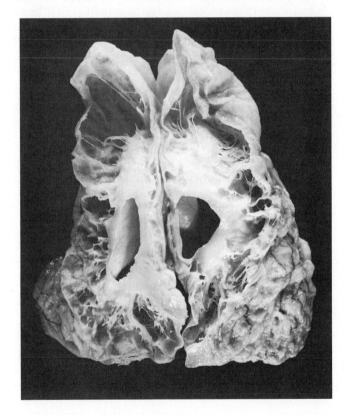

Figure 1–20C. Horizontal section of a brain from a 4-year-old child with multicystic encephalopathy.

1.21   Hydranencephaly

CLINICAL

This female infant was delivered by cesarean section because of a footling breech presentation. The newborn infant weighed 2600 grams and was meconium stained. The child was lethargic and developed tremors of the lower extremities. Transillumination of the head revealed red translucency.

PATHOLOGY

Dorsal and ventral views of the brain showed extensive loss of neural parenchyma from the cerebral hemispheres, with only portions of the inferior temporal and occipital lobes remaining intact (Figs. 1–21A and 1–21B) . In the areas of maximal destruction, the cerebral cortex was reduced to a thin membrane composed of gliotic neural parenchyma and leptomeninges that was focally adherent to the dura. The basal ganglia were partially disrupted and gliotic. Sagittal section of the brain stem (Fig. 1–21C) showed a small but relatively intact brain stem and cerebellum.

COMMENT

Hydranencephaly probably differs from multicystic encephalopathy only in the greater degree of tissue destruction. Both conditions can result from destruction of the cerebral hemispheres prior to, during, or immediately after birth. The etiology of both conditions is probably diverse, including vascular, infectious, and metabolic insults. The role of vascular insufficiency in cases of hydranencephaly is supported by the observation that the damage is generally maximal in the distribution of the carotid circulation.

The membranous remnants of the cerebral hemispheres may be densely adherent to the dura and are often disrupted during removal of the brain. The remaining components of the basal ganglia and thalamus may form a raised mass on the floor of the cavitated hemispheres. The aqueduct is usually obliterated by cellular debris and may account for the occurrence of postnatal head enlargement. In patients with early demise, the intrahemispheric cavities may contain hemorrhagic tissue debris (Fig. 1–21D). The brain stem is generally intact except for tract degeneration. The cerebellum is usually relatively well preserved.

REFERENCE

Larroche J-C: Perinatal brain damage. In Adams JH, Corsellis JAN, Duchen LW (eds): Greenfield's Neuropathology, 4th ed. New York, Wiley, 1984, pp 451-490.

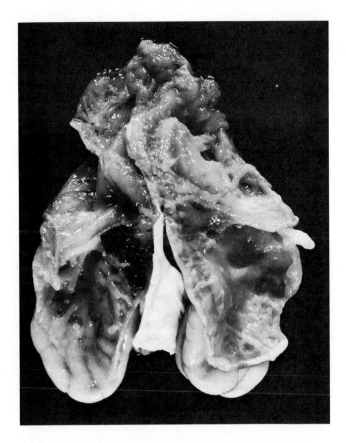

Figure 1–21A. Dorsal view of brain from infant with hydranencephaly.

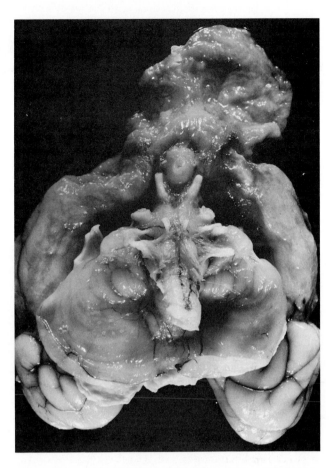

Figure 1–21B. Base of brain from infant with hydranencephaly. Note relative preservation of posterior temporal and occipital lobes.

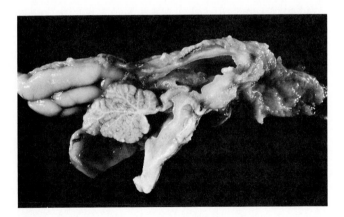

Figure 1–21C. Sagittal section of brain from infant with hydranencephaly. Note the preservation of the cerebellum.

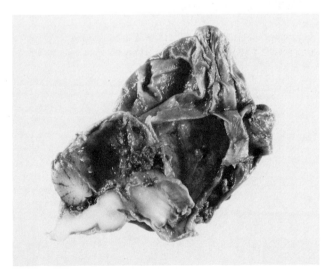

Figure 1–21D. Sagittal section showing hemorrhagic debris in a hydranencephalic brain following early demise.

1.22   Porencephaly

CLINICAL

This girl had a seizure disorder, spastic quadriparesis, and blindness since birth. She developed hydrocephalus and had multiple shunt procedures. She died at 26 months of age.

PATHOLOGY

There were massive bilateral but asymmetrical porencephalic cavities in both cerebral hemispheres (Figs. 1–22A and 1–22B). The cystic spaces extended from the lateral ventricles to the subarachnoid space (Fig. 1–22C). Externally, the cavities were covered by thin membranes composed of gliotic neural parenchyma and leptomeninges. Some of the gyri surrounding the porencephalic cavities were shrunken and irregular but did not display polymicrogyria. The ventricles were enlarged and covered by fine ependymal granulations.

COMMENT

Generally, defects in the cerebral hemispheres that extend from the ventricular system to the sub-arachnoid space are designated as porencephaly. Traditionally, two categories have been recognized. The more common encephaloclastic porencephaly is attributed to focal destruction of neural parenchyma usually during the perinatal period. Gyri surrounding these defects may be deformed and gliotic but do not show features suggestive of errors in cell migration. By contrast, the so-called schizencephalies are rare lesions that have been attributed to abnormalities in the development of the cerebral mantle. These lesions are usually bilateral and often symmetrical. They may be cystic defects or merely deep clefts in the lateral aspects of the cerebral hemispheres. Gyri surrounding the lesions are often radially oriented and show histological features of polymicrogyria. More recently, even these lesions have been attributed to tissue destruction.

REFERENCES

Dekaban A: Large defects in cerebral hemispheres associated with cortical dysgenesis. J Neuropathol Exp Neurol 1965; 24:512-530.

Warkany J, Lemire RJ, Cohen MM Jr: Mental Retardation and Congenital Malformations of the Central Nervous System. Chicago, Year Book, 1981, chap 8, pp 191-199.

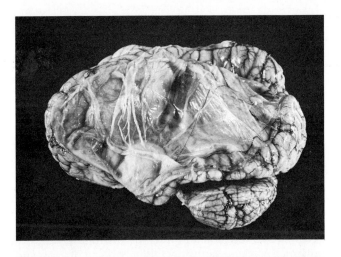

Figure 1–22A. Left lateral view of brain with bilateral porencephaly.

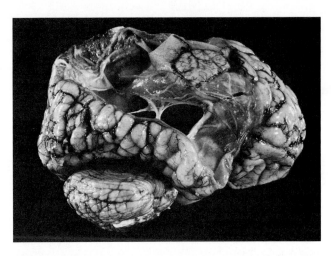

Figure 1–22B. Right lateral view of brain with bilateral porencephaly.

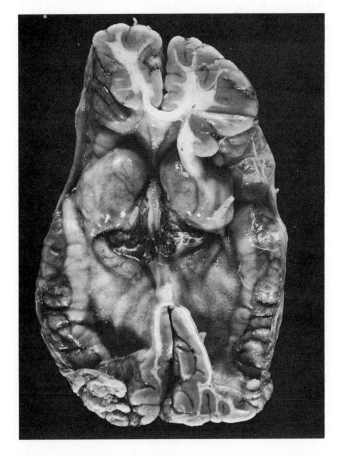

Figure 1–22C. Horizontal section of brain with bilateral poren-cephaly.

1.23 Ulegyria

CLINICAL

This 12-year-old girl had been born with an imperforate anus. A colostomy was performed at 18 hours of age and was revised at age 14 months. During the second procedure she suffered a cardiac arrest. Subsequently, she developed seizures and had psychomotor retardation.

PATHOLOGY

The brain was small and weighed only 464 grams. The cerebral hemispheres were symmetrical but abnormally firm. The gyri were narrowed and somewhat irregular (Fig. 1–23A). The gyral alterations were most apparent on the dorsal aspects of the frontal, parietal and occipital lobes (Fig. 1–23B). Horizontal sections of the cerebral hemispheres demonstrated the cortex to be thinned especially in the depths of sulci with more nearly normal gyral apices. The white matter was reduced in volume and the ventricular system was enlarged (Fig. 1–23C).

COMMENT

Hypoxic cerebral injury during early post-natal life may lead to cortical damage that is maximal in the depths of sulci and along the banks of the convolutions. The resulting sclerotic gyri have bulbous apices resembling mushrooms (Fig. 1–23D). This condition is described as ulegyria and must be distinguished from polymicrogyria, a condition that is thought to result from errors in migration or from hypoxic–ischemic insults occurring earlier in development. Less commonly, similar changes may be seen in the cerebellum (Fig. 1–23E).

REFERENCES

Friede RL: Developmental Neuropathology. New York, Springer Verlag, 1975, pp 57-63.

Menkes JH: Textbook of Child Neurology. Philadelphia, Lea & Febiger, 1985, chap 5, pp 271-315.

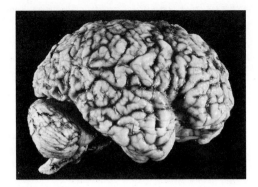

Figure 1–23A. Lateral view of brain with sclerotic ulegyria.

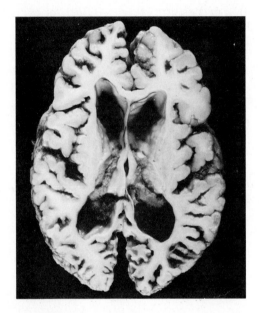

Figure 1–23C. Horizontal section of brain with sclerotic ulegyria. Note the especially severe involvement of the left frontal and both occipital lobes.

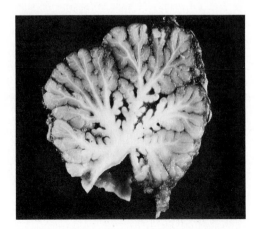

Figure 1–23E. Sagittal section of cerebellum showing sclerotic ulegyria.

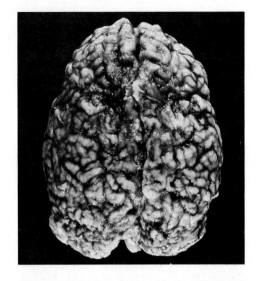

Figure 1–23B. Dorsal view of brain with sclerotic ulegyria.

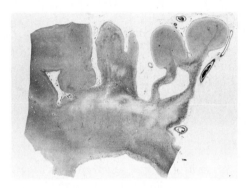

Figure 1–23D. Macrosection showing the maximal loss of tissue from the depths of sulci with relative preservation of gyral apices.

1.24   Cerebral Hemiatrophy

CLINICAL

This 58-year-old man died of pulmonary emboli. He had a lifelong history of mental retardation, seizures, and right hemiplegia. The right side of his body was smaller than the left.

PATHOLOGY

At the time of autopsy, it was noted that the base of his skull was somewhat asymmetrical. The left frontal fossa was smaller than the right and the left frontal sinuses were unusually prominent. The brain weighed only 921 grams and showed atrophy of the entire left hemisphere (Fig. 1–24A). Coronal sections of the cerebral hemispheres showed the gyri on the left to be narrowed with widened sulci (Fig. 1–24B). The subcortical and central white matter were reduced in volume (Fig. 1–24C). The basal ganglia had a mottled appearance but were nearly symmetrical. Transverse sections of the brain stem showed atrophy of the left mesencephalic peduncle, basis pontis, and medullary pyramid.

COMMENT

This patient with hemiplegia, atrophy of the right side of the body, and seizures had diffuse atrophy of the left cerebral hemisphere. This condition has been designated as "progressive sclerosing cortical atrophy of Schob." The pathogenesis of this condition is unsettled. Many of the individuals appear normal during the perinatal period but develop seizures in early childhood, often at the time of a febrile illness. Subsequently, they develop progressive hemiparesis. It has been suggested that the cerebral hemiatrophy is secondary to the recurrent seizures. Histological examination of the cortex reveals diffuse loss of neurons and gliosis.

The asymmetry of the skull with hypertrophy of the frontal bone and enlargement of the frontal sinuses comprises the so-called Dyke–Davidoff–Masson syndrome and merely reflects the early occurrence of the cerebral damage.

REFERENCES

Dyke CG, Davidoff LM, Masson CB: Cerebral hemiatrophy with homolateral hypertrophy of the skull and sinuses. Surg Gynecol Obstet 1933; 57:588-600.

Friede RL: Developmental Neuropathology. New York, Springer Verlag, 1975, pp 93-100.

Josephy H: Cerebral hemiatrophy (Diffuse sclerotic type of Schob). J Neuropathol Exp Neurol 1945; 4:250-261.

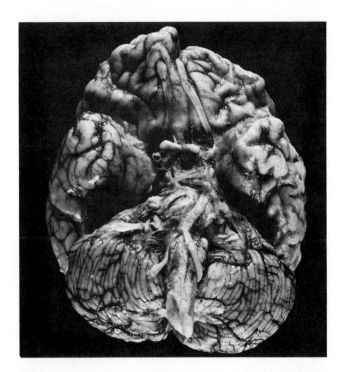

Figure 1–24A. Base of brain with hemiatrophy affecting the left cerebral hemisphere.

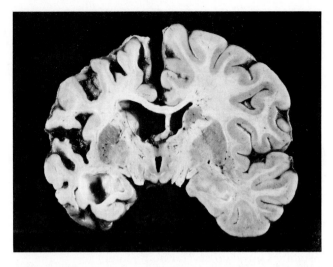

Figure 1–24B. Coronal section at level of mammillary bodies showing atrophy of left cerebral hemisphere.

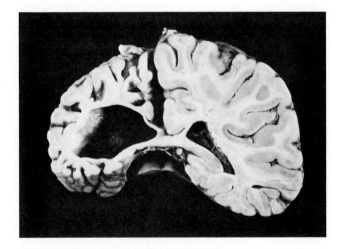

Figure 1–24C. Coronal section showing more severe atrophy in the caudal portion of the left cerebral hemisphere.

1.25 Hypotensive Brain Stem Necrosis

CLINICAL

This infant girl was delivered by emergency cesarean section when the mother developed profuse bleeding. Heart monitoring revealed severe fetal distress. At birth, the infant was pale and without pulse or spontaneous respirations. The infant was successfully resuscitated but died several hours later.

PATHOLOGY

The most striking grossly discernible abnormality in this brain was the presence of symmetrical discolored areas of hemorrhagic necrosis in the brain stem (Figs. 1–25A and 1–25B). Also present, but only evident microscopically, were areas of ischemic necrosis in the basis pontis.

COMMENT

Bilateral symmetrical foci of necrosis in the brain stem have been described as a complication of severe transient hypotension. The sites of predilection include neuronal nuclei in the mesencephalic tectum and the mesencephalic, pontine, and medullary tegmentum. These lesions may be accompanied by varying degrees of cortical necrosis in the cerebrum and cerebellum. Other infants with isolated asphyxial events may show foci of thalamic and brain stem necrosis.

Still other infants may show pontosubicular necrosis. This pattern of hypoxic injury is characterized by neuronal necrosis selectively involving the subiculum and adjacent entorhinal cortex along with gray matter in the basis pontis. Pontosubicular necrosis was originally described in infants whose ages were greater than 30 weeks of gestation but less than two postnatal months.

REFERENCES

Dambska M, Laure-Kamionowska M, Liebhart M: Brainstem lesions in the course of chronic fetal asphyxia. Clin Neuropathol 1987; 6:110-115.

Friede RL: Ponto-subicular lesions in perinatal anoxia. Arch Pathol 1972; 94:343-354.

Gilles FH: Hypotensive brain stem necrosis: Selective symmetrical necrosis of tegmental neuronal aggregates following cardiac arrest. Arch Pathol 1969; 88:32-41.

Rorke LB: Pathology of Perinatal Brain Injury. New York, Raven Press, 1982, pp 115-125.

Rowland EH, Hill A, Norman MG, et al: Selective brainstem injury in an asphyxiated newborn. Ann Neurol 1988; 23:89-92.

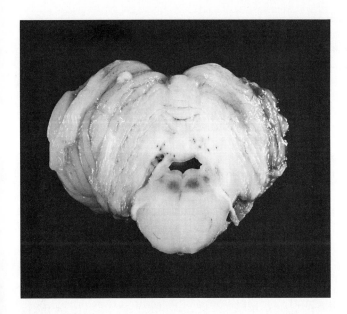

Figure 1–25A. Transverse section of brain stem showing foci of hemorrhagic necrosis in pontine tegmentum.

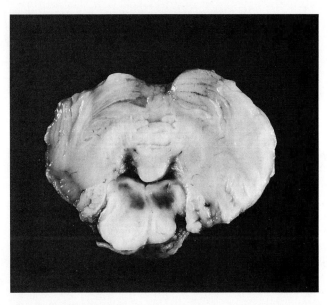

Figure 1–25B. Transverse section of brain stem showing foci of hemorrhagic necrosis in medullary tegmentum.

1.26 Neonatal Infarct

CLINICAL

Shortly after delivery, this full-term male infant became cyanotic, bradycardic, and hypotonic. Despite supportive measures, the infant died on the third postnatal day.

PATHOLOGY

The lateral aspect of the left frontal and parietal lobes was slightly swollen and softer than the rest of the brain. Coronal sections disclosed a lentiform area of softening and discoloration in the distribution of a portion of the left middle cerebral artery (Fig. 1–26A). Further examination of the vessels from the base of the brain disclosed thromboembolic material in the bifurcation of this artery.

COMMENT

In recent years there has been increased recognition of cerebral infarcts due to arterial occlusion in brains of neonates. In contrast to older individuals, the affected infants generally show only nonlocalizing manifestations such as lethargy, hypotonia, respiratory distress, bradycardia, and hypotension. Most of the patients are full-term infants and many die soon after the occurrence of the infarct. The majority of the infarcts are in the distribution of the middle cerebral arteries. Figures 1–26B and 1–26C illustrate a hemorrhagic infarct in the right occipital lobe of a full-term male infant who was the product of a normal gestation in a healthy young woman. The infant developed respiratory distress soon after an uneventful delivery and died the following day.

A widely patent ductus arteriosus was identified at autopsy. In this case, it seems possible that the occipital lobe infarct was secondary to cerebral swelling and compression of the right posterior cerebral artery. This hypothesis is supported by the coexistence of an additional infarct in the border zone between the left anterior and middle cerebral artery perfusion beds and hypotensive brain stem necrosis. No thromboembolic material was identified in any of the vessels.

REFERENCES

Barmada MA, Moossy J, Shuman RM: Cerebral infarcts with arterial occlusion in neonates. Ann Neurol 1979; 6:495-502.

Ment LR, Duncan CC, Ehrenkranz RA: Perinatal cerebral infarction. Ann Neurol 1984; 16:559-568.

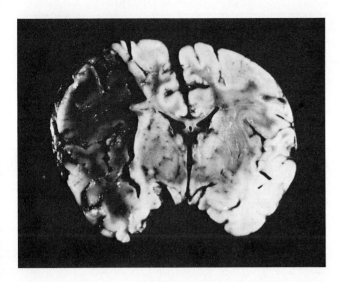

Figure 1–26A. Coronal section of infant brain showing a hemorrhagic infarct in the distribution of left middle cerebral artery.

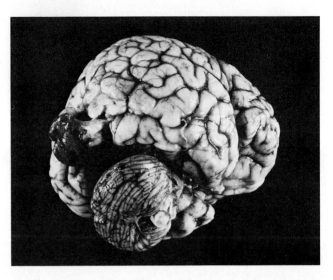

Figure 1–26B. Inferolateral view of right cerebral hemisphere showing hemorrhagic infarct in distribution of right posterior cerebral artery.

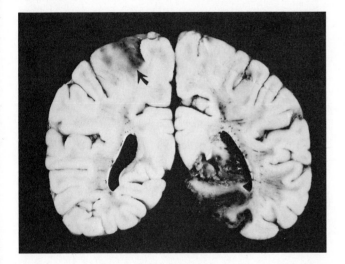

Figure 1–26C. Coronal section showing hemorrhagic infarct in distribution of right posterior cerebral artery. Note also border zone infarct (arrow) in left cerebral hemisphere.

2

Infections

2.1 Neonatal Meningitis

Group B Streptococci

CLINICAL

This infant was the product of a full-term gestation and weighed 3657 grams at the time of birth. At age 10 days, he was evaluated because of extreme irritability, poor feeding, and fever. A lumbar puncture revealed numerous polymorphonuclear leukocytes but no visible organisms. Cultures of cerebrospinal fluid grew group B streptococci. The child was treated with antibiotics. A second lumbar puncture 10 days after initiation of therapy disclosed rare polymorphonuclear leukocytes but no organisms could be seen or recovered by culture. Despite apparent improvement, the child died unexpectedly at age 50 days.

PATHOLOGY

The brain was mildly swollen and had a small amount of yellow-gray exudate in the subarachnoid space. This was maximal along the interhemispheric fissure on the dorsal aspect of the frontal lobes and on the ventromedial aspect of the left temporal lobe (Fig. 2–1A). Histological examination disclosed an admixture of lymphocytes, macrophages, and occasional polymorphonuclear leukocytes in the subarachnoid space (Fig. 2–1B).

COMMENT

Although a wide variety of bacteria have been reported to cause pyogenic meningitis, the majority of cases are actually due to a relatively small number of different organisms. These vary significantly with the age of the patient. During the neonatal period most cases of meningitis are due to *Escherichia coli* or group B streptococci. Predisposing factors include prematurity, prolonged rupture of membranes, maternal infections, and congenital malformations. *Escherichia coli*, especially strains with the K1 capsular antigen, have long been the most commonly identified organism. In recent years, group B streptococci have emerged as an important cause of neonatal meningitis and, in some areas, are even more common than *E. coli*. Group B streptococci produce two patterns of neonatal dis-

ease. The early onset form is a fulminating illness with generalized sepsis and respiratory distress. The infection is thought to be acquired intrapartum. The late onset form of group B streptococcal disease generally occurs between 2 and 6 weeks of age and is commonly manifested by meningitis. The mode of transmission in this form of the disease is unclear. Regardless of the age of the patient, most cases of streptococcal meningitis are due to organisms belonging to the group III serotype.

The color, quantity, and distribution of the exudate cannot be correlated reliably with the causative organism. The quantity of exudate is largely determined by the duration of the disease and whether the patient has been treated. Initially, abundant polymorphonuclear leukocytes and fibrin are encountered in the subarachnoid space. Later, macrophages and lymphocytes become the predominant cells. Organization of the exudate may lead to meningeal fibrosis. At least some degree of ventriculitis usually accompanies the meningitis. This may lead to aqueductal stenosis and hydrocephalus, although the latter complication is more often due to the meningeal fibrosis.

Meningitis is often accompanied by arteritis and phlebitis of the leptomeningeal vessels. Other cases may be complicated by dural sinus and venous thrombosis (Fig. 2–1C). These secondary vascular lesions produce cerebral infarcts that further contribute to the high morbidity and mortality of neonatal meningitis.

REFERENCES

Baker CJ, Barnett FF: Group B streptococcal infections in infants. The importance of the various serotypes. JAMA 1974; 230:1158-1160.

Bell WE, McCormick WF: Neurologic Infections in Children, 2nd ed. Philadelphia, Saunders, 1981, chap 3, pp 105-133.

Boyer KM, Gotoff SP: Prevention of early-onset group B streptococcal disease with selective intrapartum chemoprophylaxis. N Engl J Med 1986; 314:1665-1669.

Horn KA, Meyer WT, Wyrick BC, Zimmerman RA: Group B streptococcal neonatal infection. JAMA 1974; 230:1165-1167.

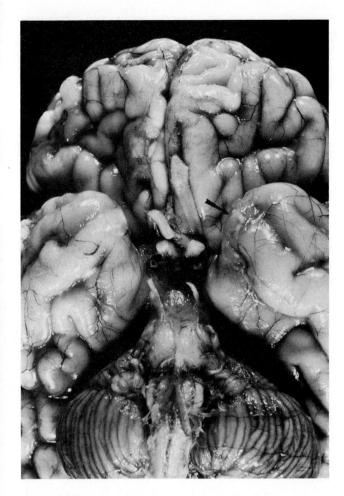

Figure 2–1A. Base of brain showing small amount of exudate best seen on ventromedial aspect of left temporal lobe (arrow).

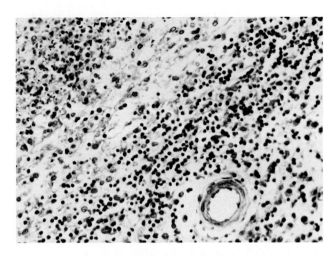

Figure 2–1B. Microscopic section showing mixed inflammatory cell infiltrate in subarachnoid space.

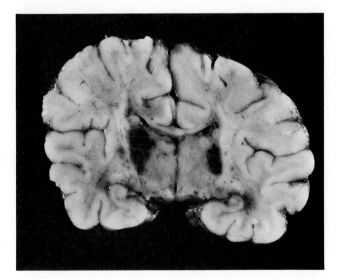

Figure 2–1C. Coronal section from another case of group B streptococcal meningitis that was complicated by venous thrombosis. Note areas of hemorrhagic infarction in lateral portions of thalami.

2.2 Neonatal Meningitis

Listeria Monocytogenes

CLINICAL

This 1100-gram female infant was the product of an estimated 28- to 30-week gestation. The pregnancy was uncomplicated except for fever 2 days prior to delivery. At birth, the neonate had no spontaneous activity but responded to resuscitation. A chest x-ray showed a fine granular appearance to the lungs. A sepsis work-up was initiated and blood cultures grew *Listeria monocytogenes*. The infant initially improved with antibiotic therapy but experienced several episodes of bradycardia and died 2 days later.

PATHOLOGY

The general autopsy revealed multiple microabscesses in the lungs, liver, and adrenals. The brain weighed only 165 grams. The leptomeningeal blood vessels were severely congested. The subarachnoid space contained exudate that was most evident over the dorsal lateral aspects of the posterior frontal and parietal lobes (Fig. 2–2A). The subarachnoid space also contained blood adjacent to the outlet foramina of the fourth ventricle. Coronal sections of the cerebral hemispheres disclosed a subependymal germinal matrix hemorrhage that had ruptured into the ventricular system. Histological examination revealed a large proportion of mononuclear cells among the inflammatory cells in the subarachnoid space (Fig. 2–2B). No necrotic foci or granulomatous lesions were present in the brain stem.

COMMENT

Listeria monocytogenes is a small pleomorphic gram-positive bacillus. It is an uncommon but well recognized cause of meningitis and meningoencephalitis. Congenital listeriosis may be acquired by transplacental spread of a mild or asymptomatic maternal infection to the fetus. This can lead to a disseminated necrotizing and granulomatous disease in the infected neonates referred to as granulomatosis infantiseptica. In other infants, especially premature infants, the infection may be acquired at the time of delivery and cause meningitis. The inflammatory response is often characterized by a relatively large proportion of mononuclear cells as in the present case.

Listeriosis also causes meningitis and meningoencephalitis in elderly and immunocompromised individuals. Rarely, adults may have rhombencephalitis in the absence of meningitis.

REFERENCES

Heck AF: *Listeria monocytogenes*. In Vinken PJ, Bruyn GW (eds): Handbook of Clinical Neurology. Amsterdam, Elsevier, 1978, vol 33, chap 7, pp 77-95.

Ishak K: Listeriosis. In Binford CH, Connor DH (eds): Pathology of Tropical and Extraordinary Diseases. Washington DC, Armed Forces Institute of Pathology, 1976, vol 1, chap 7, pp 178-186.

Weinstein AJ, Schiavone WA, Furlan AJ: Listeria rhombencephalitis. Report of a case. Arch Neurol 1982; 39:514-516.

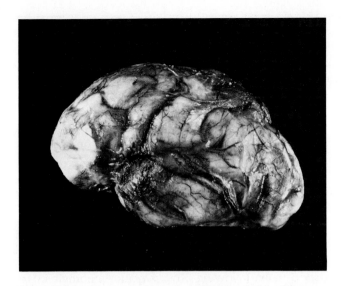

Figure 2–2A. Dorsolateral view of cerebral hemispheres from an infant with *Listeria monocytogenes* meningitis.

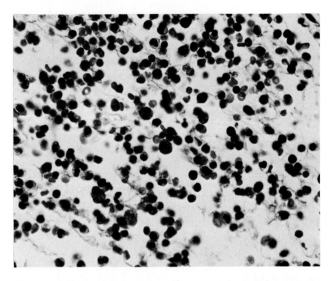

Figure 2–2B. Microscopic section showing the large proportion of mononuclear cells in the subarachnoid exudate.

2.3 Childhood Meningitis

Hemophilus influenzae

CLINICAL

This 5½-month-old male infant had a 1-week history of diarrhea. He developed fever, lethargy, and dyspnea. On arrival to the emergency room, he had a cardiac arrest. Blood cultures subsequently grew *Hemophilus influenzae*.

PATHOLOGY

The brain was swollen with widened gyri and narrowed sulci. The leptomeningeal blood vessels, including the very small vessels, were prominently congested (Fig. 2–3A). Yellow-green exudate was present in the subarachnoid space. This was most evident at the base of the brain (Fig. 2–3B) and along the leptomeningeal blood vessels. Coronal sections of the brain revealed diffuse edema with mild compression of the ventricular system. Histological examination demonstrated intact and degenerating polymorphonuclear leukocytes, macrophages, and fibrin within the subarachnoid space (Fig. 2–3C).

COMMENT

Hemophilus influenzae is the most common cause of meningitis in children between the ages of 3 months and 3 years. This selective age range is the result of diminishing protection from maternal IgG prior to the development of adequate acquired immunity in the child. *Hemophilus influenzae* is a small pleomorphic gram-negative bacillus. Most of the childhood cases are due to the serotype B organisms.

Despite the declining mortality rate, *Hemophilus influenzae* meningitis is often followed by a number of neurological sequelae. These include sensorineural hearing loss and focal deficits secondary to infarcts from the accompanying vasculitis. Subdural effusions (Fig. 2–3D) are commonly regarded as a complication of *Hemophilus influenzae* meningitis. However, they may be seen following other types of meningitis that involve children in this age group.

Hemophilus influenzae occasionally causes meningitis in adults. Frequently, these individuals have structural cranial defects or underlying debilitating diseases. In adults, the infections are less consistently due to type B organisms.

REFERENCES

Bell WE, McCormick WF: Neurologic Infections in Children, 2nd ed. Philadelphia, Saunders, 1981, chap 4, pp 134-154.

Drayna CJ: *Haemophilus influenzae* type C meningitis with sepsis. JAMA 1980; 244:1476.

Dunn DW, Daum RS, Weisberg L, Vargas R: Ischemic cerebrovascular complications of *Haemophilus influenzae* meningitis: The value of computed tomography. Arch Neurol 1982; 39:650-652.

MacDonald JT, Feinstein S: Hearing loss following *Hemophilus influenzae* meningitis in infancy. Arch Neurol 1984; 41:1058-1059.

Schlech WF III, Ward JI, Band JD, et al: Bacterial meningitis in the United States, 1978 through 1981. JAMA 1985; 253:1749-1754.

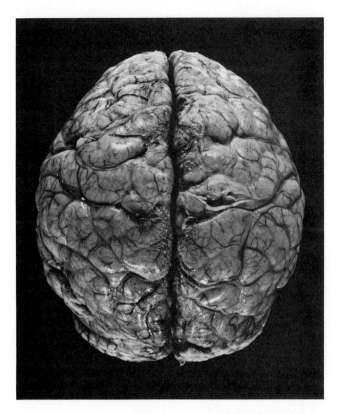

Figure 2–3A. Dorsal view of brain from child with *Haemophilus influenzae* meningitis showing exudate in subarachnoid space.

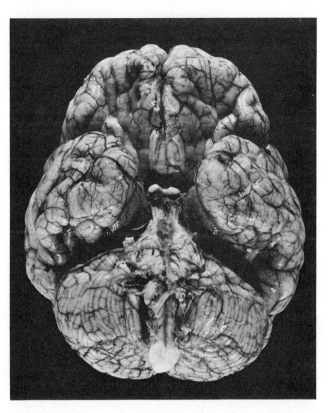

Figure 2–3B. Base of brain showing exudate in subarachnoid space and intense congestion of leptomeningeal blood vessels.

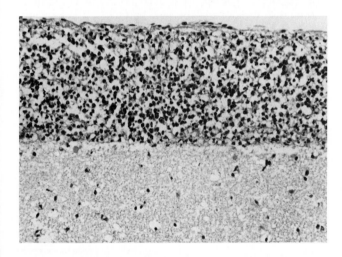

Figure 2–3C. Microscopic section showing exudate in subarachnoid space.

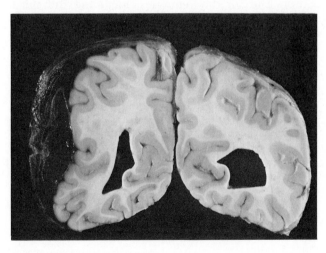

Figure 2–3D. Coronal section from a case of meningitis complicated by a subdural effusion.

2.4 Childhood Meningitis

Pneumococcal Meningitis

CLINICAL

This previously healthy, 9-year-old girl developed back, head, and eye pain. Shortly thereafter, she became febrile, confused, and combative. Nuchal rigidity was noted on examination. A lumbar puncture yielded grossly cloudy fluid with more than 10,000 white cells and numerous gram-positive diplococci. The cerebrospinal fluid glucose was markedly depressed and the protein was elevated. Despite intensive treatment, the girl died while still in the emergency room.

PATHOLOGY

The brain was markedly swollen and the leptomeningeal blood vessels were prominently congested (Fig. 2–4A). Scanty gray to yellow exudate was present throughout the subarachnoid space. The cerebral swelling caused deep grooving of both unci (Fig. 2–4B), mild parahippocampal herniation, and cerebellar tonsillar herniation (Fig. 2–4C). Coronal sections of the cerebral hemispheres revealed marked edema, with compression of the ventricles, including the third ventricle, and central herniation manifested by ventral displacement of the hypothalamus (Fig. 2–4D). Histological examination revealed numerous acute inflammatory cells within the subarachnoid space, within the Virchow–Robin spaces, and diffusely infiltrating the superficial layers of the cerebral cortex (Fig. 2–4E).

COMMENT

Pneumococcal meningitis is one of the most common causes of meningitis at all ages beyond early childhood. The disease is caused by *Streptococcus pneumoniae* , a gram-positive coccus. The organisms are often encountered as encapsulated pairs, accounting for the former name of *Diplococcus pneumoniae* .

Pneumococcal meningitis is often a complication of pneumonia, sinusitis, or otitis. The disease occurs with increased frequency among individuals with sickle cell disease and in patients who have had splenectomy during childhood. Alcoholism, skull fractures, and underlying neoplastic diseases are important predisposing factors in adults. Pneumococcal meningitis is frequently followed by neurological sequelae and the disease has a relatively high mortality. As in the present case, cerebral edema and herniation contribute to the unfavorable outcome.

REFERENCES

Bell WE, McCormick WF: Neurologic Infections in Children, 2nd ed. Philadelphia, Saunders, 1981, chap 6, pp 176-187.

Bohr V, Paulson OB, Rasmussen N: Pneumococcal meningitis: Late neurologic sequelae and features of prognostic impact. Arch Neurol 1984; 41:1045-1049.

Horwitz SJ, Boxerbaum B, O'Bell J: Cerebral herniation in bacterial meningitis in childhood. Ann Neurol 1980; 7:524-528.

Schlech WF III, Ward JI, Band JD, et al: Bacterial meningitis in the United States, 1978 through 1981. JAMA 1985; 253:1749-1754.

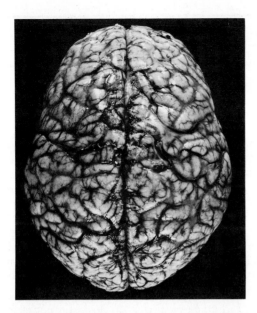

Figure 2–4A. Dorsal view of brain from child with pneumococcal meningitis. Note exudate in subarachnoid space best seen along congested leptomeningeal vessels.

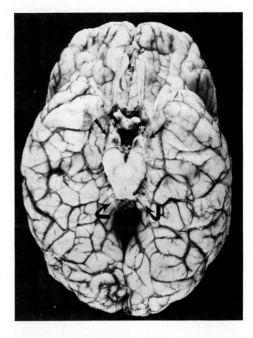

Figure 2–4B. Base of brain showing bilateral uncal herniation (arrows) and parahippocampal herniation (curved arrows).

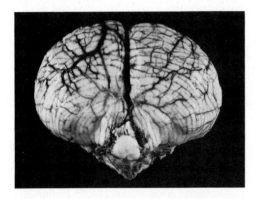

Figure 2–4C. Cerebellum showing subarachnoid exudate and cerebellar tonsillar herniation.

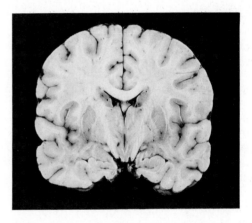

Figure 2–4D. Coronal section showing severe cerebral edema with bilateral uncal herniation and central herniation.

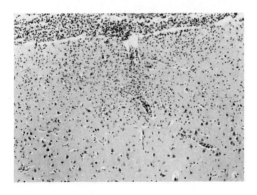

Figure 2–4E. Microscopic section showing inflammatory cells in superficial layer of cerebral cortex as well as subarachnoid space and Virchow–Robin spaces.

2.5 Pneumococcal Meningitis

Complicated by Venous Thrombosis

CLINICAL

This 40-year-old man had a history of recurrent otitis media and right ear pain. When found unresponsive to stimuli, he was suspected of having meningitis. The right external auditory canal contained blood and the tympanic membrane was bulging and had perforated. A computerized tomogram of the head revealed edema of the left cerebral hemisphere. Examination of the cerebrospinal fluid revealed 660 polymorphonuclear leukocytes, reduced glucose, and elevated protein. Gram-positive cocci, in pairs and chains, were seen in a smear and *Streptococcus pneumoniae* was cultured from the cerebrospinal fluid. Despite antibiotic therapy, the patient died 2 weeks after hospitalization.

PATHOLOGY

The brain was swollen and the meningeal blood vessels were congested. There was abundant gray to yellow exudate in the subarachnoid space. This was maximal on the dorsal surface of the cerebral hemispheres adjacent to the sagittal fissure (Fig. 2–5A). Coronal sections of the cerebral hemispheres showed thrombosed cortical veins (Fig. 2–5B) in areas where the subarachnoid exudate was most abundant. The cerebral cortex adjacent to the thrombosed veins showed early hemorrhagic infarction. In addition, a yellow-gray mass of partially organized thrombus (Fig. 2–5C) was found in the caudal portion of the sagittal sinus, adjacent to the torcula. Histological examination revealed purulent material in the lumen and walls of veins entering this portion of the dural sinus (Fig. 2–5D).

COMMENT

This case illustrates thrombosis of cortical veins and focal septic thrombosis of the sagittal sinus as a complication of pneumococcal meningitis. In the present case, the exudate is especially abundant over the dorsal surfaces of the cerebral hemispheres. This distribution of the exudate has been attributed to involvement of arachnoid granulations during the early stages of pneumococcal meningitis. Nevertheless, the distribution and appearance of the purulent exudate do not reliably reflect which organism is responsible for the meningitis.

REFERENCES

Cairns H, Russell DS: Cerebral arteritis and phlebitis in pneumococcal meningitis. J Pathol Bact 1946; 58:649-665.

Harris AA, Sokalski SJ, Levin S: Pneumococcal meningitis. In Vinken PJ, Bruyn GW (eds): Handbook of Clinical Neurology. Amsterdam, Elsevier, 1978, vol 33, chap 3, pp 35-52.

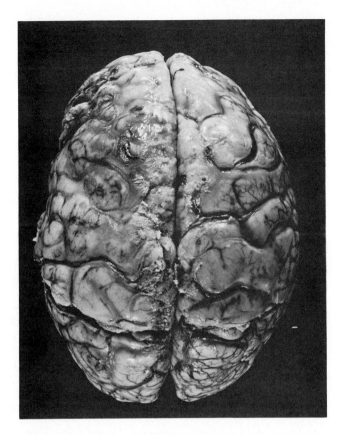

Figure 2–5A. Dorsal surface of brain showing copious exudate on dorsal surface of cerebral hemispheres.

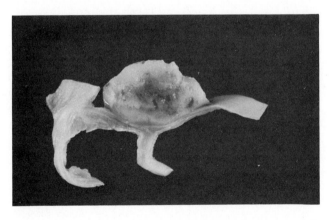

Figure 2–5C. Mass of partially organized thrombus in the interior of the sagittal sinus.

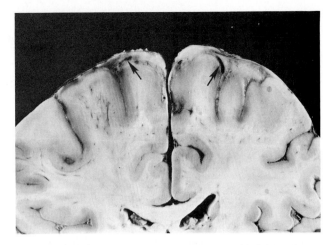

Figure 2–5B. Coronal sections showing thrombosed leptomeningeal veins (arrows) surrounded by copious subarachnoid exudate.

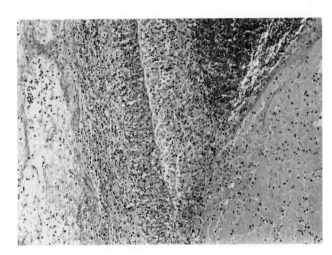

Figure 2–5D. Microscopic section showing purulent material in the wall and lumen of thrombosed meningeal vein.

2.6 Meningococcal Meningitis

CLINICAL

This 54-year-old woman with a 1-year history of systemic lupus erythematosus developed fever, chills, and exacerbation of joint pain. Later the same day, she was found unresponsive to verbal stimuli. A lumbar puncture revealed 1678 white blood cells (predominantly polymorphonuclear leukocytes), depressed glucose, and elevated protein. Numerous gram-negative diplococci were seen in a smear of the cerebrospinal fluid and *Neisseria meningitidis* was cultured from the cerebrospinal fluid. She died from systemic complications 1 week later.

PATHOLOGY

Examination of the brain revealed mild cerebral edema but copious amounts of gray exudate within the subarachnoid space (Fig. 2–6). Histologically the inflammatory exudate consisted of an admixture of acute and chronic inflammatory cells.

COMMENT

Nasopharyngeal colonization by *Neisseria meningitidis* is common and usually asymptomatic. By contrast, meningococcemia is infrequent and results from tissue invasion and hematogenous dissemination of the organism. When severe, the bacteremia and endotoxemia can lead to disseminated intravascular coagulation and rapid death. Most of the fatal cases have hemorrhagic lesions on the skin, mucous membranes, and serosal surfaces. The Waterhouse–Friderichsen syndrome, characterized by adrenal hemorrhages and infarcts, occurs in about one half of the fatal cases. Nearly 80 percent show foci of myocarditis. More recently, the shock and rapid demise have been attributed to microvascular thrombi in the lungs and acute development of cor pulmonale.

Many of the patients dying rapidly with meningococcemia have cerebral congestion and edema but only minimal subarachnoid exudate. Others may have hemorrhagic lesions reflecting the disseminated intravascular coagulation. Still others have meningitis and microscopic foci of cerebritis. Rarely, older patients or patients with intercurrent diseases develop a subacute meningitis with copious exudate. In the present case, the deficiency of complement components associated with lupus erythematosus, probably promoted the development of the subacute form of the disease.

REFERENCES

Artenstein MS: Meningococcal meningitis. In Vinken PJ, Bruyn GW (eds): Handbook of Clinical Neurology. Amsterdam, Elsevier, 1978, vol 33, chap 2 pp 21-33.

Bell WE, McCormick WF: Neurologic Infections in Children, 2nd ed. Philadelphia, Saunders, 1981, chap 5, pp 155-175.

Dalldorf FG, Jennette C: Fatal meningococcal septicemia. Arch Pathol Lab Med 1977; 101:6-9.

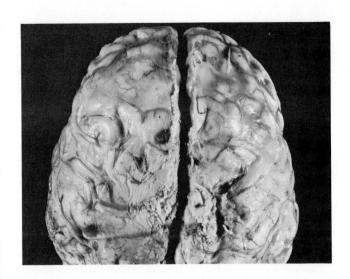

Figure 2-6. Dorsal view of brain showing copious subarachnoid exudate due to chronic meningococcal meningitis in a patient with lupus erythematosus.

2.7   Subdural Empyema

CLINICAL

This 40-year-old man was involved in a motor vehicle accident. He sustained a left frontal laceration and bilateral mandibular and ethmoid fractures. He remained unresponsive to pain from the time of the accident. His hospital course was complicated by pneumonia and diabetes insipidus. A left subdural hygroma (Fig. 2–7A) was evacuated. He died 3 weeks after the accident.

PATHOLOGY

Copious gray-white exudate was present in the subdural space over the dorsolateral surface of the left frontal lobe. Much of the semifluid purulent material was lost at the time of brain removal. However, sufficient exudate remained adherent to the outer surface of the leptomeninges to obscure the details of the underlying frontal lobe (Fig. 2–7B). The patient also had leptomeningitis, cortical vein thrombosis, and venous infarcts. The thrombosed cortical veins were accompanied by gray-white exudate over the dorsal aspect of the cerebral hemispheres. Coronal sections showed the exudate on the outer surface of the meninges over the left frontal lobe, leptomeningitis, foci of hemorrhagic necrosis, and foci of cerebritis (Fig. 2–7C). Histological examination of sections from the left frontal lobe showed the exudate to be maximal on the outer surface of the leptomeninges (Fig. 2–7D).

COMMENT

Subdural abscesses or empyemas are uncommon but serious infections that are most often a complication of sinusitis or otitis. Occasionally, they result from penetrating wounds or complicated surgical procedures. Some develop from secondary infection of chronic subdural hematomas. Rarely, they may be the result of hematogenous spread from a distant site of infection such as a lung abscess. In about 25 percent of cases, subdural empyemas are bilateral. The lesions may be difficult to detect by computerized tomography. A wide variety of organisms have been isolated from subdural empyemas. Most often they are aerobic or microaerophilic Streptococci, anaerobic cocci, or Staphylococci. Spinal subdural empyemas are much less common than cranial subdural empyemas and are usually the result of hematogenous dissemination.

REFERENCES

Dunker RD, Khakoo RA: Failure of computed tomographic scanning to demonstrate subdural empyema. JAMA 1981; 246:1116-1118.

Kaufman DM, Litman N, Miller MH: Sinusitis: Induced subdural empyema. Neurology 1983; 33:123-132.

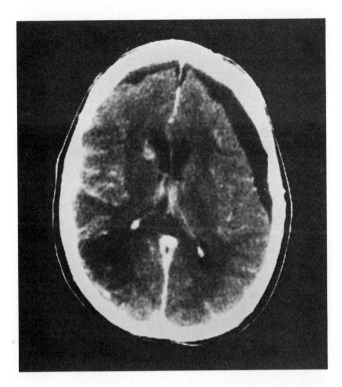

Figure 2–7A. Computerized tomogram showing large subdural hygroma over left frontal lobe and smaller hygroma over right frontal pole.

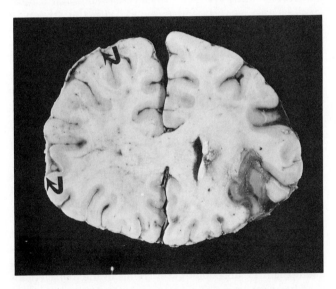

Figure 2–7C. Coronal section showing subdural exudate over left frontal lobe (between arrows) and hemorrhagic necrosis in inferolateral portion of right frontal lobe.

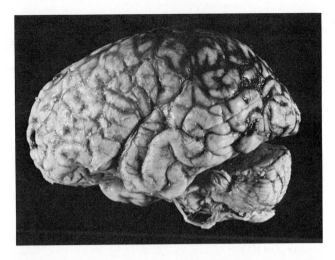

Figure 2–7B. Lateral surface of brain showing shaggy, gray-white purulent exudate adherent to outer surface of leptomeninges over left frontal lobe.

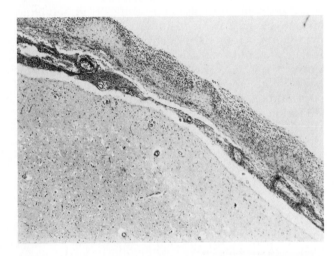

Figure 2–7D. Microscopic section showing abundant subdural exudate.

2.8　Brain Abscess

CLINICAL

When initially seen, this 14-year-old girl was mildly febrile and complained of headaches. She was thought to have sinusitis. She died 1 week later, shortly after being brought to an emergency room for a seizure.

PATHOLOGY

Coronal sections of the cerebral hemispheres revealed a poorly encapsulated cerebral abscess in the left frontal lobe surrounded by edematous white matter (Fig. 2–8A). The contents of the abscess were semifluid and gray-green in color. Histological examination demonstrated necrotic tissue debris, polymorphonuclear leukocytes, and numerous macrophages in the interior of the lesion. The wall of the abscess was composed of inflamed granulation tissue (Fig. 2–8B). The surrounding neural parenchyma was edematous and gliotic.

COMMENT

There are multiple circumstances that predispose individuals to brain abscesses. Formerly, a large proportion of abscesses arose as complications of otitis, mastoiditis, or sinusitis. Abscesses associated with otitis and mastoiditis were commonly in the temporal lobes or cerebellum while those complicating sinusitis were more often in the frontal lobes. In these cases, the infection may gain access to the nervous system by retrograde thrombophlebitis.

Other abscesses are the result of hematogenous dissemination from more distant sites. Formerly, bronchopulmonary infections such as bronchiectasis and lung abscesses were major causes of brain abscesses. Cyanotic congenital heart disease is still an important predisposing circumstance in children. In more recent years, opportunistic infections associated with the acquired immune deficiency syndrome have emerged as major problems. Abscesses secondary to hematogenous dissemination may arise anywhere in the central nervous system but are most often found within the distribution of the middle cerebral arteries. They are usually multiple and can be visualized by computerized tomography (Fig. 2–8C).

Less commonly, abscesses may complicate surgical procedures or penetrating head wounds. Especially when there is retained foreign material, a cerebral abscess may become symptomatic long after the injury. This is illustrated by an abscess containing a fragment of shrapnel (Figs. 2–8D and 2–8E) that became symptomatic 25 years after the injury.

Herniation from the mass effect of the associated cerebral edema is usually the most serious feature of brain abscesses. The edema is thought to occur because the proliferating endothelial cells in the abscess capsule do not form a competent blood–brain barrier. Less often, the abscesses may rupture into the ventricular system.

Brain abscesses are caused by a wide variety of organisms, including anaerobic and microaerophilic species among the most common of which are anaerobic streptococci, staphylococci, *Bacteroides*, and various gram-negative bacilli. With the advent of the acquired immune deficiency syndrome, various mycobacteria, fungi, and parasites have been encountered with increased frequency.

REFERENCES

Brook I: Bacteriology of intracranial abscess in children. J Neurosurg 1981; 54:484-488.

Garfield J: Brain abscesses and focal suppurative infections. In Vinken PJ, Bruyn GW (eds). Handbook of Clinical Neurology. Amsterdam, Elsevier, 1978, vol 33, chap 9, pp 107-147.

Kagawa M, Takeshita M, Yato S, Kitamura K: Brain abscess in congenital cyanotic heart disease. J Neurosurg 1983; 58:913-917.

Mampalam TJ, Rosenblum ML: Trends in the management of bacterial brain abscesses: A review of 102 cases over 17 years. Neurosurgery 1988; 23:451-458.

Yang S-Y: Brain abscess: A review of 400 cases. J Neurosurg 1981; 55:794-799.

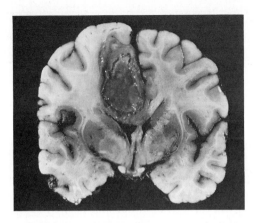

Figure 2–8A. Coronal section showing pyogenic abscess in left frontal lobe.

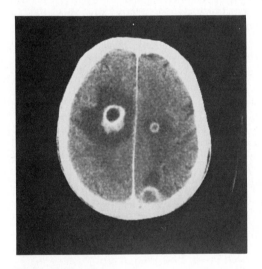

Figure 2–8C. Computerized tomogram showing multiple abscesses.

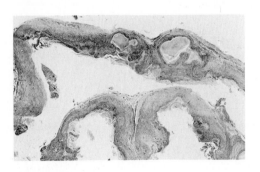

Figure 2–8E. Microscopic section showing the densely fibrotic wall of the chronic abscess.

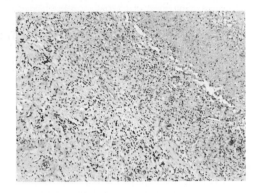

Figure 2–8B. Microscopic section showing the inflamed granulation tissue comprising the wall of the abscess.

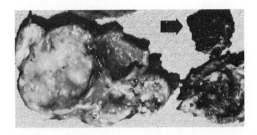

Figure 2–8D. Chronic abscess containing fragment of shrapnel (arrow). *(Schochet, SS Jr: Infectious diseases. In RN Rosenberg (ed.):* The Clinical Neurosciences. *New York: Churchill Livingstone, vol 3, chapter 5, pp III:195–III:240, 1983.)*

2.9   Nocardiosis

CLINICAL

This 73-year-old man had a history of autoimmune hemolytic anemia and had been on chronic steroid therapy. He was admitted to the hospital with a fever of unknown origin. Pulmonary lesions developed and he died a few weeks after admission.

PATHOLOGY

Coronal sections of the cerebral hemispheres revealed multiple abscesses (Figs. 2–9A and 2–9B). The abscesses contained yellow to gray necrotic, purulent material and were poorly encapsulated. The surrounding neural parenchyma displayed little edema. Sections of the brain stem disclosed an additional abscess in the pontine tegmentum (Fig. 2–9C). Histological examination of the abscesses disclosed numerous thin, branched filaments. These were gram-positive, weakly acid-fast and best demonstrated with the methenamine silver technique (Fig. 2–9D).

COMMENT

Disseminated nocardiosis is becoming more prevalent as an opportunistic infection in immunocompromised individuals. The disease is caused by an aerobic filamentous bacteria that is classified among the actinomycetes. Although there are several pathogenic species, most of the disseminated infections are due to *Nocardia asteroides*. The lungs are the usual site of primary infection and may lead to pulmonary abscesses or empyema. The cerebral abscesses are the result of hematogenous dissemination and occur in 25 to 30 percent of cases of systemic nocardiosis. As in the present case, the abscesses are often multiple and show minimal encapsulation. Meningitis is rare. The organisms are best demonstrated by the use of overstained methenamine silver preparations. We have used this technique on smears and aspirates from abscesses as well as tissue sections.

REFERENCES

Adair JC, Beck AC, Apfelbaum RI, Baringer R: Nocardial cerebral abscesses in the acquired immunodeficiency syndrome. Arch Neurol 1987; 44:548-550.

Frazier AR, Rosenow ED, Roberts GD: Nocardiosis: A review of 25 cases occurring in 24 months. Mayo Clin Proc 1975; 50:657-663.

Myerowitz RL: The Pathology of Opportunistic Infections: With Pathogenetic, Diagnostic, and Clinical Correlations. New York, Raven Press, 1983, chap 8, pp 77-82.

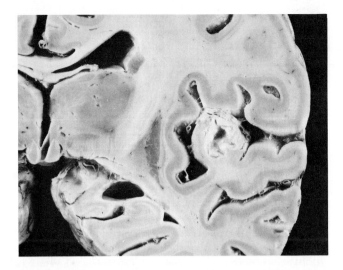

Figure 2–9A. Coronal section showing an abscess in the right insula due to *Nocardia*.

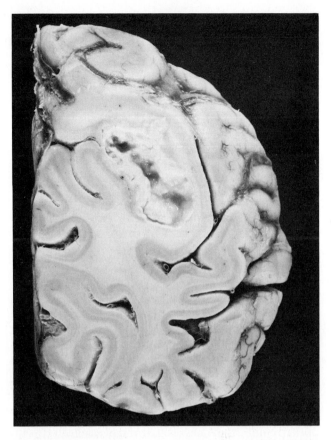

Figure 2–9B. Coronal section showing an abscess in the right parietal lobe due to *Nocardia*.

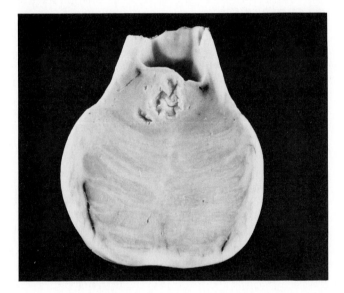

Figure 2–9C. Abscess in brain stem due to *Nocardia*.

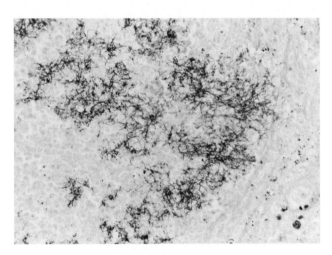

Figure 2–9D. Microscopic section, stained by the Gomori methenamine silver technique, showing the thin, branched filaments characteristic of *Nocardia*.

2.10   Epidural Abscess

Spinal

CLINICAL

This 45-year-old woman had moderately well differentiated carcinoma of the colon. She developed pelvic metastases and received abdominal and pelvic radiation as well as chemotherapy. She died shortly after developing bony metastases.

PATHOLOGY

At autopsy, gray-white purulent material was encountered in the lumbar epidural space (Fig. 2–10A). This was maximal on the dorsal surface of the spinal dura. Histological examination revealed acute inflammation and necrosis of the epidural adipose tissue (Fig. 2–10B). Tissue gram stains revealed gram-positive cocci that were consistent with staphylococci.

COMMENT

Spinal epidural abscesses are often associated with vertebral osteomyelitis. Most involve the thoracic and lumbar regions. The inflammatory exudate tends to be most abundant on the dorsal surface of the spinal cord where the epidural space is larger. Common antecedent events include back trauma and cutaneous infections. Epidural abscesses are also associated with bacteremia in intravenous drug users. Most are due to *Staphylococcus aureus*. However, among drug users, the causative organisms are varied and may include gram-negative bacteria. Tuberculosis was formerly a common cause of epidural abscesses.

REFERENCES

Baker AS, Ojemann RG, Swartz MN, Richardson EP Jr: Spinal epidural abscess. N Engl J Med 1975; 293:463-468.

Kaufman DM, Kaplan JG, Litman N: Infectious agents in spinal epidural abscesses. Neurology 1980; 30:844-850.

Lasker BR, Harter DH: Cervical epidural abscess. Neurology 1987; 37:1747-1753.

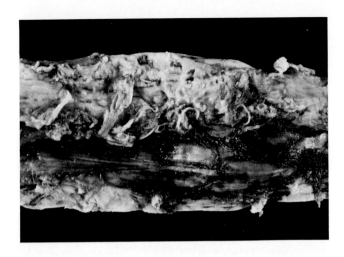

Figure 2–10A. Purulent material on epidural surface of spinal dura.

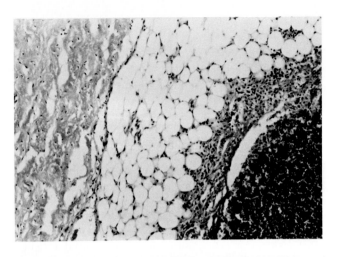

Figure 2–10B. Microscopic section showing purulent exudate and adipose tissue in the epidural space.

2.11 Tuberculous Meningitis

Mycobacterium tuberculosis

CLINICAL

This 45-year-old alcoholic man had a history of headache, fever, and night sweats. When admitted to the hospital he was disoriented and confused. A chest x-ray demonstrated multiple pulmonary calcifications and pleural thickening. The following day, he lapsed into coma and was noted to have nuchal rigidity. Lumbar puncture revealed 169 white blood cells (predominantly lymphocytes), a normal glucose, and a markedly elevated protein. He was treated for presumed tuberculous meningitis but died shortly after admission.

PATHOLOGY

The brain was diffusely swollen. There was copious exudate within the basal cisterns (Fig. 2–11A) and surrounding the brain stem in the ambient cistern (Fig. 2–11B). Blood vessels and nerves on the ventral surface of the brain stem were obscured by the exudate. There were discrete granulomas on the dorsal and lateral aspects of the cerebrum (Fig. 2–11C). Coronal sections of the cerebral hemispheres disclosed moderate dilatation of the lateral ventricles and an infarct in the left caudate nucleus (Fig. 2–11D). Transverse sections of the brain stem showed moderate dilatation of the fourth ventricle. The cranial nerves, basilar artery, and vertebral arteries were encased by exudate (Fig. 2–11E). Histological examination revealed foci of caseous necrosis within the granulomatous exudate (Fig. 2–11F). Vessels traversing

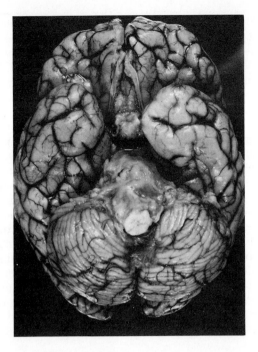

Figure 2–11A. Base of brain showing abundant, relatively firm exudate that obscured vessels and cranial nerves.

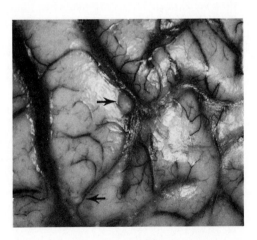

Figure 2–11C. Individual miliary granulomas (arrows) could be seen on the cerebral convexities.

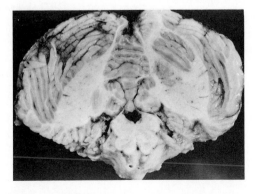

Figure 2–11E. Transverse section of brain stem and cerebellum showing encasement of vessels and cranial nerves by exudate.

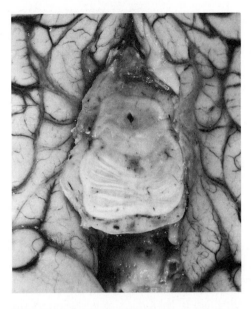

Figure 2–11B. The exudate filled the ambient cistern.

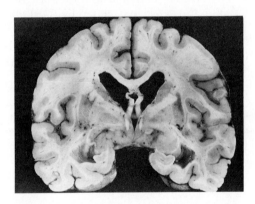

Figure 2–11D. Coronal section showing hydrocephalus, an infarct of the left caudate nucleus, and abundant exudate at the base of the brain.

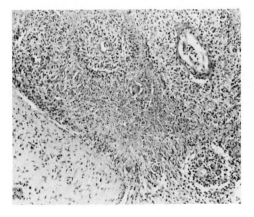

Figure 2–11F. Microscopic section showing foci of caseous necrosis within the granulomatous subarachnoid exudate.

the subarachnoid space showed proliferative arteritis (Fig. 2–11G). In addition, there was a small tuberculoma within the basis pontis (Fig. 2–11H).

COMMENT

Since about 1940, the incidence of tuberculous meningitis in the United States has declined markedly, and most cases are seen in adults. Tuberculous meningitis is much more common in Asia, Africa, Central America, and South America, where it is predominantly a disease of childhood. The mortality is especially high in young children, the elderly, and pregnant women.

Involvement of the central nervous system is the result of hematogenous dissemination. In adults, tuberculous meningitis is commonly associated with active extrapulmonary disease. In children, the meningitis usually develops while the primary complex and other foci of hematogenous dissemination are in advanced stages of healing. The meningitis usually results from subarachnoid extension of meningeal or superficial intraparenchymal granulomas. As in the present case, the exudate is generally most abundant at the base of the brain.

The histological appearance of the meningeal reaction varies with the stage of the disease. Initially, there may be fibrinous exudate with occasional polymorphonuclear leukocytes. This is replaced by abundant caseous exudate with mononuclear inflammatory cells and occasional giant cells. Acid-fast mycobacteria are best seen in the areas of caseation. Partially treated and chronic cases may show a highly cellular infiltrate with abundant fibrosis, but few if any organisms. Hydrocephalus may occur and is the result of impeded flow of cerebrospinal fluid. This results from meningeal fibrosis and involvement of ependymal surfaces.

Arteries that are encased by exudate in the subarachnoid space may develop obliterative endarteritis. This leads to cerebral infarcts and contributes significantly to the morbidity and mortality of the disease. Similar vascular changes may occur with other chronic bacterial, mycotic, and parasitic infections. In patients with syphilis, the arteritis is known as Heubner's endarteritis (see Fig. 2–11I, from a case of meningovascular syphilis).

The intraparenchymal granulomas are usually areas of caseous necrosis surrounded by mononuclear inflammatory cells, epithelioid cells, and giant cells. Occasionally, tuberculomas undergo liquefaction or mineralization. Tuberculomas account for a large proportion of intracranial space-occupying lesions in parts of the world where tuberculosis is still common.

REFERENCES

Dastur KD, Lalitha VS: The many facets of neurotuberculosis: An epitome of neuropathology. In Zimmerman HM (ed): Progress in Neuropathology. New York, Grune and Stratton, 1973, vol 2, chap 11, pp 351-408.

Kennedy DH, Fallon JR: Tuberculous meningitis. JAMA 1979; 241:264-268.

Tandon PN: Tuberculous meningitis (cranial and spinal). In Vinken PJ, Bruyn GW (eds): Handbook of Clinical Neurology. Amsterdam, Elsevier, 1978, vol 33, chap 12, pp 195-262.

Vengsarkar US, Pisipaty RP, Parkekh B, et al: Intracranial tuberculoma and the CT scan. J Neurosurg 1986; 64:568-574.

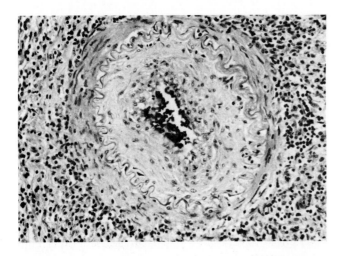

Figure 2–11G. Microscopic section showing proliferative endarteritis.

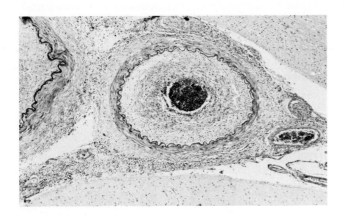

Figure 2–11I. Microscopic section showing Heubner's proliferative endarteritis in a patient with meningovascular syphilis.

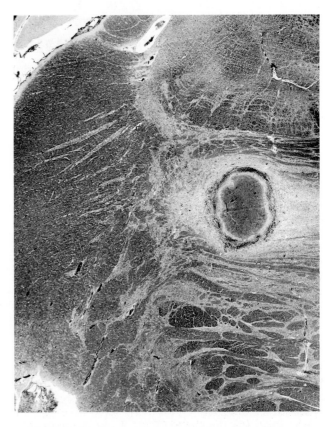

Figure 2–11H. Macroscopic section of pons showing a small tuberculoma.

2.12 Sarcoidosis

CLINICAL

This 60-year-old black woman had a history of non-insulin dependent diabetes mellitus, pernicious anemia, and facial sarcoid. She was doing well until she was found on the floor having a generalized tonic clonic seizure. While being evaluated in the emergency room, she had focal seizures. A chest x-ray revealed hilar adenopathy but no active infiltrates. Her hospital course was complicated by respiratory distress, hypothermia, intermittent focal seizures, and congestive heart failure.

PATHOLOGY

Examination of the brain revealed patches of relatively firm gray-white exudate in the leptomeninges at the base of the brain. These were most prominent at the cervicomedullary junction, on the ventral surface of the basilar artery, and on the ventral surface of the gyri recti (Fig. 2–12A). Coronal sections of the cerebral hemispheres disclosed additional deposits of granulomas in the superficial layers of the cerebral cortex (Fig. 2–12B). Histologically, the lesions were composed of noncaseating granulomas that were often closely approximated to veins (Fig. 2–12C).

COMMENT

Sarcoidosis is a systemic granulomatous disease that is encountered more commonly among the black population. The etiology and pathogenesis have not been established. The disorder is variously regarded as an infectious disease caused by an unidentified agent, possibly related to tuberculosis, or a reaction to diverse immunologic stimuli. Sarcoidosis affects many organ systems including lungs, lymph nodes, skin, salivary glands, skeletal muscles, and eyes. Central nervous system involvement is less common and usually consists of granulomatous meningitis and small intraparenchymal granulomas. These have a predilection for the base of the brain (Fig. 2–12D) and often result in hypothalamic–pituitary dysfunction and cranial nerve palsies. Rarely, the intraparenchymal granulomas present as space-occupying masses.

The individual granulomas are frequently adjacent to small blood vessels and are composed of compact aggregates of epithelioid cells with occasional giant cells. The granulomas are surrounded by lymphocytes and plasma cells. The lesions may show foci of central necrosis but do not undergo caseation. Upon healing, the granulomas may undergo fibrosis and hyalinization. Mycobacteria and fungi must be excluded by appropriate stains before the diagnosis of sarcoidosis can be considered.

REFERENCES

Clark WC, Acker JD, Dohan FC Jr, Robertson JH: Presentation of central nervous system sarcoidosis as intracranial tumors. J Neurosurg 1985; 63:851-856.

Delaney P: Neurologic manifestations in sarcoidosis: Review of the literature, with a report of 23 cases. Ann Intern Med 1977; 87:336-345.

Rosen Y, Vuletin JC, Pertschuk LP, Silverstein E: Sarcoidosis: From the pathologist's vantage point. In Sommers SC, Rosen PP: Pathology Annual, New York, Appleton-Century-Crofts 1979, part 1, pp 405-439.

Stern BJ, Krumholz A, Johns C, et al: Sarcoidosis and its neurological manifestations. Arch Neurol 1985; 42:909-917.

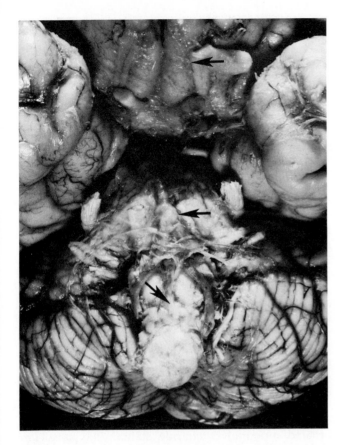

Figure 2–12A. Base of brain showing patches of firm, granulomatous exudate (arrows) in a patient with sarcoidosis.

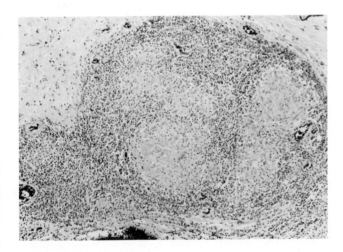

Figure 2–12C. Microscopic section showing confluent noncaseating granulomas.

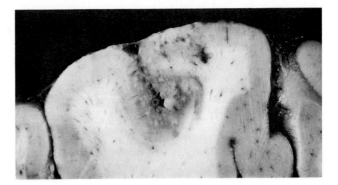

Figure 2–12B. Coronal section showing granulomas in meninges and underlying cerebral cortex.

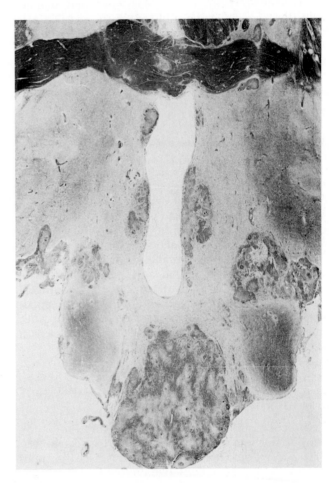

Figure 2–12D. Macroscopic section from another case of sarcoidosis showing multiple confluent granulomas in the hypothalamus and infundibular stalk.

2.13   Cryptococcosis

CLINICAL

This 64-year-old man, with long-standing chronic obstructive pulmonary disease, had a 1-month history of weight loss, frontal headaches, and a staggering gait. He became confused and incontinent of urine. Examination of the cerebrospinal fluid (CSF) disclosed a markedly depressed glucose, normal protein, and one white blood cell. A CSF cytology specimen, stained with the periodic acid–Schiff technique revealed numerous budding yeast, morphologically consistent with cryptococci. Despite therapy, the patient died a few days later.

PATHOLOGY

The leptomeningeal blood vessels were moderately congested. The subarachnoid space contained gray gelatinous exudate and a small amount of blood (Fig. 2–13A). The exudate was sufficiently abundant to obscure details of the underlying gyri. In coronal sections, the exudate caused widening of the sulci in the absence of gyral atrophy (Fig. 2–13B). A similar widening of the interfolial sulci was evident in a frontal section of the cerebellum. In addition, there were small cystic spaces in and about the dentate nucleus (Fig. 2–13C). Histologically, the meningeal exudate and the cysts contained numerous encapsulated budding yeasts. These could be seen with hematoxylin–eosin but were better demonstrated with the mucicarmine stain (Fig. 2–13D).

COMMENT

Cryptococcosis is a common mycotic infection of the central nervous system. The disease is caused by *Cryptococcus neoformans*. This organism can be found in soil that has been contaminated with bird excreta. The primary infection is in the lung; however, this is often inapparent because the pulmonary lesions often do not calcify. Hematogenous dissemination commonly leads to involvement of the central nervous system, usually in the form of meningitis. The nature and intensity of the meningeal inflammatory response are highly variable but often consist of only scanty mononuclear cells. Extension of the infection along Virchow–Robin spaces give rise to superficial intraparenchymal cysts, the so-called soap bubbles. Cystic spaces deeper in the brain are more likely the result of hematogenous spread. Rarely, the infection may give rise to multiple small meningeal granulomas (Fig. 2–13E) or even large space-occupying intraparenchymal granulomas.

The organisms generally appear as budding yeast, 5 to 25 µm in diameter. They are only faintly stained with hematoxylin–eosin but are intensely stained with methenamine silver and periodic acid–Schiff techniques. The latter stain can be effectively employed to facilitate the recognition of the organisms in cerebrospinal fluid cytology preparations. The mucoid capsules that surround the yeast are responsible for the "halos" seen in india ink preparations of CSF. The capsules can be stained selectively with mucicarmine or acid mucopolysaccharide stains such as alcian blue (Fig. 2–13F) or colloidal iron.

Although cryptococcal meningitis can occur in apparently immunocompetent individuals, a relatively large percentage of the patients have lymphoproliferative disorders, such as Hodgkin's disease. Other predisposing conditions include diabetes, prolonged corticosteroid therapy, and, more recently, the acquired immune deficiency syndrome.

REFERENCES

Anders KH, Guerra WF, Tomiyasu U, et al: The neuropathology of AIDS: UCLA experience and review. Am J Pathol 1986; 124:537-558.

Myerowitz RL: The Pathology of Opportunistic Infections: With Pathogenetic, Diagnostic, and Clinical Correlations. New York, Raven Press, 1983, pp 145-160.

Salaki JS, Louria DB, Chmel H: Fungal and yeast infections of the central nervous system: A clinical review. Medicine 1984; 63:108-132.

Stockstill MT, Kauffman CA: Comparison of cryptococcal and tuberculous meningitis. Arch Neurol 1983; 40:81-85.

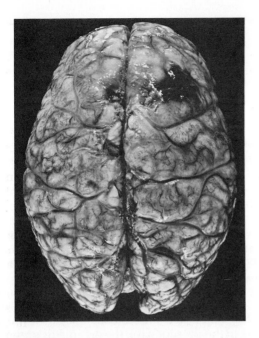

Figure 2–13A. Dorsal surface of brain showing abundant gray gelatinous exudate.

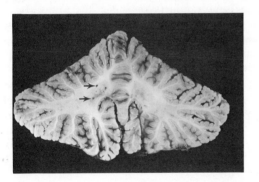

Figure 2–13C. Frontal section of cerebellum showing widening of the interfolial sulci and small cysts (arrows) in the white matter and dentate nucleus.

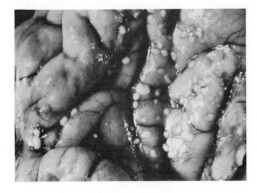

Figure 2–13E. Base of brain showing multiple discrete granulomas due to cryptococcosis.

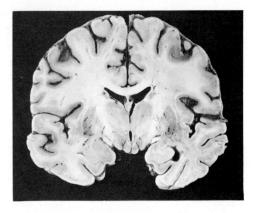

Figure 2–13B. Coronal section showing widening of sulci in the absence of significant gyral atrophy due to the abundant gelatinous exudate.

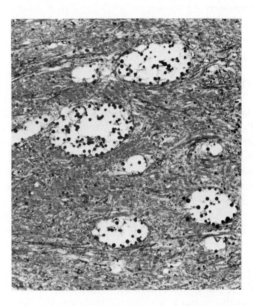

Figure 2–13D. Microscopic section, stained with a mucicarmine stain, showing small intraparenchymal cysts containing yeasts.

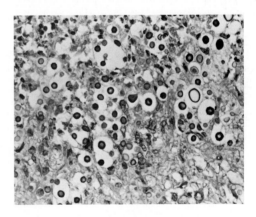

Figure 2–13F. Microscopic section showing staining of the mucopolysaccharide capsules with alcian blue. The "empty" spaces around the stained capsules result from contraction during tissue processing.

2.14 Candidiasis

CLINICAL

This 61-year-old man with non-insulin dependent diabetes mellitus was admitted to the hospital with Fournier's gangrene involving the perianal region. He underwent multiple surgical debridement procedures. The patient's prolonged hospital course was complicated by renal failure, adult respiratory distress syndrome, and sepsis. A computerized tomogram of the head revealed a remote infarct of the right basal ganglia and multiple areas of decreased attenuation. *Candida* species were cultured from the blood shortly before his death.

PATHOLOGY

Coronal sections of the cerebral hemispheres showed a large area of remote, cystic encephalomalacia involving the right internal capsule and basal ganglia and small, poorly defined areas of recent infarction involving the left frontal and both temporal lobes (Fig. 2–14A).

Histological examination disclosed many other necrotic areas (for example, the left basal ganglia as seen in Fig. 2–14B). There were collections of acute inflammatory cells within many of the areas. Yeast and pseudohyphae infiltrated the inflammatory foci and the surrounding necrotic neural tissue. Although the organisms were barely visible with hematoxylin–eosin, they were intensely stained by periodic acid–Shiff (Fig. 2–14C) and methenamine silver (Fig. 2–14D) techniques.

COMMENT

Candida species are commonly present in the flora of the skin, gastrointestinal tract, and genitourinary tract.

Relatively minor alterations in the host defenses can lead to local overgrowths. More severe injuries can lead to tissue invasion and hematogenous dissemination. *Candida* is probably the most common opportunistic mycotic infection and is frequently encountered in the nervous system at the time of autopsy. Among the many conditions that predispose patients to candidiasis are prolonged treatment with broad- spectrum antibiotics, corticosteroids, or cytotoxic drugs, prolonged use of intravenous catheters, intravenous drug abuse, diabetes, and neoplastic diseases, especially leukemias and lymphomas. In more recent years, candidiasis has also been seen in individuals with the acquired immune deficiency syndrome.

As in the present case, the organisms often can be cultured from the blood, although they are not readily recovered from the cerebrospinal fluid. The lesions in the central nervous system are usually small, widely disseminated microabscesses but may be granulomatous (Fig. 2–14E) in more chronic cases. Meningitis is much less common than parenchymal involvement. Candidiasis may coexist with other opportunistic infections.

REFERENCES

Anders KH, Guerra WF, Tomiyasu U, et al: The neuropathology of AIDS: UCLA experience and review. Am J Pathol 1986; 124:537-558.

Lipton SA, Hickey WF, Morris JH, Loscalzo J: Candidal infections in the central nervous system. Am J Med 1984; 76:101-108.

Myerowitz RL: The Pathology of Opportunistic Infections: With Pathogenetic, Diagnostic, and Clinical Correlations. New York, Raven Press, 1983, chap 10, pp 95-114.

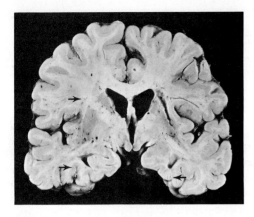

Figure 2–14A. Coronal section showing a large area of remote cystic encephalomalacia in the right internal capsule and multiple small, poorly defined areas of recent infarction (arrows).

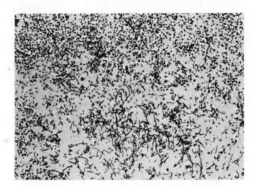

Figure 2–14C. Microscopic section, stained by the periodic acid–Schiff technique, showing acute inflammatory cells with yeast and pseudohyphae in the surrounding tissue.

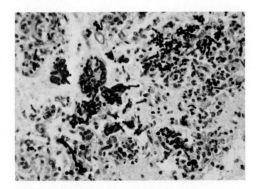

Figure 2–14E. Microscopic section, stained by the periodic acid–Schiff technique, showing a granulomatous response to *Candida*.

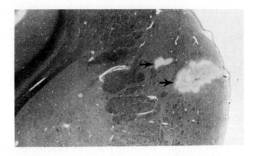

Figure 2–14B. Macrosection showing necrotic foci (arrows) in the left caudate nucleus that were not evident grossly.

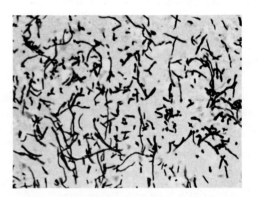

Figure 2–14D. Microscopic section, stained by the Gomori methenamine silver technique, showing yeast and pseudohyphae.

2.15 Aspergillosis

CLINICAL

This 55-year-old man was hospitalized for congestive heart failure secondary to a cardiomyopathy. Three days after admission, he became combative. This was attributed to liver dysfunction and an elevated serum ammonia. His course was complicated by renal failure requiring dialysis, peritonitis, pneumonia, and sepsis. He died after a prolonged hospitalization.

PATHOLOGY

Examination of the dura revealed a thin organizing subdural hematoma that had not deformed the underlying cortex. Coronal sections of the cerebral hemispheres revealed an area of hemorrhagic necrosis in the left occipital lobe, partially involving the visual cortex (Fig. 2–15A). The white matter immediately surrounding the lesion had a faint green color. A macrosection revealed central necrosis with petechial hemorrhages surrounding the blood vessels at the periphery of the lesion (Fig. 2–15B). Histological examination of sections stained with methenamine silver showed dichotomously branching septate hyphae that were morphologically consistent with aspergillosis (Fig. 2–15C).

COMMENT

Aspergillosis is another opportunistic mycotic infection that may involve the nervous system. The infection is most often due to *Aspergillus fumigatus*. However, in the absence of cultures, even a diagnosis of aspergillosis is presumptive. This opportunistic infection is encountered predominantly in immunosuppressed individuals and in patients with various neoplastic diseases. Neutropenia and prolonged use of corticosteroids or cytotoxic agents are important predisposing factors.

The infection is usually acquired from inhaled spores. The lungs are the most common site of primary infection. The disease is also encountered in individuals who have had cardiac surgery or cardiac transplants. In these cases, direct contamination from airborne spores has been suggested. Central nervous system involvement is usually the result of hematogenous dissemination. The fungal hyphae readily invade vessel walls and the cerebral lesions typically appear as areas of hemorrhagic infarction (see Fig. 2–15D, from another patient). The hyphae are septate and characteristically branch at acute angles. They may be seen with hematoxylin–eosin but are much better demonstrated with periodic acid–Schiff or methenamine silver techniques.

REFERENCES

Britt RH, Enzmann DR, Remington JS: Intracranial infection in cardiac transplant recipients. Ann Neurol 1981; 9:107-119.

Myerowitz RL: The Pathology of Opportunistic Infections: With Pathogenetic, Diagnostic, and Clinical Correlations. New York, Raven Press, 1983, chap 11, pp 115-128.

Walsh TJ, Hier DB, Chaplan LR: Aspergillosis of the central nervous system: Clinicopathological analysis of 17 patients. Ann Neurol 1985; 18:574-582.

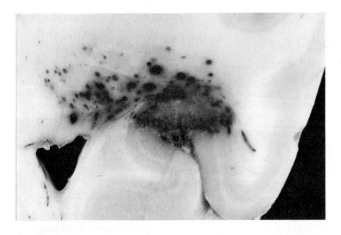

Figure 2–15A. Coronal section showing an area of hemorrhagic necrosis in the left occipital lobe.

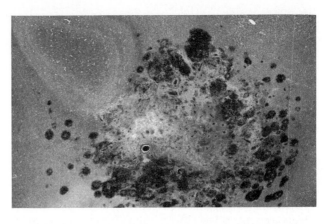

Figure 2–15B. Macrosection showing the area of hemorrhagic necrosis.

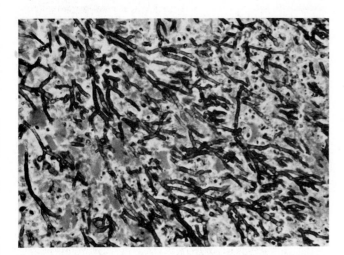

Figure 2–15C. Microscopic section, stained by the Gomori methenamine silver technique, showing dichotomously branching, septate hyphae in the necrotic lesions.

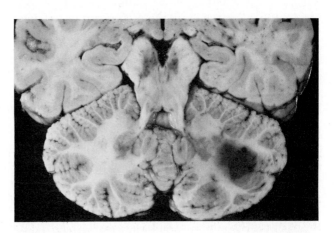

Figure 2–15D. Section of cerebellum showing a hemorrhagic, necrotic lesion due to aspergillosis.

2.16   Mucormycosis

CLINICAL

This 9-year-old girl had a 6-month history of acute nonlymphocytic leukemia. Despite numerous chemotherapeutic regimens, a lasting remission was never achieved. During her last hospitalization, she developed fever, diarrhea, and a nonproductive cough. A chest x-ray showed a right middle lobe infiltrate that was refractory to antibiotic therapy. During her prolonged hospitalization she developed periods of confusion, incontinence, and bilateral focal neurological deficits. A computerized tomogram showed multiple areas of decreased attenuation (Fig. 2–16A). She died 6 weeks after admission.

PATHOLOGY

The leptomeninges were mildly fibrotic. The subarachnoid space was free of grossly discernible exudate. The occipital lobes were softened and faintly discolored. Horizontal sections of the cerebral hemispheres revealed large areas of necrosis involving the white matter of the occipital lobes, the splenium of the corpus callosum, and the basal ganglia (Fig. 2–16B). The necrotic lesions were gray to green in color. The lesions in the basal ganglia were focally hemorrhagic. There was no distinct encapsulation and the surrounding neural parenchyma was not significantly edematous. Histological sections showed numerous hyphae in and about blood vessels. The hyphae were weakly stained with hematoxylin–eosin but were more clearly seen with periodic acid–Schiff (Fig. 2–16C) and methenamine silver techniques (Fig. 2–16D). The hyphae were variable in diameter, branched at obtuse angles, and were wrinkled but nonseptate. The organisms were histologically consistent with mucormycosis. Some of the lesions also contained yeast and pseudohyphae that were morphologically consistent with a *Candida* species.

COMMENT

The term mucormycosis is commonly employed to designate opportunistic infections caused by various fungi belonging to the order *Mucorales*. These fungi are ordinarily saprophytes found in the soil and on decaying vegetable matter. In patients with rhinocerebral mucormycosis, the infection begins in the nose and paranasal sinuses and then spreads to the orbit and brain, usually involving the frontal and temporal lobes. This form of the disease occurs most often in poorly controlled diabetic patients. Cerebral mucormycosis can also result from hematogenous dissemination. This is encountered predominantly in individuals with malignant neoplasms such as leukemias and lymphomas. It has also been seen following cardiac surgery and in intravenous drug abusers.

The fungi readily invade and occlude blood vessels. The resulting cerebral lesions generally appear as hemorrhagic infarcts, cerebritis, or abscesses. The hyphae are variable in diameter, are nonseptate, and branch at obtuse angles. The hyphae may permeate necrotic tissue with a minimal inflammatory reaction or may be accompanied by numerous polymorphonuclear leukocytes.

REFERENCES

Masucci EF, Fabara JA, Saini N, Kurtzke JF: Cerebral mucormycosis (Phycomycosis) in a heroin addict. Arch Neurol 1982; 39:304-306.

Myerowitz RL: The Pathology of Opportunistic Infections: With Pathogenetic, Diagnostic, and Clinical Correlations. New York, Raven Press, 1983, chap 12, pp 129-135.

Rangel-Geurra R, Martinez H, Saenz C: Mucormycosis: Report of 11 cases. Arch Neurol 1985; 42:578-581.

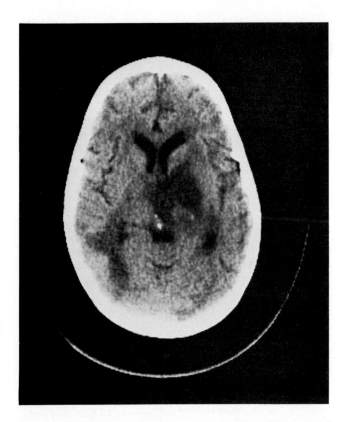

Figure 2–16A. Computerized tomogram showing multiple areas of decreased attenuation including the thalamus and both occipital lobes.

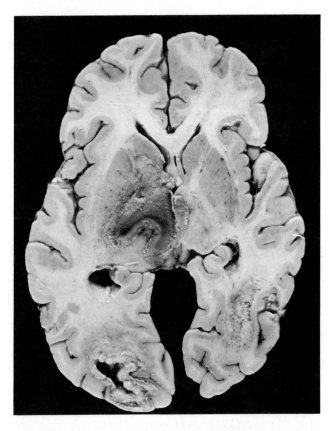

Figure 2–16B. Horizontal section showing necrotic lesions in the basal ganglia, thalamus, and both occipital lobes.

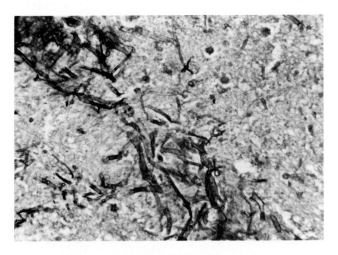

Figure 2–16C. Microscopic section, stained by the periodic acid–Schiff technique, showing irregular, nonseptate, branched hyphae that were consistent with mucormycosis.

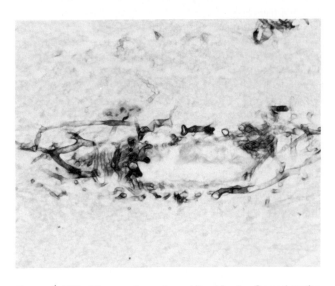

Figure 2–16D. Microscopic section, stained by the Gomori methenamine silver technique, showing the hyphae around a blood vessel.

2.17 Histoplasmosis

CLINICAL

This 28-year-old male intravenous drug abuser with AIDS was hospitalized for a productive cough, fever, chills, and night sweats. *Histoplasma capsulatum* was isolated from blood and sputum cultures. Shortly thereafter, he became confused and lethargic but showed no focal neurological deficits. He developed pneumonia and septicemia prior to death.

PATHOLOGY

The cerebral hemispheres were symmetrical. The leptomeninges were mildly fibrotic and contained a small number of petechial hemorrhages. Coronal sections of the cerebral hemispheres disclosed multiple large demyelinated and focally necrotic areas that were due to progressive multifocal leukoencephalopathy. In addition, there were small necrotic areas with petechial hemorrhages in the cortex on the medial aspect of the right frontal lobe (Fig. 2–17A) and on the inferior surface of the right temporal lobe. Histological examination disclosed additional necrotic foci in the brain stem. All of these necrotic areas contained macrophages that were filled with small yeast. In sections stained with hematoxylin–eosin or by the periodic acid–Schiff technique, the individual organisms were seen to be surrounded by a capsule (Fig. 2–17B). They appeared as clusters of small dark spheres in sections stained with the methenamine silver technique (Fig. 2–17C).

COMMENT

Histoplasmosis is common in the central part of the United States, especially in the Ohio and Mississippi river valleys. Spores from contaminated soil are inhaled and give rise to pulmonary lesions. This is often followed by hematogenous dissemination. The pulmonary and miliary extrapulmonary lesions frequently undergo fibrosis and mineralization. Despite the prevalence of histoplasmosis, involvement of the central nervous system is uncommon. Cerebral lesions, when present, may be in the form of meningitis, miliary granulomas, or histoplasmomas. Histoplasmomas are larger granulomas that may present as mass lesions. An example of a surgically resected cerebral histoplasmoma is shown in Fig. 2–17D. Microscopically the necrotic center and surrounding capsule contained myriads of the yeast within the cytoplasm of macrophages and giant cells (Fig. 2–17E).

Although the disease is generally not regarded as an opportunistic infection, both disseminated cerebral lesions and focal granulomas have been reported in immunocompromised individuals. These include patients with diabetes, connective tissue diseases, tuberculosis, leukemia, or myeloma, individuals receiving corticosteroids or cytotoxic agents, and more recently, in patients with the acquired immune deficiency syndrome.

REFERENCES

Anders KH, Guerra WF, Tomiyasu U, et al: The neuropathology of AIDS: UCLA experience and review. Am J Pathol 1986; 124:537-558.

Schochet SS Jr, Sarwar M, Kelly PJ, Masel BE: Symptomatic cerebral histoplasmoma: Case report. J Neurosurg 1980; 52:273-275.

Vakill ST, Eble JN, Richmond BD, Yount RA: Cerebral histoplasmoma: Case report. J Neurosurg 1983; 59:332-336.

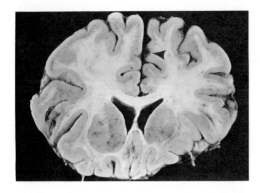

Figure 2–17A. Coronal section showing a focus of hemorrhagic necrosis (arrowhead) on the medial aspect of the right frontal lobe. There were also multiple lesions attributable to progressive multifocal leukoencephalopathy, for example, below right putamen.

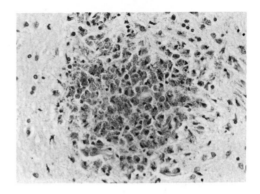

Figure 2–17B. Microscopic section, stained by the periodic acid–Schiff technique, showing a collection of macrophages filled with small yeast, consistent with *Histoplasma*. They were located near the hemorrhagic areas.

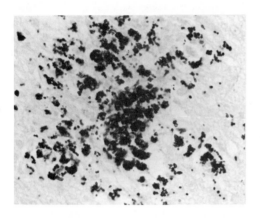

Figure 2–17C. Microscopic section, stained by the Gomori methenamine silver technique showing yeast, consistent with *Histoplasma*.

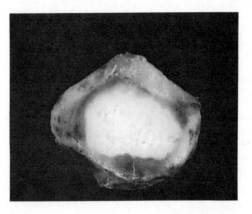

Figure 2–17D. Surgically resected histoplasmoma.

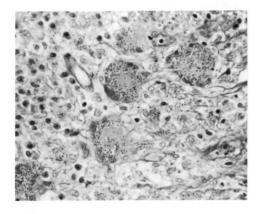

Figure 2–17E. Microscopic section showing the *Histoplasma* yeast in macrophages and giant cells.

2.18   Toxoplasmosis

Congenital

CLINICAL

This female infant was the product of an uncomplicated full-term pregnancy and delivery. When the infant was seen at age 1 week, the mother described excessive crying. By the age of 2 weeks, the head circumference had increased markedly, prompting further evaluation. Radiological studies revealed hydrocephalus but no intracerebral calcifications. Cerebrospinal fluid examination revealed 1000 white blood cells and a protein content of 4.2 grams/dL. TORCH titers were negative except for toxoplasma which was positive at a dilution of 1:256. The child died at age 6 weeks.

PATHOLOGY

Upon opening the skull, the brain was found to be severely hydrocephalic (Fig. 2–18A). The normal gyral markings on the dorsal surface of the left cerebral hemisphere were effaced and the remaining tissue was focally discolored yellow and gray. The dorsal aspect of the right cerebral hemisphere was reduced to a thin membrane covering viscous, amber-colored ventricular fluid. Partially organized, fibrinous exudate was evident at the base of the brain (Fig. 2–18B). Coronal sections of the formalin-fixed brain revealed a proteinaceous coagulum within the dilated ventricular cavities (Fig. 2–18C). The cerebellum and brain stem were also affected, but less severely than the cerebrum (Fig. 2–18D). Histological examination disclosed necrosis of the neural parenchyma with scattered mineralized concretions but no identifiable toxoplasma cysts or trophozoites. The left eye was smaller than the right and the contents of the globe were disorganized (Fig. 2–18E).

COMMENT

Toxoplasmosis is a common parasitic infection caused by a coccidian, *Toxoplasma gondii*. Infections are usually acquired from contamination with cat feces or consumption of inadequately cooked meat. Antibodies, indicative of prior infection, are found in 5 to 85 percent of the population. Fetal infections are thought to complicate 30 to 40 percent of primary infections in pregnant women. Although many are subclinical, fetal death or severe congenital disease may occur when the maternal infection is contracted during the second to sixth month of gestation.

Severely affected brains show multifocal or confluent areas of parenchymal necrosis that are most extensive in periventricular regions. The brains may develop hydrocephalus or even hydranencephaly. The cerebrospinal fluid typically has a markedly elevated protein content. Frenkel has attributed much of the tissue destruction to vasculitis mediated by the interaction between antigens diffusing into the tissue from the ventricular system and passively transferred maternal antibody. Toxoplasma, either free or encysted, may be very sparse and difficult to distinguish from foci of mineralization. The mineral deposits may be scattered widely throughout the neural parenchyma and may become large enough to be demonstrated by radiological studies. As in the present case, the eyes commonly show chorioretinitis and the intraocular structures may be severely disorganized.

REFERENCES

Desmonts G, Couvreur J: Congenital toxoplasmosis. A prospective study of 378 pregnancies. N Engl J Med 1974; 290:1110-1116.

Frenkel JK: Toxoplasmosis. In Binford CH, Connor DH (eds): Pathology of Tropical and Extraordinary Diseases. Washington DC, Armed Forces Institute of Pathology, 1976, vol 1, chap 6, pp 284-300.

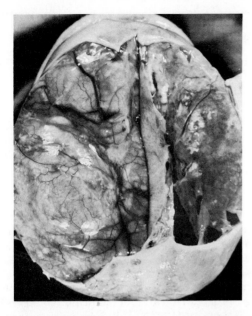

Figure 2–18A. Dorsal view of brain, in situ, showing hydrocephalus and marked thinning of cortex.

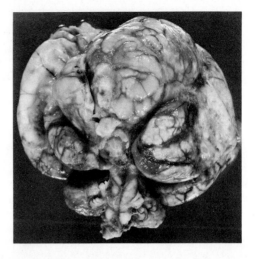

Figure 2–18B. Base of brain showing partially organized fibrinous exudate.

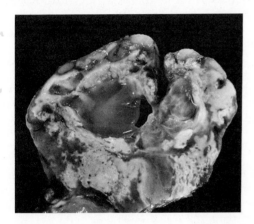

Figure 2–18C. Section of cerebral hemisphere showing extensive destruction of neural parenchyma and proteinaceous coagulum in ventricular cavities.

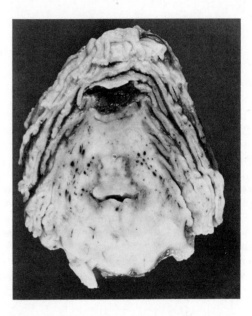

Figure 2–18D. Section of cerebellum and brain stem showing less severe destruction. Note the proteinaceous material in the cavity of the fourth ventricle.

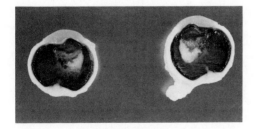

Figure 2–18E. Bisected small left eye showing disorganization of internal structures.

2.19 Toxoplasmosis

Immunocompromised Adult

CLINICAL

This 49-year-old man had a long history of Hodgkin's disease for which he had been treated with various chemotherapeutic regimens. His final admission was for general debility and slurred speech. He progressively became confused and lethargic and developed paresis of the right upper extremity shortly before death.

PATHOLOGY

Coronal sections of the brain revealed multiple focally necrotic lesions, especially in the left basal ganglia and internal capsule (Fig. 2–19A). Histological examination of the neural parenchyma immediately surrounding these areas disclosed free and encysted *Toxoplasma* (Fig. 2–19B).

COMMENT

Immunocompromised adults are at risk of developing symptomatic toxoplasmosis. Formerly, this was relatively uncommon and encountered predominantly in individuals with lymphoreticular neoplasms and organ transplant recipients who were receiving immunosuppressive therapy. In recent years, toxoplasmosis has become one of the most common causes of cerebritis and cerebral abscesses in patients with the acquired immune deficiency syndrome. In these cases, computerized tomography generally shows focal hypodense lesions with peripheral ring enhancement (Fig. 2–19C).

Cerebral toxoplasmosis in the immunocompromised adult is thought to result from reactivation of latent infections. In contrast to the congenitally infected infants, the organisms are generally readily demonstrated in the surrounding tissue where the inflammatory response is less intense. Identification of the organisms can be confirmed by the use of immunohistochemical techniques. This is demonstrated in an aspirate from a brain abscess in a patient with AIDS. The smear has been stained with an immunoperoxidase method for toxoplasma (Fig. 2–19D).

REFERENCES

Krick JA, Remington JS: Toxoplasmosis in the adult—An overview. N Engl J Med 1978; 298:550-553.

Myerowitz RL: The Pathology of Opportunistic Infections: With Pathogenetic, Diagnostic, and Clinical Correlations. New York, Raven Press, 1983, pp 225-233.

Navia BA, Petito CK, Gold JWM, et al: Cerebral toxoplasmosis complicating the acquired immune deficiency syndrome: Clinical and neuropathological findings in 27 patients. Ann Neurol 1986; 19:224-238.

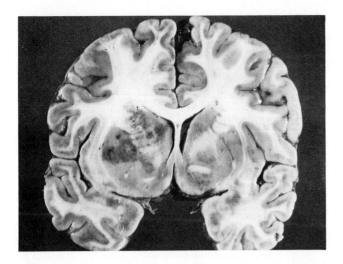

Figure 2–19A. Coronal section showing multiple focally necrotic lesions in the left basal ganglia.

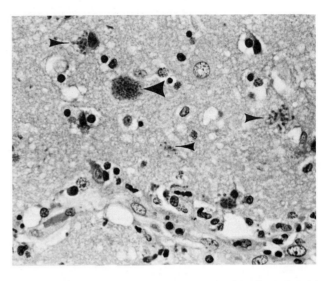

Figure 2–19B. Microscopic section showing free (small arrowheads) and encysted (large arrowhead) *Toxoplasma*.

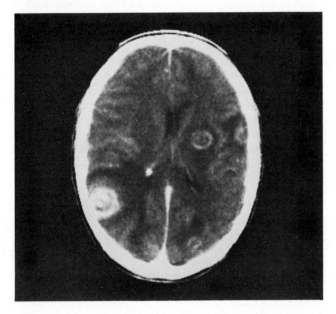

Figure 2–19C. Computerized tomogram showing multiple ring- enhancing lesions in the brain of a patient with AIDS.

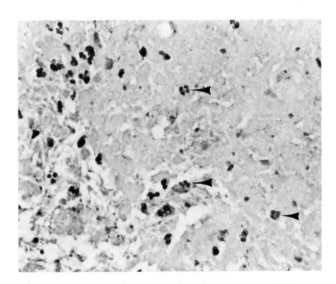

Figure 2–19D. Microscopic section, stained by immunoperoxidase technique for *Toxoplasma* , showing the organisms (arrowheads) in material aspirated from one of the cerebral abscesses.

2.20 Cysticercosis

CLINICAL

This 14-year-old girl had a 3- to 4-week history of intermittent headaches. She had at least one sensory visual cortical seizure. She denied any other neurological or constitutional symptoms. Travel history is significant for a vacation to southern California and a trip to Mexico. A computerized tomogram (Fig. 2–20A) revealed a ring enhancing lesion in the right occipital region. A craniotomy was performed for removal of a mass lesion.

PATHOLOGY

A macrosection of the surgical specimen revealed a sharply demarcated partially cystic lesion (Fig. 2–20B). The inner part of the cyst wall was sparsely cellular and hyalinized. This was surrounded by chronically inflamed connective tissue. The surrounding neural parenchyma was gliotic. Examination of the cyst contents with partial polarization revealed a partially necrotic scolex with attached refractile hooklets (Fig. 2–20C).

COMMENT

Cysticercosis is caused by encysted larvae of the pork tapeworm, *Taenia solium*. Ordinarily, man is definitive host, harboring the adult tapeworm in his small intestine with minimal complications. Periodically, proglottids containing ova are shed from the terminal segment of the adult worm. When these are ingested by an intermediate host, usually a pig, the resulting embryos become disseminated throughout the body and develop into cystic larvae. The usual life cycle is completed when man consumes pork containing viable larvae and develops the adult tapeworm.

Human cysticercosis develops when man serves as the intermediate host and harbors the cystic larvae of this parasite. This is relatively uncommon in the United States but is more prevalent and a major cause of neurological disease in many other parts of the world. The disease is usually acquired from ingestion of ova in fecally contaminated food or water. Autoinfection, from fecal contamination or reverse peristalsis, may occur in individuals who harbor the adult tapeworms. The cysticerci are especially common in subcutaneous tissue, skeletal muscle, brain, and eye.

Within the nervous system, one to hundreds of the encysted larvae may be found in the meninges, cerebral parenchyma or ventricular system. The intraparenchymal cysticerci are fluid filled vesicles 1 to 2 centimeters in diameter. Each cysticercus contains a single invaginated scolex with a rostellum, 4 suckers, and 22 to 32 hooklets. The cyst wall is multilayered and sparsely cellular and contains fine mineralized concretions. The surrounding neural parenchyma shows minimal reaction while the larvae are alive. Dead and degenerating larvae elicit more intense inflammation and some eventually undergo mineralization. The clinical manifestations are due to a combination of mass effects, inflammation, and obstruction of cerebrospinal fluid pathways.

Racemose cysticerci are large multiloculated forms of the cystic larvae that lack the invaginated scolex but have the typical multilayer cyst walls (Fig. 2–20D). They are most commonly found in the basal cisterns about the brain stem. Arachnoiditis and a prominent vasculitis may occur especially in association with degenerating racemose cysticerci (Fig. 2–20E).

REFERENCES

McCormick GF, Zee C-S, Heiden J: Cysticercosis cerebri: Review of 127 cases. Arch Neurol 1982; 39:534-539.

Sotelo J, Margin C: Hydrocephalus secondary to cysticercotic arachnoiditis: A long-term follow-up review of 92 cases. J Neurosurg 1987; 66:686-689.

Stern WE: Neurosurgical considerations of cysticercosis of the central nervous system. J Neurosurg 1981; 55:382-389.

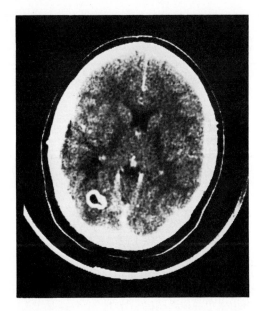

Figure 2–20A. Computerized tomogram showing a ring-enhancing lesion in right occipital region.

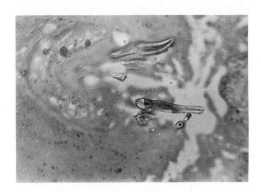

Figure 2–20C. Microscopic section of the cyst contents, viewed with partially polarized light, showing refractile hooklets.

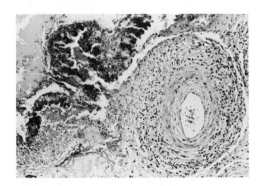

Figure 2–20E. Microscopic section showing vasculitis in the vicinity of a degenerating cysticercus.

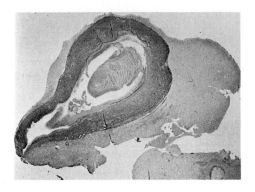

Figure 2–20B. Macrosection showing the partially cystic, surgically resected lesion.

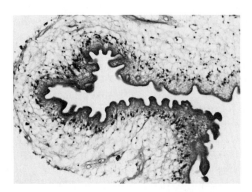

Figure 2–20D. Microscopic section showing the multilayered wall of a racemose cysticercus.

2.21   Other Parasitic Infections

Malaria
Paragonimiasis
Amebic Meningoencephalitis
Visceral Larva Migrans

On a worldwide basis, malaria is generally considered to be the most common parasitic disease. Cerebral involvement is encountered predominantly, if not exclusively, in cases caused by *Plasmodium falciparum*. The neurological manifestations are generally attributed to impaired perfusion from capillary obstruction. An immunologically mediated vasculopathy also has been suggested. Brains from fatal cases are edematous and some show a slate gray discoloration. Microscopically, blood vessels are congested and may be surrounded by ring hemorrhages. The parasitized erythrocytes contain small granules of a dark brown, birefringent pigment that is similar to formalin pigment (Fig. 2–21A).

Paragonimiasis is caused by various lung flukes, of which *Paragonimus westermani* is the most common. The disease is encountered predominantly in southeast Asia. The parasites have a complex life cycle. The adult flukes are found in the lungs of the infected patients while snails and various crustaceans serve as intermediate hosts. Cerebral involvement is uncommon but can include meningitis, necrotizing cerebritis, or granulomas. In endemic areas, paragonimiasis is an important cause of intracerebral mass lesions. Ova and, rarely, adult flukes can be seen in the cerebral lesions. The ova measure approximately 50 by 100 microns and have a terminal operculum (Fig. 2–21B). The pathway by which the nervous system becomes involved is uncertain.

Naegleria fowleri is a free-living ameba, found in soil and water, that can cause a hemorrhagic meningoencephalitis. Most of the patients are previously healthy adults and children who have a history of recently swimming in freshwater. The amebae are thought to enter the nervous system directly through the cribriform plate. Brains from fatal cases often show hemorrhage and exudate in the basal subarachnoid space. The olfactory bulbs and tracts are usually extensively necrotic. Additional areas of hemorrhagic necrosis are found in the ventral portions of the frontal and temporal lobes and along the brain stem. The amebae can be seen within the subarachnoid space, along vessels in the Virchow–Robin spaces (Fig. 2–21C), and within the necrotic intra-parenchymal lesions. The organisms can be distinguished from macrophages by their very prominent nucleoli. Other free-living amebae belonging to the genus *Acanthamoebae* may cause a granulomatous encephalitis. This disorder has been encountered predominantly in immunosuppressed individuals.

Visceral larva migrans is the result of human parasitism by the larvae of various nematodes such as *Toxocara* . These normally parasitize other animals. Human infection is usually acquired by ingestion of ova from fecally contaminated soil. In the unnatural human host, these nematodes cannot complete their life cycle and the larvae migrate for months through various tissues. The liver and other abdominal viscera are the principal sites of involvement but, on rare occasions, the brain and eye are also involved. Usually only foci of granulomatous inflammation and necrosis, corresponding to the tracts produced by the migrating larvae, are found. It is very uncommon to find the larvae, especially in the brain. Figure 2–21D illustrates a granuloma containing an ascarid larva. This lesion was found in the mesencephalon of a child who died in a fire. The child also had intestinal parasitism by *Ascaris lumbricoides*. Most cases of visceral larva migrans are attributed to the dog ascarid, *Toxocara canis*. However, the raccoon ascarid, *Baylisascaris procyonis*, has also been reported to produce human visceral larva migrans with a fatal meningoencephalitis.

REFERENCES

Martinez AJ, dos Santos Neto JG, Nelson EC, et al: Primary amebic meningoencephalitis. In Sommers SC, Rosen PP: Pathology Annual, New York, Appleton-Century-Crofts, 1977, part 2, pp 225–250.

Meyers WM, Neafie RN: Paragonimiasis. In Binford CH, Conner DH (eds): Pathology of Tropical and Extraordinary Diseases. Washington DC, Armed Forces Institute of Pathology, 1976, vol 2, chap 3, pp 517-523.

Oo MM, Aikawa M, Than T, et al: Human cerebral malaria: A pathological study. J Neuropathol Exp Neurol 1987; 46:223-231.

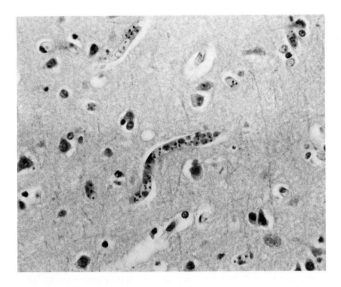

Figure 2–21A. Microscopic section showing intracerebral capillaries in a patient with malaria. Note the dark granules in the parasitized erythrocytes.

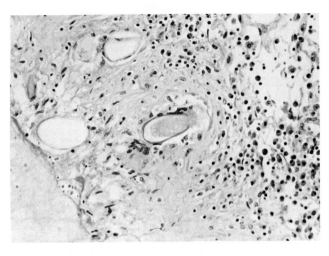

Figure 2–21B. Microscopic section showing operculated ova in an intracerebral mass lesion from a patient with paragonimiasis.

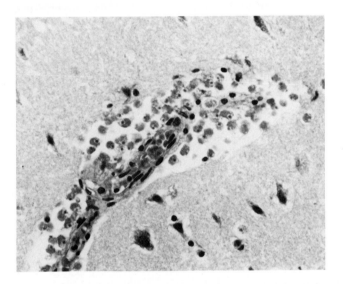

Figure 2–21C. Microscopic section showing *Naegleria fowleri* amebae in a Virchow–Robin space.

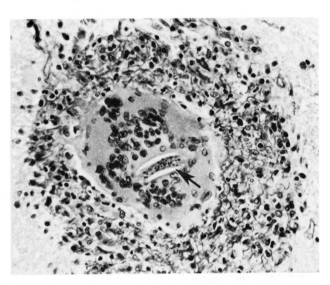

Figure 2–21D. Microscopic section showing a granuloma with a portion of an ascarid larva (arrow) within a giant cell in the brain of a child with visceral larva migrans.

2.22 Coxsackievirus Infection

Neonatal Encephalomyocarditis

CLINICAL

This full-term male infant was the product of an apparently uncomplicated gestation and delivery. The infant did well until 2 days of age when he developed cyanosis and respiratory distress. A lumbar puncture revealed 363 white blood cells (predominantly lymphocytes) a glucose of 51 mg/dL, and a protein of 151 mg/dL. No organisms were seen on CSF smear or isolated from blood cultures. The infant subsequently developed tachycardia and tachypnea and died at 10 days of age.

PATHOLOGY

The brain was mildly swollen and weighed 400 grams. The leptomeninges were slightly clouded and the leptomeningeal vessels were congested (Fig. 2–22A). Coronal sections of the cerebral hemispheres and transverse sections of the brain stem and cerebellum failed to reveal any grossly discernible abnormalities other than mild congestion. Histological examination disclosed abundant mononuclear cells in the subarachnoid space over the cerebral hemispheres (Fig. 2–22B). Sections of the brain stem revealed scattered foci of neuronal necrosis and nodular mononuclear cells infiltrates that were most numerous in the inferior olivary nuclei (Fig. 2–22C). The heart showed interstitial inflammation and foci of myofiber necrosis (Fig. 2–22D). A group B coxsackievirus was isolated postmortem from the heart.

COMMENT

The coxsackieviruses are a common cause of aseptic meningitis and, occasionally, encephalitis. In adults, they usually produce relatively mild central nervous system illnesses. However, certain group B strains can produce a severe encephalomyocarditis in neonates.

Brains from these infants typically show mononuclear cells in the meninges and focally in the brain and spinal cord. The brain stem is generally more severely affected than the cerebral hemispheres. As in this case, the infiltrates may be especially prominent in the inferior olivary nuclei. Rarely, foci of noninflammatory liquefactive necrosis have been observed in the cerebral hemispheres. These may be responsible for neurological deficits in infants who survive this illness. The heart is commonly involved, along with the brain, in neonatal coxsackievirus infections and is the optimal tissue for recovery of the virus at the time of postmortem examination.

Occasionally, older children or adults with coxsackievirus infections develop paralytic encephalomyelitis. Clinically, this is similar to the paralytic disease that was formerly caused by the polioviruses. Although cases caused by the coxsackieviruses are rarely fatal, pathological studies have shown similar lesions in both conditions. Inflammatory cell infiltrates and foci of neuronophagia are encountered predominantly in the brain stem and in the anterior horns of the spinal cord. The same histological features are seen in a spinal cord from an adult with coxsackie encephalomyelitis (Fig. 2–22E) and in a spinal cord from a child with acute paralytic poliomyelitis (Fig. 2–22F). In the adult, the coxsackieviruses are also an important cause of viral myocarditis.

REFERENCES

Estes ML, Rorke LB: Liquefactive necrosis in coxsackie B encephalitis. Arch Pathol Lab Med 1986; 110:1090-1092.

Fechner RE, Smith MG, Middlekamp JN: Coxsackie B virus infection of the newborn. Am J Pathol 1963; 42:493-503.

Hanshaw JB, Budgeon JA: Viral Diseases of the Fetus and Newborn. Philadelphia, Saunders, 1978, pp 185-187.

Price RW, Plum F: Poliomyelitis. In Vinken PJ, Bruyn GW (eds): Handbook of Clinical Neurology. Amsterdam, Elsevier, 1978, vol 34, chap 6, pp 93-132.

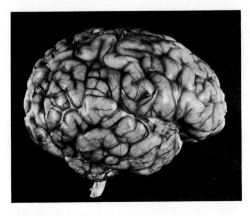

Figure 2–22A. Lateral view of brain from an infant with coxsackie meningoencephalitis showing mild clouding of meninges.

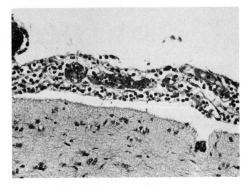

Figure 2–22B. Microscopic section showing mononuclear cell infiltrate in the subarachnoid space.

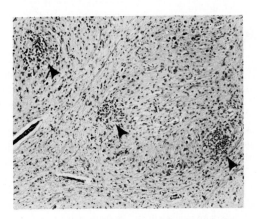

Figure 2–22C. Microscopic section showing nodular mononuclear cell infiltrates in the inferior olivary nucleus.

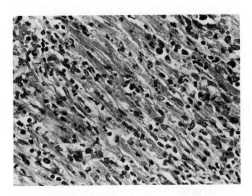

Figure 2–22D. Microscopic section of heart showing interstitial inflammation and foci of myofiber necrosis.

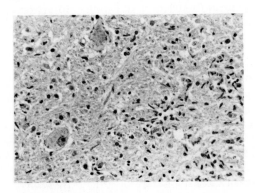

Figure 2–22E. Microscopic section of spinal cord from an adult with coxasackie encephalomyelitis.

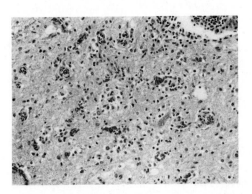

Figure 2–22F. Microscopic section of spinal cord from a child with paralytic poliomyelitis.

2.23 Herpes Simplex Encephalitis

CLINICAL

This 19-year-old man complained of headaches, nausea, and vomiting. He was brought to the hospital 4 days later when he became disoriented and incontinent. At that time, his speech was slurred and facility in his left hand was decreased. He had bilateral Babinski reflexes.

A computerized tomogram revealed an area of decreased attenuation with minimal nonhomogenous enhancement in the right temporal lobe. Lumbar puncture disclosed a normal opening pressure. The cerebrospinal fluid contained 50 red blood cells, 23 mononuclear cells, and 3 polymorphonuclear leukocytes per microliter. The glucose level was 86 mg/dL and the protein content was 37 mg/dL. The clinical diagnosis of herpes encephalitis was confirmed by brain biopsy. Despite therapy with adenine arabinoside (Ara-A), the patient died 3 weeks after hospitalization.

PATHOLOGY

A small portion of the biopsy specimen was used to make smear preparations as well as more conventional frozen sections. The smears, stained with hematoxylin–eosin, permit rapid identification of perivascular inflammatory cell infiltrates (Fig. 2–23A) and may demonstrate intranuclear inclusions somewhat more clearly than the frozen sections.

The routine paraffin-embedded sections of the biopsy specimen showed mononuclear cells in the overlying subarachnoid space and around vessels in the edematous, focally necrotic cortex (Fig. 2–23B). Intranuclear inclusions were found predominantly in glial cells. The inclusions were eosinophilic and surrounded by a halo that resulted from margination of the chromatin (Fig. 2–23C). Although these histological findings were consistent with herpes simplex encephalitis, the definitive diagnosis in this case was established by isolation of the virus from the biopsy specimen.

At autopsy, the brain was diffusely swollen and weighed 1520 grams. The cerebral hemispheres were symmetrical except for the focal area of herniation at the biopsy site (Fig. 2–23D). Coronal sections showed multiple areas in which the cerebral cortex was thinned, softened, and focally hemorrhagic. These foci of cortical necrosis were most prominent on the ventromedial aspects of the frontal and temporal lobes and on the insular cortices (Figs. 2–23E and 2–23F). The white matter was diffusely swollen and focally necrotic. The basal ganglia and hypothalamus were intact.

COMMENT

Herpes simplex encephalitis is the most common form of sporadic, severe encephalitis. In adults and older children, the disease is due to the type 1 herpes simplex virus. The initial infection with this virus is usually acquired in childhood and manifested by gingivostomatitis or may be asymptomatic. Serological studies have shown antibodies to type 1 herpes simplex virus in 40 to 90 percent of the population, reflecting the widespread dissemination of this virus. In many individuals, virus is harbored in a latent state in the trigeminal ganglia. Reactivation of these latent infections may cause recurrent attacks of herpes labialis ("fever blisters"). Most cases of encephalitis are also thought to result from reactivation of latent infections. In these individuals, the virus is thought to spread from the trigeminal ganglia along nerves to the meninges of the frontal and middle cranial fossae prior to entering the brain. In other cases, the infection appears to spread to the central nervous system along olfactory pathways.

As in the present case, the cerebral lesions are generally most severe in the ventromedial portions of the frontal and temporal lobes. Histologically, they are characterized by foci of necrosis and varying degrees of inflammation. The infected cells may contain so-called Cowdry type A inclusions. These are relatively large, eosinophilic intranuclear inclusions that may be surrounded by a halo produced by margination of the chromatin. They are often most readily seen inglial cells. Immunoperoxidase techniques are more sensitive than conventional histological techniques and may demonstrate the presence of viral antigens,

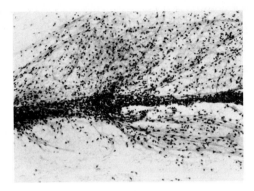

Figure 2–23A. Smear prepared from a portion of biopsy specimen from a patient with Herpes simplex encephalitis. Note the perivascular mononuclear inflammatory cell infiltrate.

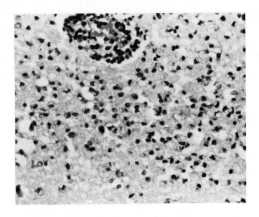

Figure 2–23B. Microscopic section of biopsy specimen showing edema, necrosis, and mononuclear cell infiltrates.

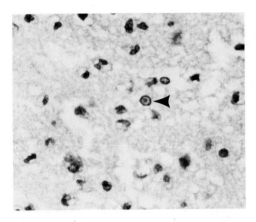

Figure 2–23C. Microscopic section showing an eosinophilic intranuclear inclusion (arrowheads).

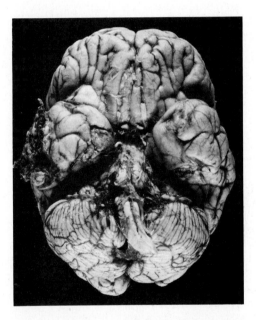

Figure 2–23D. Base of brain showing swelling, herniation and biopsy site on right temporal lobe.

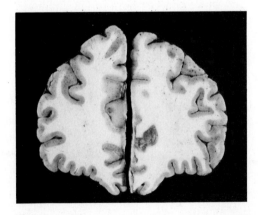

Figure 2–23E. Coronal section through frontal lobes showing cortical necrosis on medial aspect of right frontal lobe.

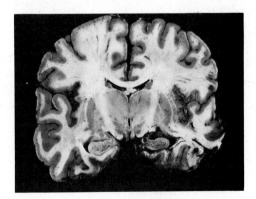

Figure 2–23F. Coronal section showing cortical necrosis on the inferiomedial aspects of the temporal lobes and insulae. Note also the biopsy site on the right temporal lobe.

even in cells that do not contain obvious inclusions (Fig. 2–23G). Nevertheless, isolation of the virus from brain tissue continues to provide the most definitive diagnosis. The virus cannot be recovered from the cerebrospinal fluid in the majority of adults with disease due to type 1 herpes simplex virus.

REFERENCES

Corey L, Spear PG: Infections with herpes simplex viruses. N Engl J Med 1986; 314:686-691, and 1986; 314:749-757.

Davis LE, Johnson RT: An explanation for the localization of herpes simplex encephalitis? Ann Neurol 1979; 5:2-5.

Esiri MM: Herpes simplex encephalitis: An immunohistological study of the distribution of viral antigen within the brain. J Neurol Sci 1982; 54:209-226.

Schroth G, Gawehn J, Thorn A, et al: Early diagnosis of herpes simplex encephalitis by MRI. Neurology 1987; 37:179-183.

Whitley R, Lakeman AD, Nahmias A, Roizman B: DNA restriction-enzyme analysis of herpes simplex virus isolates obtained from patients with encephalitis. N Engl J Med 1982; 307:1060-1062.

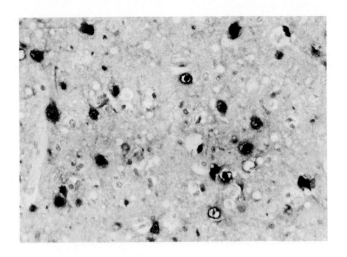

Figure 2–23G. Microscopic section, stained by immunoperoxidase technique for herpes virus, showing staining of intranuclear inclusions and cells without obvious inclusions.

2.24 Neonatal Herpes Simplex

CLINICAL

This 1200-gram male infant was born to an 18-year-old primigravida woman at approximately 30 weeks of gestation. The infant developed respiratory distress and hyperbilirubinemia requiring exchange transfusion. On the 11th day, a small vesicle was noted on the right shin. This subsequently grew herpes simplex virus. Despite treatment with adenine arabinoside (Ara-A), the child developed further respiratory problems, acidosis, and intravascular coagulation and died.

PATHOLOGY

The general autopsy revealed hepatic and adrenal necrosis. Histological examination of the liver revealed multiple small foci of necrosis with intranuclear inclusions in many of the hepatocytes (Fig. 2–24A). Staining with an immunoperoxidase technique demonstrated herpes virus antigens.

The brain was soft and swollen (Fig. 2–24B). There were petechial hemorrhages in the frontal and temporal lobes and especially in the cerebellum. Coronal sections disclosed additional petechial hemorrhages in the thalamus. Histological examination revealed multiple foci of hemorrhagic necrosis. Many of the glial cells had vesicular nuclei and some contained intranuclear inclusions (Fig. 2–24C). Staining with the immunoperoxidase technique demonstrated widespread dissemination of the viral antigen even in cells that contained no inclusions.

COMMENT

Most cases of neonatal herpes simplex encephalitis are due to the type 2 herpes simplex virus. This virus is spread venerally and may be harbored in a latent state in sacral ganglia. Reactivation of the latent infection results in recurrent genital herpes. Neonatal infections are generally acquired at the time of delivery from contact with genital secretions. The risk of neonatal infection is greater among infants born to women with primary genital herpes than among infants born to women with recurrent infections. The risk is especially high when the primary maternal infection is acquired during the third trimester of pregnancy.

The neonatal infections commonly become disseminated. As in the present case, skin vesicles, hepatic necrosis, and foci of adrenal necrosis are frequent extracranial lesions. Cerebral involvement may lead to extensive destruction of neural parenchyma. Even with treatment, infants with encephalitis have a high mortality and the survivors may have serious sequelae.

In adults, the type 2 herpes simplex virus may cause aseptic meningitis, radiculopathy, and, rarely, myelitis or encephalitis. In these individuals, the virus may be recovered from the cerebrospinal fluid.

REFERENCES

Brown ZA, Vontver LA, Bebedetti J, et al: Effects on infants of a first episode of genital herpes during pregnancy. N Engl J Med 1987; 317:1246-1251.

Corey L, Spear PG: Infections with herpes simplex viruses. N Engl J Med 1986; 314:686-691, and 1986; 314:749-757.

Dix RD, Bredesen DE, Erlich KS, Mills J: Recovery of herpesviruses from cerebrospinal fluid in immunodeficient homosexual men. Ann Neurol 1985; 18:611-614.

Prober CG, Sullender WM, Yasukawa LL, et al: Low risk of herpes simplex virus infections in neonates exposed to the virus at the time of vaginal delivery to mothers with recurrent genital herpes simplex infections. N Engl J Med 1987; 316:240-244.

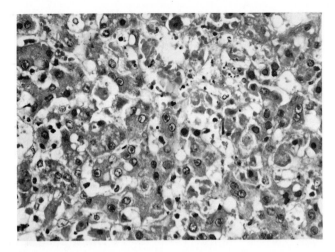

Figure 2–24A. Microscopic section of liver from a child with disseminated herpes showing small foci of necrosis and intranuclear inclusions in hepatocytes.

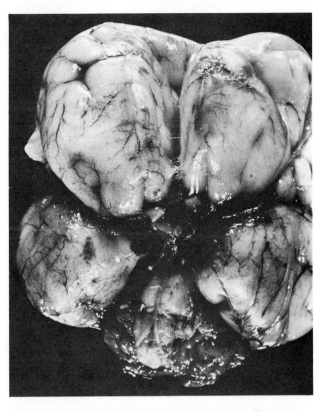

Figure 2–24B. Base of brain showing swelling and hemorrhage about cerebellum.

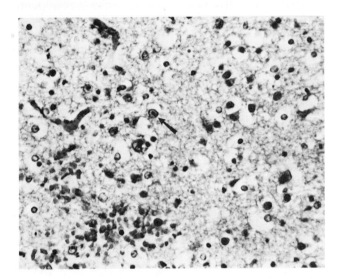

Figure 2–24C. Microscopic section showing foci of hemorrhagic necrosis and occasional cells with intranuclear inclusions (arrow).

2.25 Cytomegalovirus Encephalitis

CLINICAL

This 443-gram fetus was the product of a 19-week gestation in a 23-year-old woman. Although there was no history of maternal illness during the pregnancy, an ultrasound study was interpreted as showing hydrocephalus.

PATHOLOGY

The fetus was found to have disseminated cytomegalovirus infection with involvement of many visceral organs, including the lungs, liver, pancreas, testes, and heart. The brain was immature and weighed only 57 grams. Only primary sulci were demarcated. Blood was present in the subarachnoid space. Coronal sections of the cerebral hemispheres demonstrated mild ventricular dilatation. There was extensive hemorrhagic and nonhemorrhagic necrosis of the neural parenchyma surrounding the ventricular system (Fig. 2–25A). Histological examination of these areas disclosed numerous enlarged cells with prominent intranuclear inclusions and copious granular cytoplasm (Fig. 2–25B).

COMMENT

Antibodies to the cytomegalovirus have been found in as many as 80 percent of adults in various survey populations. Most of the infections in immunocompetent adults and older children are asymptomatic. Some may produce mild forms of hepatitis, pneumonitis or myocarditis. In other individuals, the Guillain–Barré syndrome has been associated with cytomegalovirus infections.

Congenital cytomegalovirus infections are common and may result from primary or recurrent maternal disease. Infection has been reported in 0.2 to 2.2 percent of all newborn infants. However, the majority of the congenitally infected neonates are asymptomatic. Nevertheless, some of these infants later develop mental retardation and hearing loss. Fetal disease is more severe when it is the result of primary maternal infection acquired during the first half of pregnancy. The severely affected infants may have hepatosplenomegaly, thrombocytopenia, chorioretinitis, and microcephaly. Brains from infants with fulminating disease often show necrotizing encephalitis with a predilection for the periventricular structures. These areas later undergo mineralization.

Immunosuppressed adults may have disseminated cytomegalovirus infections with cerebral involvement. Microglial nodules and occasional enlarged inclusion bearing cells have been reported in brains from renal transplant recipients. More recently, the cytomegalovirus has emerged as an important cause of encephalitis in individuals with the acquired immune deficiency syndrome. Figure 2–25C illustrates the characteristic cytomegalic cells in the hypothalamus of a man with AIDS.

REFERENCES

Anders KH, Guerra WF, Tomiyasu U, et al: The neuropathology of AIDS: UCLA experience and review. Am J Pathol 1986; 124:537-558.

Bale JF Jr: Human cytomegalovirus infection and disorders of the nervous system. Arch Neurol 1984; 41:310-320.

Stagno S, Pass RF, Cloud G, et al: Primary cytomegalovirus infection in pregnancy: Incidence, transmission to fetus, and clinical outcome. JAMA 1986; 256:1904-1908.

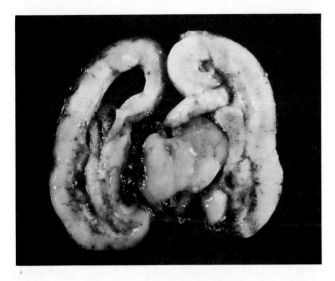

Figure 2–25A. Coronal section of brain from a fetus with cytomegalovirus infection showing periventricular necrosis.

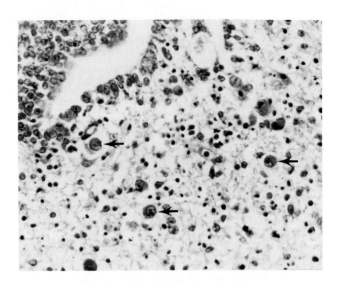

Figure 2–25B. Microscopic section showing multiple enlarged cells with prominent intranuclear inclusions (arrows) in subependymal region.

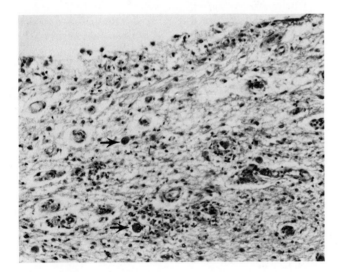

Figure 2–25C. Microscopic section showing cytomegalic cells (arrows) in the hypothalamus of a man with AIDS.

2.26 Subacute Sclerosing Panencephalitis

CLINICAL

This 14-year-old boy was admitted to the hospital with a history of seizures and personality changes. His past medical history included measles at age 3 years and chickenpox at age 5 years.

On physical examination he was found to have slurred speech and a short attention span. The cranial nerves were intact. He had decreased strength in the right hand, arm, and shoulder. He tended to fall to the right and had impaired rapid alternating movements. Palatomental and glabellar reflexes were present. Lumbar puncture yielded cerebrospinal fluid with normal glucose and total protein content; however, the proportion of gamma globulin was increased.

His course was characterized by progressive deterioration with increased emotional lability, decreased orientation, and increased right sided weakness. He developed a tremor and became dysarthric and progressively obtunded. He died 3 weeks after hospitalization.

PATHOLOGY

The brain was mildly swollen and the leptomeningeal blood vessels were moderately congested (Fig. 2–26A). Coronal sections disclosed grossly intact cerebral cortex and white matter. Histological examination revealed scattered mononuclear cells in the subarachnoid space. Scattered neurons and glial cells in the isocortex, basal ganglia, and brain stem (Fig. 2–26B) contained eosinophilic intranuclear inclusions. The inclusions were especially prominent and numerous in the pyramidal neurons of the hippocampi (Fig. 2–26C). Multiple inclusions were also present in oligodendroglial cells in the white matter. Electron microscopy demonstrated the inclusions to be composed of randomly oriented filamentous structures.

COMMENT

The morphological findings in this case are consistent with subacute sclerosing panencephalitis. This disorder is due to persistent infection by the measles virus.

The disease is rare and has an incidence of about one per million. Most cases have the onset of symptoms between the ages of 6 and 12 years. The initial manifestations are commonly mental deterioration and behavioral changes. These may be followed by motor dysfunction, seizures, myoclonus, and visual impairment. Many of the patients display a characteristic encephalographic pattern. The cerebrospinal fluid contains increased gamma globulin with oligoclonal bands and measles antibodies. The course of the disease is generally 1 to 3 years but may be longer or much shorter, as in this patient.

Brains from individuals with subacute sclerosing panencephalitis may be grossly normal or severely atrophic with ventricular dilatation and extensive demyelination of the white matter. Generally, more severe changes are encountered in cases with a protracted course. Histologically, prominent intranuclear inclusions are seen in neurons and glia. They are composed of smooth paramyxovirus nucleocapsids. The cytoplasm may contain coated or "fuzzy" nucleocapsids that have a somewhat larger diameter. Occasionally, neurons display neurofibrillary tangles. There is also prominent astrocytosis and proliferation of microglia in the form of elongated rod cells.

The pathogenesis of subacute sclerosing panencephalitis is incompletely elucidated. The persistence of the measles virus infection has been attributed to deficient production of M protein, a viral protein involved in the assembly of mature viral particles.

REFERENCES

Hall WW, Choppin PW: Measles-virus proteins in the brain tissue of patients with subacute sclerosing panencephalitis. Absence of the M protein. N Engl J Med 1981; 304:1152-1155.

Krawiecki NS, Kyken PR, El Gammal T, et al: Computed tomography of the brain in subacute sclerosing panencephalitis. Ann Neurol 1984; 15:489-493.

Ohya T, Martinez J, Jabbour JT, et al: Subacute sclerosing panencephalitis: Correlation of clinical, neurophysiologic and neuropathologic findings. Neurology 1974; 24:211-218.

Silva CA, Paula-Barbosa MM, Pereira S, Cruz C: Two cases of rapidly progressive subacute sclerosing panencephalitis: Neuropathological findings. Arch Neurol 1981; 38:109-113.

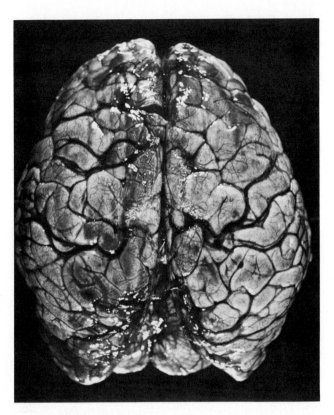

Figure 2–26A. Dorsal surface of brain showing swelling and congestion of leptomeningeal blood vessels.

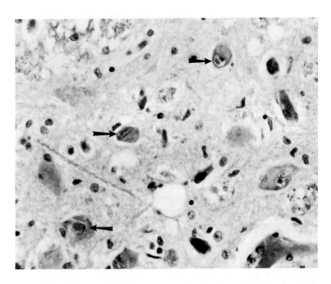

Figure 2–26B. Microscopic section showing prominent eosinophilic intranuclear inclusions (arrows) in brain stem nuclei.

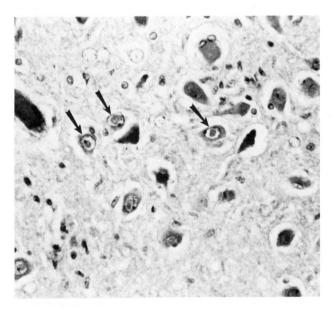

Figure 2–26C. Microscopic section showing intranuclear inclusions in pyramidal neurons of the hippocampus (arrows).

2.27 Progressive Multifocal Leukoencephalopathy

CLINICAL

This 66-year-old man had a long history of rheumatoid arthritis, recently treated with methotrexate. He developed a left hemiplegia, dementia, and dyspraxia. His neurological status further deteriorated over the next 2 months until he was unable to converse or feed and dress himself. He was hospitalized for further evaluation but suffered a respiratory arrest.

PATHOLOGY

The brain weighed 1387 grams and the cerebral hemispheres were symmetrical. Gyri and sulci were of normal proportions except for mild gyral atrophy over the frontal poles. Coronal sections of the cerebral hemispheres revealed extensive demyelination and partial necrosis of the white matter in the frontal lobes and genu of the corpus callosum (Figs. 2–27A, 2–27B). In the maximally affected areas, the cut surface of the white matter was soft and pitted. Additional smaller foci of demyelination were evident in the brain stem and white matter of the cerebellum. The cerebral cortex and nuclear gray matter were grossly intact but contained minute foci of demyelination.

Histologically, the lesions showed varying proportions of demyelination, partial necrosis, and gliosis. The larger lesions contained numerous lipid-laden macrophages and reactive astrocytes (Fig. 2–27C). Occasionally, the astrocytes were very large and harbored grotesque nuclei. Some of the oligodendrocytes contained enlarged hyperchromatic nuclei that were filled by acidophilic, amphophilic, or even basophilic inclusions (Fig. 2–27D). These were most numerous in smaller lesions and around the periphery of larger lesions evolved from coalescence of the smaller lesions.

COMMENT

Progressive multifocal leukoencephalopathy is a demyelinating disorder caused by certain papovaviruses. The disease is usually encountered in adults with impaired cell-mediated immunity. Many of the patients have had lymphomas, leukemias, or granulomatous infections. Other cases have occurred in individuals who were therapeutically immunosuppressed or organ transplant recipients. More recently, the disease has been encountered in patients with the acquired immune deficiency syndrome. Rare cases have occurred in children.

Clinical manifestations are protean but usually include weakness, impairment of speech and vision, and mental deterioration. The disease is gradually progressive and most of the patients die in 4 to 6 months. The demyelinating lesions can be visualized by computerized tomography or magnetic resonance imaging. Cerebrospinal fluid changes are nonspecific.

Most cases from which the virus has been isolated have been attributed to the JC virus. Two cases have been due to an SV40-like agent. Another papovavirus, the BK virus, has been isolated from urine but not the brain of patients with progressive multifocal leukoencephalopathy. Although the disease is relatively uncommon, antibodies to the JC and BK agents have been detected in a large proportion of the survey populations.

The demyelination has been attributed to infection and cytolysis of oligodendroglial cells. The papovavirus, in the form of spheres 35 to 45 nm in diameter or filaments 20 to 30 nm in diameter, can be demonstrated ultrastructurally in the nuclei of the infected oligodendrocytes. Astrocytes may contain large bizarre nuclei that are often more conspicuous than the inclusion-bearing oligodendroglial nuclei. Virions have not been demonstrated ultrastructurally in the astrocytic nuclei. Astrocytic alterations were previously interpreted as a manifestation of oncogenic transformation. However, more recent studies have suggested that they are merely an unusual form of a reactive change. Nevertheless, the JC virus has been shown to be oncogenic in certain laboratory animals.

REFERENCES

Aksamit AJ, Sever JL, Major ED: Progressive multifocal leukoencephalopathy: JC virus detection by in situ hybridization compared with immunohistochemistry. Neurology 1986; 36:499-504.

Blum LW, Chambers RA, Schwartzmann RJ, Streletz LJ: Progressive multifocal leukoencephalopathy in acquired immune deficiency syndrome. Arch Neurol 1985; 42:137-139.

Houff SA, Major ED, Katz DA, et al: Involvement of JC virus-infected mononuclear cells from the bone marrow and spleen in the pathogenesis of progressive multifocal leukoencephalopathy. N Engl J Med 1988; 318:301-305.

Krupp LB, Lipton RB, Swerdlow ML, et al: Progressive multifocal leukoencephalopathy: Clinical and radiographic features. Ann Neurol 1985; 17:344-349.

Levy JD, Cottingham KL, Campbell RJ, et al: Progressive multifocal leukoencephalopathy and magnetic resonance imaging. Ann Neurol 1986; 19:399-401.

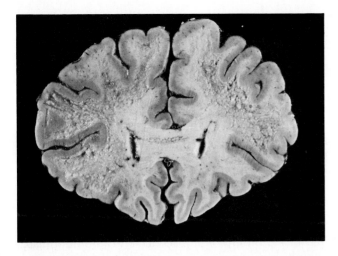

Figure 2–27A. Coronal section through genu of corpus callosum from a patient with progressive multifocal leukoencephalopathy. Note the extensive areas of demyelination and necrosis.

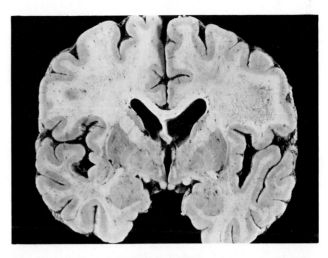

Figure 2–27B. Coronal section through mammillary bodies showing areas of demyelination and necrosis in white matter of both frontal lobes.

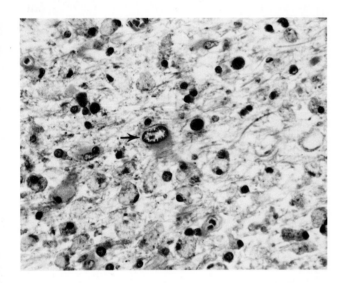

Figure 2–27C. Microscopic section showing lipid-laden macrophages and reactive astrocytes (arrow) in a demyelinated lesion.

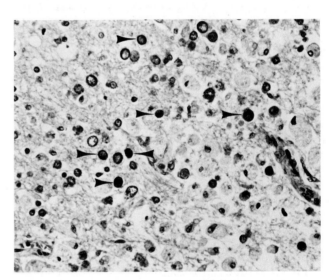

Figure 2–27D. Microscopic section showing enlarged, hyperchromatic nuclei containing intranuclear inclusions (arrowheads).

2.28   Rabies

Rabies is caused by a virus belonging to the rhabdovirus group. The major reservoirs are in wild carnivores, of which skunks, foxes, and raccoons are of particular importance, and in bats. Although bites from dogs and cats are responsible for most rabies treatments, domestic animals are of little importance in perpetuating the disease. Human infection generally results from a bite by an animal in the advanced stages of the disease. However, occasional cases have been the result of inhalation of airborne virus in bat caves. Rare cases have also resulted from corneal transplants and laboratory accidents. The incubation period is generally 30 to 60 days. The initial clinical manifestations are often pain and paresthesias at the site of the previous bite. Abnormal behavior, hyperactivity, laryngeal, and pharyngeal muscle spasms and autonomic dysfunction are common features. The disease is almost invariably fatal.

The virus replicates in skeletal muscles near the site of injury prior to transport through peripheral nerves to the central nervous system. The spinal cord, brain stem, cerebellum, septal nuclei, limbic cortex, and hippocampi are preferentially involved. These structures may contain perivascular and intraparenchymal mononuclear cell infiltrates. The intraparenchymal microglial nodules in cases of rabies are designated as Babes nodes. In addition, about 70 percent of the cases will harbor Negri bodies. These are eosinophilic intracytoplasmic inclusions. They are encountered most often in the pyramidal layer neurons of the hippocampi (Fig. 2–28A) and in the Purkinje cells of the cerebellum (Fig. 2–28B). Ultrastructurally, they are composed of a fibrillar matrix containing viral particles. Immunofluorescent and immunohistochemical techniques can be used for the diagnosis of rabies.

REFERENCES

Baer GM, Shaddock JH, Houff SA, et al: Human rabies transmitted by corneal transplant. Arch Neurol 1982; 39:103-107.

Iwasaki Y, Liu D-S, Yamamoto T, Konno H: On the replication and spread of rabies virus in the human central nervous system. J Neuropathol Exp Neurol 1985; 44:185-195.

Johnson RT: Viral Infections of the Nervous System. New York, Raven Press, 1982, chap 7, pp 159-167.

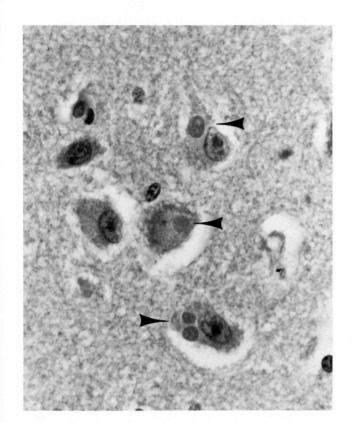

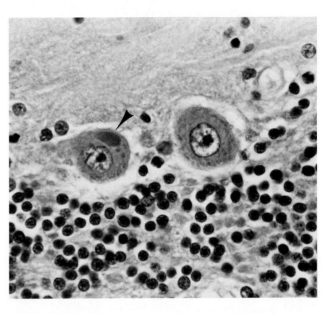

Figure 2–28B. Microscopic section showing a Negri body (arrow-head) in a Purkinje cell.

Figure 2–28A. Microscopic section from brain of an adult with rabies. Note the intracytoplasmic Negri bodies (arrowheads) in hippocampal neurons.

3

Vascular Disease

3.1   Border Zone Infarcts

Clinical

This 59-year-old man had a long history of hypertension and severe rheumatoid arthritis. Prosthetic devices had been placed in both hips, both knees, and in the left hand. Eight years previously, he had a right hemiparesis and aphasia that resolved over a 3 month period. The patient died of congestive heart failure.

PATHOLOGY

The dorsal surface of the cerebrum displayed bilateral, linear depressions that extended from the frontal through the parietal lobes (Fig. 3–1A). The lesions were roughly symmetrical and somewhat broader on the parietal lobes as compared to the frontal lobes. Coronal sections showed old infarcts underlying the depressed areas (Figs. 3–1B and 3–1C). The lesions showed loss of cortical gray matter, and to a lesser extent white matter, in areas that corresponded to the border zones between the anterior and middle cerebral artery perfusion beds. In addition, there was a smaller area of cortical infarction in the border zone between the perfusion beds of the left middle and posterior cerebral arteries (Fig. 3–1C).

COMMENT

Over the years, increased emphasis has been given to the role of extracranial vascular disease in the pathogenesis of cerebral infarcts. Extracranial atherosclerotic disease tends to be most severe at the carotid bifurcations. This is followed by the cavernous portions of the internal carotid arteries, the origins of the great vessels from the aortic arch, and the origins of the vertebral arteries. Atherosclerotic disease of the carotids can lead to stenosis or precipitate thrombosis. The extracranial lesions can serve as the source of emboli that can be composed of fragments of thrombus or atheromatous material.

Individuals with asymptomatic carotid artery stenosis may develop border zone infarcts if they suffer marked hypotension. This may occur as a result of myocardial infarcts, overly aggressive treatment of hypertension, or during surgical procedures. The lesions are often bilateral but may be more severe on one side than the other, depending on the distribution of accompanying intra- and extracranial vascular disease. Alternatively, it has been suggested that some border zone infarcts are caused by microemboli occluding leptomeningeal arteries in the watershed areas. Regardless of the mechanism, the lesions are generally most prominent in the border zones between the anterior and middle cerebral artery perfusion beds.

REFERENCES

Bogousslavsky J, Regli F: Borderzone infarctions distal to internal carotid artery occlusion. Ann Neurol 1986; 20:346-350.

Howard R, Trend P, Russell RWR: Clinical features of ischemia in cerebral arterial border zones after periods of reduced cerebral blood flow. Arch Neurol 1988; 44:934-940.

Torvik A, Skullerud K: Watershed infarcts in the brain caused by microemboli. Clin Neuropathol 1982; 1:99-105.

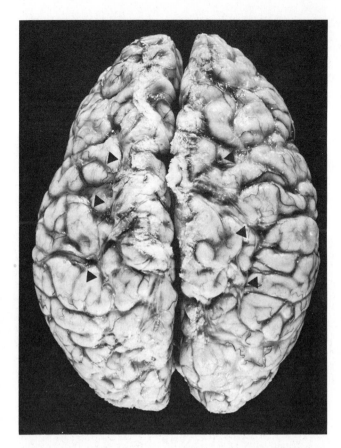

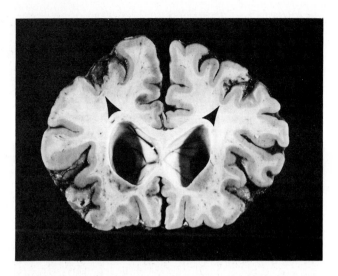

Figure 3–1B. Coronal section at genu of corpus callosum showing bilateral border zone infarcts (arrowheads).

Figure 3–1A. Dorsal surface of brain showing bilateral border zone infarcts (arrowheads).

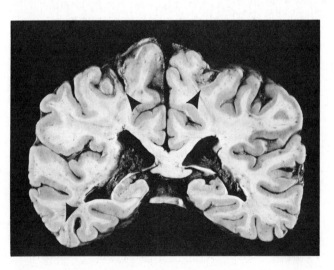

Figure 3–1C. Coronal section at splenium of corpus callosum showing bilateral border zone infarcts (arrowheads).

3.2 Middle Cerebral Infarct

Internal Carotid Artery Thrombosis

CLINICAL

This 67-year-old woman awoke on the morning of admission unable to speak or get out of bed. When hospitalized she was somnolent, aphasic, and had a dense right hemiparesis. She had a past medical history of hypertension and hypothyroidism. She died 4 days later.

PATHOLOGY

Autopsy revealed thrombosis of the left internal carotid artery. The brain was diffusely swollen but asymmetrical due to fullness of the left cerebral hemisphere (Fig. 3–2A). Coronal sections of the cerebral hemispheres show the swelling to be maximal in the distribution of the left middle cerebral artery (Figs. 3–2B and 3–2C). Within the area of infarction, the cortex was expanded and faintly discolored. Demarcation between the infarcted cortex and subcortical white matter was less distinct than in the intact contralateral hemisphere. The central white matter was expanded, mildly softened, and friable. The left cingulate gyrus was herniated beneath the falx (Fig. 3–2B). The left basal ganglia were shifted to the right. The left lateral ventricle was compressed while the right lateral ventricle was enlarged (Fig. 3–2C). The third ventricle was bowed to the right.

COMMENT

Thrombosis of the carotid arteries is recognized as a major cause of cerebral infarction. The resulting infarcts are most commonly in the distribution of the middle cerebral artery but may include all or portions of the distribution of the anterior and posterior cerebral arteries as well. It is now recognized that middle cerebral infarcts are relatively infrequently due to atherosclerosis and thrombosis of the middle cerebral artery itself.

The appearance of the infarcted cerebral tissue is influenced by the period of time that has elapsed between arterial occlusion and examination of the brain. When 18 to 24 hours have elapsed, the infarcted tissue is swollen and softened and the gray matter is faintly discolored. Occasional petechial hemorrhages may be seen in the gray matter. After 36 to 48 hours the so-called cracking artifact tends to accentuate the demarcation between the friable infarcted tissue and the surrounding viable tissue. The increased volume of the edematous necrotic tissue results in distortion of the ventricular system and herniation. Cavitation does not begin to appear until after 4 or 5 days.

REFERENCES

McCormick WF: Vascular diseases. In Rosenberg RN (ed): The Clinical Neurosciences. New York, Churchill Livingstone, 1983, vol 3, chap 2, pp III:35–III:83.

Mohr JP, Kase CS: Cerebrovascular disease. In Rosenberg RN (ed): The Clinical Neurosciences. New York, Churchill Livingstone, 1983, vol 1, chap 3, pp I:167–I:231.

Pessin MS, Hinton RC, Davis KR, et al: Mechanisms of acute carotid stroke. Ann Neurol 1979; 6:245-252.

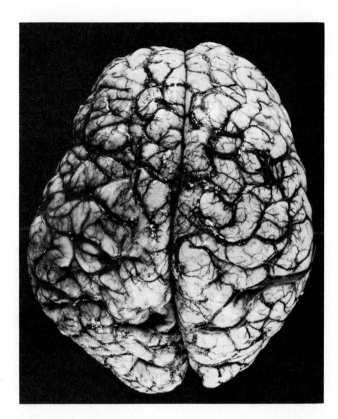

Figure 3–2A. Dorsal surface of brain showing infarct with swelling in the left cerebral hemsiphere.

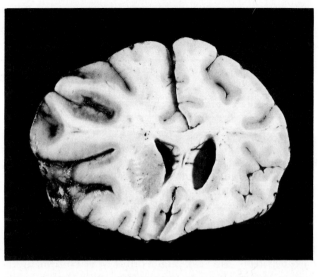

Figure 3–2B. Coronal section at genu of corpus callosum showing recent infarction in distribution of left middle cerebral artery.

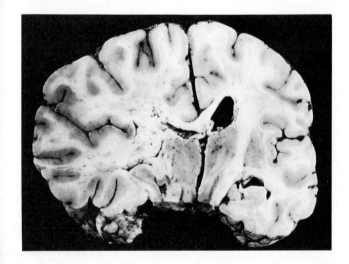

Figure 3–2C. Coronal section at a more caudal level showing recent infarction in distribution of left middle cerebral artery and associated mass effect.

3.3 Middle Cerebral Infarct

Middle Cerebral Artery Thrombosis

CLINICAL

This 71-year-old woman, who was previously in good health, was found by her family in an obtunded condition. On examination, she was found to have a dense left hemiparesis. She had decreased pain perception on the left but no sensory extinction or neglect. Her eyes deviated to the right. She had no carotid bruits. Her hospital course was complicated by a myocardial infarct and cardiac arrhythmias. She died 3 weeks later.

PATHOLOGY

Examination of the brain showed severe arteriosclerosis with numerous atheromatous plaques in the walls of the major intracranial blood vessels. Coronal sections demonstrated a subacute infarct within the distribution of the right middle cerebral artery. Rostrally, the infarct involved the basal ganglia, internal capsule, and insula (Fig. 3–3A). More caudally, the posterior frontal and parietal cortex were also infarcted (Fig. 3–3B). The lumen of the proximal right middle cerebral artery was distended by reddish-tan thrombus (Fig. 3–3A, curved arrow). The infarcted tissue was diffusely softened and discolored. Rostrally, the white matter showed early cavitation.

COMMENT

This case illustrates cerebral infarction secondary to thrombosis of an arteriosclerotic intracranial artery. In recent years it has become recognized that infarcts in the distribution of the middle cerebral arteries are more commonly due to embolization or thrombosis of the internal carotid arteries rather than thrombosis of the middle cerebral arteries themselves. This correlates with the observation that atherosclerotic changes are usually much more severe in the extracranial vessels. As in the present case, deaths among patients with atherothrombotic strokes are most often due to the associated cardiovascular disease.

REFERENCES

Kistler JF, Ropper AH, Heros RC: Therapy of ischemic cerebral vascular disease due to atherothrombosis. N Engl J Med 1984; 311:27-34, and 1984; 311:100-105.

Lhermitte F, Gautier JC, Derouesne C: Nature of occlusions of the middle cerebral artery. Neurology 1970; 20:82-88.

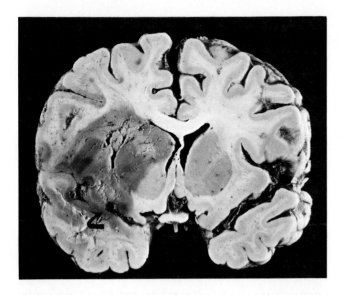

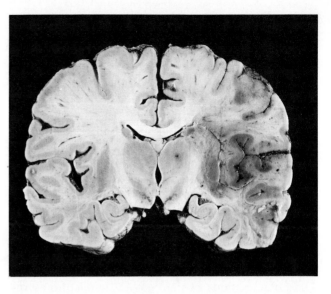

Figure 3–3A. Coronal section, viewed from the front, showing thrombus in the right middle cerebral artery (curved arrow) and associated subacute infarct.

Figure 3–3B. Coronal section, at a more caudal level, showing infarct in distribution of right middle cerebral artery.

3.4 Middle Cerebral Infarct

Old with Aphasia

CLINICAL

This 59-year-old man developed a right hemiplegia, aphasia, and a homonymous visual field defect. These deficits persisted until his death 2 months later.

PATHOLOGY

Horizontal sections of the cerebral hemispheres revealed a massive old cerebral infarct with early cavitation in the distribution of the left middle cerebral artery (Figs. 3–4A and 3–4B). In addition to disrupting the left basal ganglia and posterior limb of the internal capsule, the infarct also involved a portion of the inferior frontal convolution, the superior temporal convolution, and the inferior parietal lobule.

COMMENT

This individual had global aphasia. The posterior portion of the inferior frontal convolution (Brodmann's area 44) is designated as Broca's area and is involved with the motor control of speech. The posterior portion of the superior temporal convolution (Brodmann's area 41 and 42) is designated as Wernicke's area and is involved with the perception of speech. The inferior parietal lobule harbors the angular gyrus (Brodmann's area 39) and is involved with the comprehension of written information. All of these centers and the arcuate fasciculus interconnecting these areas were disrupted by this massive infarct. The visual field defect resulted from interruption of the optic radiation on the left.

REFERENCES

Mohr JP: Acquired language disorders. In Asbury AK, McKhann GM, McDonald WI (eds): Diseases of the Nervous System. Philadelphia, Saunders, 1986, vol II, chap 64, pp 816–827.

Ross ED, Geschwind N: Disorders of higher brain functions. In Rosenberg RN (ed): The Clinical Neurosciences. New York, Churchill Livingstone, 1983, vol 2, chap 19, pp I:777–I:796.

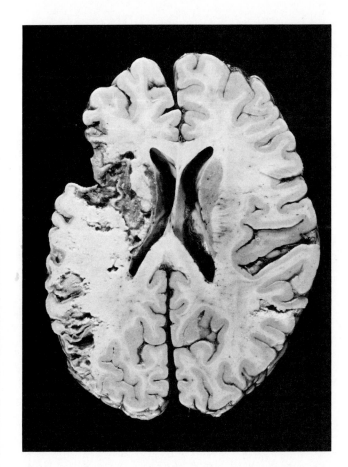

Figure 3–4A. Horizontal section showing a massive remote infarct in the distribution of the left middle cerebral artery.

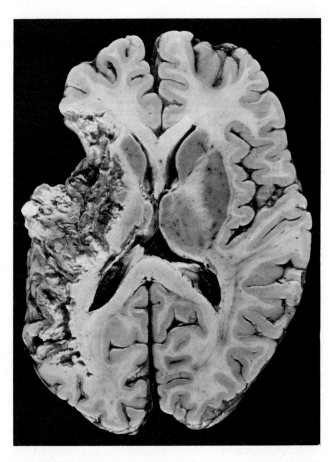

Figure 3–4B. Horizontal section showing the massive remote infarct responsible for the patient's aphasia.

3.5   Middle Cerebral Infarct

Remote with Tract Degeneration

CLINICAL

This 60-year-old man had a large left hemispheric cerebral infarct 6 years prior to his death from a heart attack.

PATHOLOGY

The lateral surface of the left cerebral hemisphere displayed an unusually deep indentation along the Sylvian fissure (Fig. 3–5A). Horizontal sections of the cerebral hemispheres disclosed a large remote infarct involving the left basal ganglia, internal capsule, and the insular cortex (Fig. 3–5B). The resulting degeneration of the pyramidal tract caused atrophy of the left mesencephalic crus cerebri (Fig. 3–5C), left half of the basis pontis (Fig. 3–5D), and left medullary pyramid (Fig. 3–5E).

COMMENT

The cerebral infarct had disrupted the pyramidal tract contained in the rostral portion of the posterior limb of the internal capsule. The distal portion of the disrupted tract subsequently underwent Wallerian degeneration. This process occurs slowly, and grossly discernible atrophy would not have been evident for several months.

Within the mesencephalon, the fibers of the pyramidal tract are found predominantly in the middle two thirds of the crus cerebri. Within the pons, the fibers are more widely dispersed among the pontine nuclei and the unilateral atrophy is somewhat less conspicuous. The fibers are reaggregated in the medullary pyramids resulting in a striking contrast between the atrophic and nonatrophic sides.

REFERENCE

Brodal A: Neurological Anatomy. New York, Oxford University Press, 1981, pp 180-194.

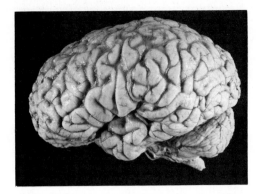

Figure 3–5A. Lateral surface of brain showing a deep indentation from a remote infarct along sylvian fissure.

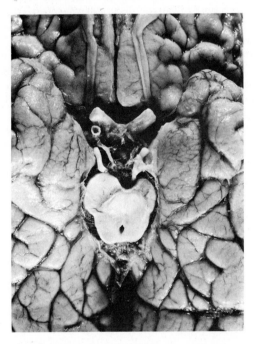

Figure 3–5C. Base of brain showing tract degeneration manifested by atrophy of the left mesencephalic crus cerebri.

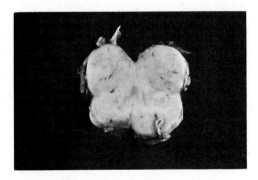

Figure 3–5E. Transverse section of brain stem showing tract degeneration with severe atrophy of left medullary pyramid.

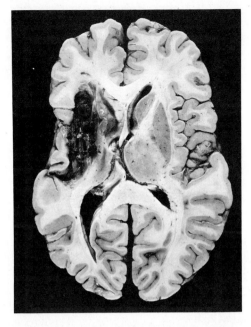

Figure 3–5B. Horizontal section showing a remote infarct involving insula, left basal ganglia, and left internal capsule.

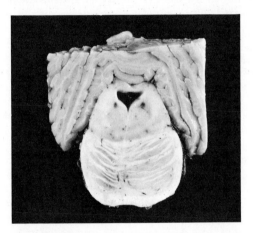

Figure 3–5D. Transverse section of brain stem showing tract degeneration with atrophy of left half of basis pontis.

3.6 Pontine Infarct

Basilar Artery Thrombosis

CLINICAL

This 65-year-old man developed slurred speech and difficulty with walking. He was hospitalized and found to have dysarthria, disconjugate gaze, and flaccid paralysis of the right side of his body. This progressed within a few hours to a flaccid quadriplegia. A computerized tomogram revealed a pontine infarct. His hospital course was complicated by atrial fibrillation and aspiration pneumonia. He died 3 weeks later.

PATHOLOGY

The cerebral hemispheres were symmetrical. Gyri on the inferior surfaces of the temporal lobes and the occipital lobes were swollen, softened, and focally discolored. The ventral surface of the pons also was softened and slightly discolored. The vessels at the base of the brain formed a normal circle of Willis except for hypoplasia of the posterior communicating arteries. The right vertebral artery was also hypoplastic. The vessels showed arteriosclerotic changes that were most severe in the distal internal carotid arteries, the posterior cerebral arteries, and the vertebrobasilar system (Fig. 3–6A). The mid-portion of the basilar artery was discolored (Fig. 3–6B). Cross sections of the basilar artery showed the proximal portion to be markedly narrowed by atheromatous changes while the discolored mid-portion was distended by thrombus (Fig. 3–6C). Transverse sections of the pons disclosed bilateral infarction of the basis pontis that was slightly more extensive on the left than the right (Fig. 3–6D).

COMMENT

This case illustrates infarction of the pons secondary to thrombosis of an atherosclerotic basilar artery. In contrast to the anterior circulation, infarcts in the distribution of the vertebrobasilar system are more commonly the result of local thrombosis, rather than embolization or thrombosis of more proximal vessels. The clinical manifestations associated with basilar artery thrombosis reflect involvement of corticospinal and corticobulbar connections, ascending sensory pathways, cranial nerve nuclei, and interconnections among the various cranial nerve nuclei. The individuals may be comatose or conscious but unable to respond ("locked in"), depending upon the extent of involvement of the reticular activating system.

Individuals with basilar artery thrombosis also may have infarcts in the thalamus, posterior temporal lobes, and occipital lobes. This occurs when the posterior cerebral arteries are perfused predominantly from the vertebrobasilar system. However, infarcts in the posterior temporal and occipital lobes more commonly result from kinking of the posterior cerebral arteries during downward displacement of the brain stem by an expanding supratentorial mass lesion.

Less extensive, predominantly unilateral pontine infarcts (Fig. 3–6E) may result from occlusions involving only paramedian branches of the basilar artery rather than the entire basilar artery. These lesions produce a spectrum of overlapping clinical syndromes, reflecting the more selective involvement of the many motor and sensory pathways and cranial nerve nuclei.

REFERENCES

Caplan LR: Vertebrobasilar occlusive disease. In Barnett HJM, Mohr JP, Stein BM, Yatsu FM (eds): Stroke. Pathophysiology, Diagnosis, and Management. New York, Churchill Livingstone, 1986, vol 1, chap 29, pp 549–619.

Sears ES, Patten JP: Diseases of the cranial nerves and the brain stem. In Rosenberg RN (ed): The Clinical Neurosciences. New York, Churchill Livingstone, 1983, vol 2, chap 23, pp I:915–I:954.

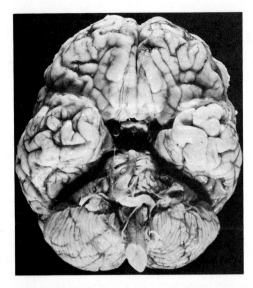

Figure 3–6A. Base of brain with severe cerebral arteriosclerosis. The midportion of the basilar artery is discolored and the right vertebral artery is hypoplastic.

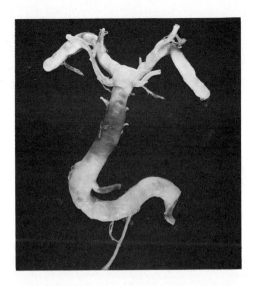

Figure 3–6B. Vessels removed from base of brain. The vessels show nearly confluent atheromatous changes. The midportion of the basilar artery is discolored and distended.

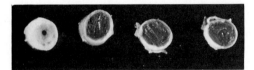

Figure 3–6C. Transverse sections of the basilar artery. Note the atheromatous stenosis and the intralumenal thrombus.

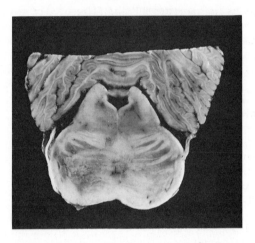

Figure 3–6D. Transverse section of the brain stem showing extensive, bilateral infarction of the basis pontis.

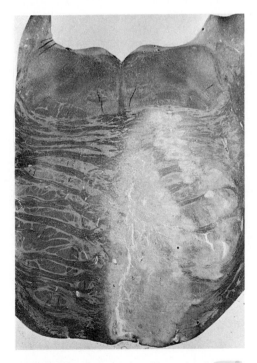

Figure 3–6E. Macrosection of pons showing a unilateral infarct.

3.7 Lateral Medullary Infarct

Wallenberg Syndrome

CLINICAL

This 64-year-old man was admitted to the hospital with an acute myocardial infarct and died 6 days later. His previous medical history was significant for hypertension, chronic atrial fibrillation, and a left lateral medullary infarct, 3 years previously. At that time, he had presented with a left Horner's syndrome, nystagmus, dysarthria, left leg and arm ataxia, and decreased pinprick sensation over the left side of his face and right side of his body.

PATHOLOGY

The vessels at the base of the brain formed an essentially normal circle of Willis. There were numerous atheromatous plaques in the walls of the vessels. The left vertebral artery had been remotely occluded and was yellow-gray in color (Fig. 3–7A). Transverse sections of the brain stem showed the dorsolateral quadrant of the medulla to be shrunken and focally cavitated (Fig. 3–7B). The cavity was traversed by strands of residual glial tissue.

COMMENT

This case illustrates the late sequelae of a lateral medullary infarct from occlusion of a vertebral artery.

Although the infarct is in the distribution of the medullary branch of the posterior inferior cerebellar artery, most of these lesions result from occlusion of the vertebral artery. The infarct had produced a so-called Wallenberg syndrome, one of the more common and probably the best known of the many brain stem syndromes that are alternatively designated by eponyms. Despite the close proximity of the many important anatomic structures in the medulla, these patients often do remarkably well and survive their infarcts. Figure 3–7C shows a macrosection of the medulla from a patient who died shortly after suffering a lateral medullary infarct. Note the necrosis and swelling in the dorsolateral quadrant of the medulla. The medullary lesions may be accompanied by cerebellar infarcts in the distribution of the posterior inferior cerebellar artery.

REFERENCES

Fisher CM, Karnes WE, Kubik CS: Lateral medullary infarction: The pattern of vascular occlusion. J Neuropathol Exp Neurol 1961; 20:323-379.

Loeb C, Meyers JS: Strokes Due to Vertebro-Basilar Disease. Springfield, Ill, Thomas, 1965, pp 52-79.

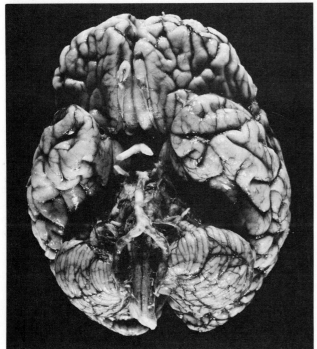

Figure 3–7A. Base of the brain with severe cerebral arteriosclerosis. The left vertebral artery had been remotely occluded and was yellow-gray in color.

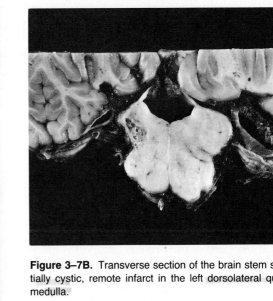

Figure 3–7B. Transverse section of the brain stem showing a partially cystic, remote infarct in the left dorsolateral quadrant of the medulla.

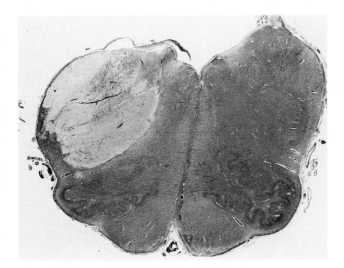

Figure 3–7C. Macrosection showing a recent infarct involving the dorsolateral quadrant of the medulla.

3.8   Cerebellar Infarct

Inferior Surface

CLINICAL

This 76-year-old man had advanced, recurrent carcinoma of the tongue. He was hospitalized with pneumonia and died a few days later.

PATHOLOGY

The vessels at the base of the brain contained numerous atherosclerotic plaques. The cerebral hemispheres showed no vascular lesions. The inferior surface of the right cerebellar hemisphere displayed irregular areas of old infarction in the distribution of the posterior inferior cerebellar artery (Fig. 3–8). No lesions were evident grossly or microscopically in the brain stem.

COMMENT

Cerebellar infarcts are encountered most commonly in elderly individuals with advanced arteriosclerosis.

Most of the infarcts are on the inferior surface of the cerebellar hemisphere in the distribution of the posterior inferior cerebellar artery. As in the present case, many of these individuals have no documented clinical deficits and may show no pathological evidence of an associated brain stem infarct. In other individuals, the infarcts may produce acute cerebellar dysfunction and signs of progressive, potentially lethal, brain stem compression.

REFERENCES

Duncan GW, Parker SW, Fisher CM: Acute cerebellar infarction in the PICA territory. Arch Neurol 1975; 32:364–368.

Scotti G, Spinnler H, Sterzi R, Vallar G: Cerebellar softening. Ann Neurol 1980; 8:133–144.

Sypert GW, Alvord EC Jr: Cerebellar infarction: A clinico-pathological study. Arch Neurol 1975; 32:357–363.

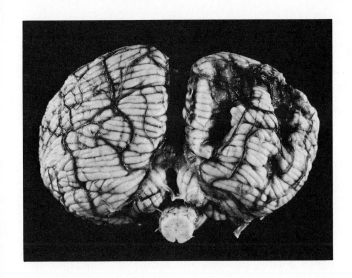

Figure 3–8. Remote infarct of inferior surface of right cerebellar hemisphere.

3.9 Cerebellar Infarct

Superior Surface
Transsynaptic Degeneration of Olives

CLINICAL

This 68-year-old man had a long history of hypertension and coronary arteriosclerosis. He had had two vessel coronary artery bypass grafts 9 years previously. He was hospitalized following the sudden onset of occipital headache and dizziness. This had been preceded by chest pain during the previous 3 or 4 days. On neurological examination he was found to have dysarthric speech, a slight intention tremor on the left, and left lateral nystagmus. An electrocardiogram revealed changes consistent with an acute diaphragmatic myocardial infarct. A computerized tomogram showed a left cerebellar hemisphere infarct and a lacunar infarct in the anterior limb of the right internal capsule. He died 7 days later.

PATHOLOGY

Examination of the heart revealed an old anteroseptal myocardial infarct with overlying mural thrombus and a recent posterolateral myocardial infarct.

Sections of the cerebral hemispheres revealed a lacunar infarct in the anterior limb of the right internal capsule and head of the right caudate nucleus. Examination of the cerebellum disclosed an area of recent softening and hemorrhagic discoloration on the superior surface of the left cerebellar hemisphere (Fig. 3–9A). On section, the lesion was found to be extensively hemorrhagic and consistent with an embolic infarct (Fig. 3–9B).

COMMENT

This case illustrates a recent infarct in the distribution of the superior cerebellar artery. Lesions in this area are less common than infarcts in the distribution of the posterior inferior cerebellar arteries. Figure 3–9C illustrates another case in which there was a remote infarct in the distribution of the superior cerebellar artery. The latter case also displayed transsynaptic degeneration of the contralateral inferior olivary nucleus. This process is characterized by enlargement and vacuolation of olivary neurons (Fig. 3–9D). Dendrites arising from the affected neurons become unusually prominent and form complex glomeruloid structures that can be seen best with silver stains (Fig. 3–9E). The affected olives also display gliosis. In some cases, the olivary nuclei are enlarged and the process is described somewhat inappropriately as "olivary hypertrophy."

Transsynaptic degeneration of the inferior olivary nuclei is seen most commonly in elderly individuals with pontine infarcts that interrupt the central tegmental tracts. However, this form of transsynaptic degeneration may be seen with disruptive lesions anywhere along the so-called Guillain–Molleret triangle. This pathway projects rostrally from the dentate nucleus through the superior cerebellar peduncle, crosses the brain stem in the commissure of Wernekink near the red nuclei, and then projects caudally through the central tegmental tract to the contralateral inferior olivary nucleus. Some of the patients with these olivary changes have palatal myoclonus.

REFERENCES

Barron KD, Dentinger MP, Koeppen AH: Fine structure of the hypertrophied human inferior olive. J Neuropathol Exp Neurol 1982; 41:186–203.

Kase CS, White JL, Joslyn JN, et al: Cerebellar infarction in the superior cerebellar artery distribution. Neurology 1985; 35:705–711.

Lapresle J, Ben Hamida, M: The dentato–olivary pathway: Somatotopic relationship between the dentate nucleus and the contralateral inferior olive. Arch Neurol 1970; 22:135-143.

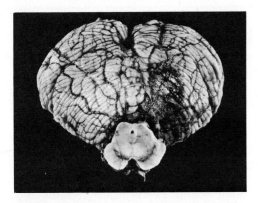

Figure 3–9A. Recent hemorrhagic infarct on superior surface of left cerebellar hemisphere.

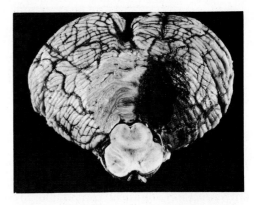

Figure 3–9B. A section through the superior cerebellar infarct shows extensive hemorrhage, consistent with an embolic infarct.

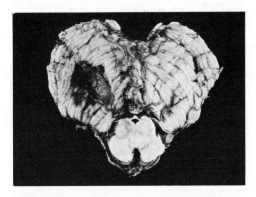

Figure 3–9C. Remote infarct on superior surface of right cerebellar hemisphere.

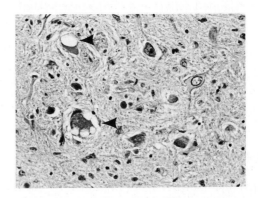

Figure 3–9D. Microscopic section of the contralateral inferior olivary nucleus demonstrating vacuolation of neurons (arrowheads) and gliosis.

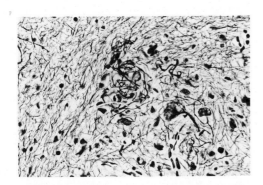

Figure 3–9E. Microscopic section, stained with the Bodian silver technique, demonstrating a dendritic glomeruloid.

3.10 Embolic Infarcts

Cardiogenic Emboli

CLINICAL

This 79-year-old woman presented with the acute onset of right sided weakness, slurred speech, and apparent confusion. Physical examination revealed right hemiparesis, decreased pain perception on the right, and aphasia. She had an irregularly irregular pulse and a holosystolic murmur. Echocardiography revealed mitral stenosis and atrial thrombi. The patient developed sepsis and died 10 days later.

PATHOLOGY

The vessels at the base of the brain formed a normal circle of Willis with only scattered, nonocclusive atheromatous plaques. Examination of the exterior of the brain showed a recent infarct on the lateral surface of the left cerebral hemisphere above the caudal end of the Sylvian fissure (Fig. 3–10A). This area was softened, faintly discolored, and contained a small number of petechial hemorrhages. Horizontal sections of the cerebral hemispheres revealed additional foci of recent infarction, predominantly in the depths of sulci, in the left superior parietal lobule (Fig. 3–10B).

COMMENT

This case is an example of cerebral infarction secondary to emboli from intracardiac thrombus. In recent years, various authors have attributed 15 to 60 percent of cerebral infarcts, especially those in the cerebral hemispheres, to embolism. Major sources of the embolic material are the heart and neck vessels. Cardiac arrhythmias, especially fibrillation, are an important predisposing factor because they tend to dislodge fragments of intracardiac thrombi associated with myocardial infarcts or valvular disease.

Embolic material may lodge in any of the intracranial vessels; however, the middle cerebral artery and its branches are the most commonly obstructed vessels. The embolic material often occludes the vessel at bifurcations. The resulting infarcts may be hemorrhagic, partially hemorrhagic or even nonhemorrhagic. The classic hemorrhagic appearance of many of these infarcts has been attributed to lysis of the embolic material followed by reperfusion of necrotic brain tissue.

Embolic infarcts are often multiple and may involve widely separated areas as seen in coronal sections from still another case with cardiogenic emboli (Figs. 3–10C and 3–10D). The infarcts also may be different ages. This can be seen in the brain from a patient who died following coronary artery bypass surgery. He had an acute hemorrhagic infarct in the distribution of the left middle cerebral artery (Fig. 3–10E) and a remote embolic infarct in the distribution of the right anterior cerebral artery (Fig. 3–10F).

REFERENCES

Cerebral Embolism Task Force (Dyken ML, Fisher M, Harrison MJG, Hart RG, Sherman DG): Cardiogenic brain embolism. Arch Neurol 1986; 43:71-84.

McCall AJ, Fletcher PJH: Pathology. In Hutchinson EC, Acheson EJ (eds): Strokes: Natural History, Pathology, and Surgical Treatment. London, Saunders, 1975, chap 3, pp 36-105.

Mohr JP, Kase CS: Cerebrovascular disease. In Rosenberg RN (ed): The Clinical Neurosciences. New York, Churchill Livingstone, 1983, vol 1, chap 3, pp I:167–I:231.

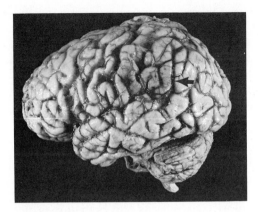

Figure 3–10A. Recent embolic infarct (arrow) on lateral surface of brain. The infarct was soft, discolored, and contained a small number of petechial hemorrhages.

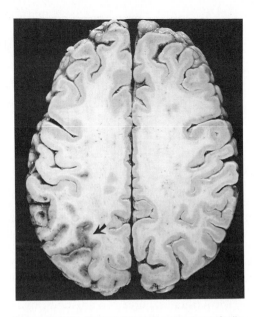

Figure 3–10B. Horizontal section showing soft, discolored cortex containing a small number of petechial hemorrhages in the infarct.

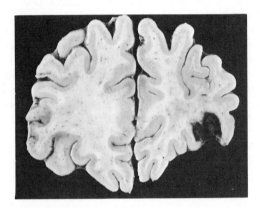

Figure 3–10C. Coronal section showing a hemorrhagic embolic infarct on the inferior surface of the right frontal lobe.

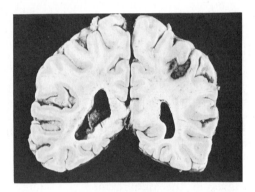

Figure 3–10D. Coronal section, at a more caudal level, showing a second hemorrhagic embolic infarct.

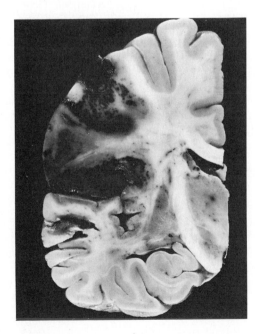

Figure 3–10E. Coronal section of the left cerebral hemisphere showing a recent hemorrhagic embolic infarct in the distribution of the left middle cerebral artery.

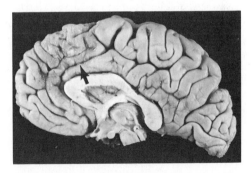

Figure 3–10F. Sagittal section showing a remote embolic infarct (arrow) in the distribution of the right anterior cerebral artery.

3.11 Embolic Infarcts

Endocarditis
Prosthetic Heart Valve

CLINICAL

This 30-year-old woman with a prosthetic aortic valve developed fever, chills, and malaise. Shortly thereafter she complained of headache, slurred speech, and impaired coordination. She was hospitalized with a diagnosis of bacterial endocarditis and septic cerebral emboli. Medications at the time of admission included prophylactic antibiotics and an oral anticoagulant. Cardiac catheterization and angiography revealed a fistula between the aorta and left atrium, a valve ring abscess, and a mycotic aneurysm of the left anterior descending coronary artery. Computerized tomograms of the head revealed hemorrhagic lesions in the brain and intraventricular blood (Fig. 3–11A). A mitral valve replacement, fistula repair, and coronary artery angioplasty were performed. The patient died 36 hours later.

PATHOLOGY

Hemorrhagic necrotic lesions were visible on the surface of the brain. The largest of these lesions was in the right inferior temporal convolution (Fig. 3–11B). Coronal sections showed hemorrhagic infarcts and hematomas in the right frontal lobe (Fig. 3–11C), posterior left frontal lobe (Fig. 3–11D), and right temporal lobe (Fig. 3–11E). The hematoma in the left frontal lobe had extended into the lateral ventricle. Microscopic examination revealed microabscesses in the cerebral cortex and white matter, in addition to the hemorrhagic infarcts and hematomas.

COMMENT

Endocarditis is a well known cause of cerebral embolic lesions. Acute bacterial endocarditis may produce small foci of cerebritis and abscesses. By contrast, subacute endocarditis rarely if ever produces abscesses but is an important cause of embolic infarcts. These may be hemorrhagic and may evolve to hematomas, especially when the patient is receiving anticoagulants at the time of embolism. The resulting hematomas tend to be more rounded than hemorrhagic infarcts and may involve central white matter as well as the cortex and subcortical white matter. The risk of secondary hemorrhage from embolic infarcts is an important consideration in the management of patients with prosthetic heart valves.

REFERENCE

Cerebral Embolism Task Force (Dyken ML, Fisher M, Harrison MJG, Hart RG, Sherman DG): Cardiogenic brain embolism. Arch Neurol 1986; 43:71-84.

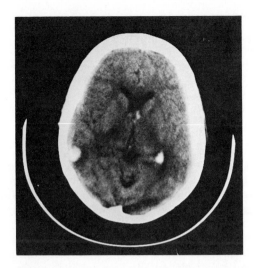

Figure 3–11A. Computerized tomogram showing multiple hemorrhagic lesions with blood extending into the ventricular system.

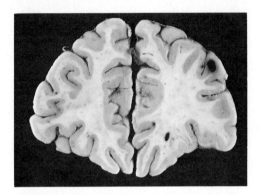

Figure 3–11C. Coronal section showing three hemorrhagic lesions in right frontal lobe.

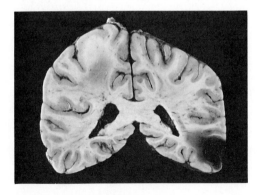

Figure 3–11E. Coronal section showing large hemorrhagic infarct that was seen from the exterior of the brain in Figure 3–11B.

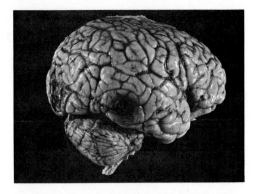

Figure 3–11B. Hemorrhagic embolic infarct in right inferior temporal gyrus.

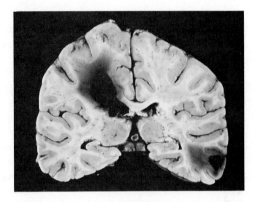

Figure 3–11D. Coronal section showing multiple hemorrhagic infarcts with hemorrhage extending into the left lateral ventricle.

3.12 Atheromatous Embolism

CLINICAL

This 72-year-old man was hospitalized with shortness of breath. He had a long history of hypertension and congestive heart failure. He died 6 days after admission.

PATHOLOGY

General autopsy revealed cardiomegaly, old and recent myocardial infarcts, and generalized severe arteriosclerosis.

The vessels at the base of the brain formed a normal circle of Willis except for relatively hypoplastic posterior communicating arteries. The vessels contained numerous atherosclerotic plaques and the distal branches of the left posterior cerebral artery had a diffuse gray white color suggesting remote occlusion. Examination of the exterior of the brain following removal of the brain stem revealed a large remote infarct in the posterior portion of the left temporal lobe and occipital lobe (Fig. 3–12A). Horizontal sections of the cerebral hemispheres showed additional infarcts in the right calcarine cortex and left caudate nucleus (Fig. 3–12B). Histological examination of the occipital lobe infarcts disclosed numerous remotely occluded small vessels that contained intraluminal acicular clefts (Fig. 3–12C).

COMMENT

The multiple remote infarcts in this brain were the result of prior embolism, although the events were not documented clinically. Emboli producing the infarcts in the posterior cerebral artery distribution can reach the brain either through the carotid or vertebrobasilar systems. In this case, the vertebrobasilar system is more likely since the posterior communicating arteries were relatively small. The acicular clefts in the occluded vessels indicated that at least a portion of the embolic material consisted of cholesterol crystals from atheromatous plaques. Embolization can result from spontaneous ulceration or iatrogenic manipulation of plaques. Atheromatous cerebral embolization is being identified with increasing frequency and is no longer regarded as an especially rare event. In some cases, transient ischemic attacks have been attributed to atheromatous emboli.

REFERENCE

Beal MF, Williams RS, Richardson EP Jr, Fisher CM: Cholesterol embolism as a cause of transient ischemic attacks and cerebral infarction. Neurology 1981; 31:860-865.

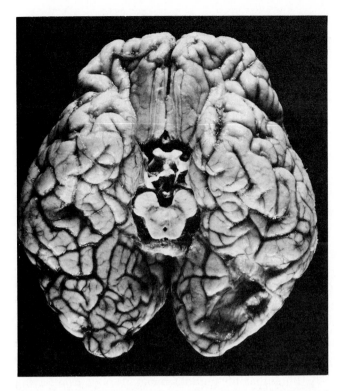

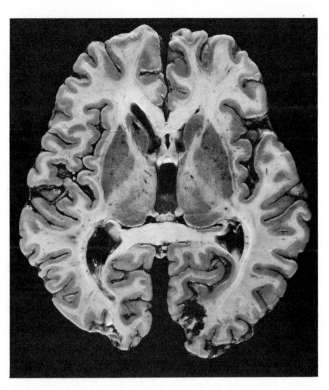

Figure 3–12A. Base of brain showing old infarcts in the left temporal and occipital lobes and a smaller infarct in the right occipital lobe.

Figure 3–12B. Horizontal section showing infarcts of left and right occipital lobe.

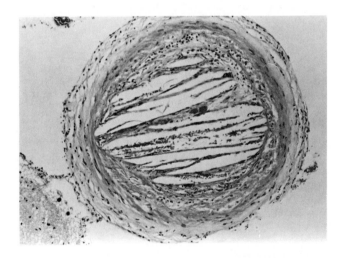

Figure 3–12C. Microscopic section showing acicular clefts, evidence of atheromatous embolism, in vessels overlying the occipital infarct.

3.13 Embolism By Nonthrombotic Material

Fat Embolism
Bone Marrow Emboli
Tumor Emboli
Mucin Emboli

CLINICAL

This 20-year-old man was involved in a motor vehicle accident. He sustained multiple fractures including the symphysis pubis, femur, and tibia. His neurological examination was normal. On the third day, he developed respiratory distress, pulmonary infiltrates, metabolic acidosis, and became comatose.

PATHOLOGY

The brain was mildly swollen but the exterior was otherwise unremarkable. Coronal sections of the cerebral hemispheres revealed petechial hemorrhages in the white matter (Fig. 3–13A). Additional petechial hemorrhages were present in the cerebellum. Histological examination disclosed foci of perivascular hemorrhage, necrosis, and inflammation (Fig. 3–13B). Some of the affected vessels contained clear intraluminal vacuoles. Frozen sections of formalin fixed brain tissue, stained with oil-red-O, showed lipid droplets within vessel lumina.

COMMENT

Fat embolism occurs very frequently following severe traumatic injuries of long bones and soft tissues. Most of the emboli are trapped in the lungs but some enter the systemic circulation through alveolar capillaries or paradoxically through a patent foramen ovale. Only a small percentage of the cases become symptomatic. The clinical manifestations generally do not appear until 2 to 3 days after injury and include respiratory distress, pulmonary infiltrates, cutaneous petechiae, alterations in mental status, and, occasionally, focal neurological deficits.

The cerebral damage has been attributed to mechanical occlusion of capillaries by the fat droplets, or, more recently, to injury by fatty acids derived from the embolized fat droplets by pulmonary lipase. As in the present case, the brain may show petechial hemorrhages that are most numerous in the cerebral white matter and cerebellum. The petechial hemorrhages in the cerebral white matter must be distinguished from

similar lesions that can result from closed head trauma.

Histologically, the white matter lesions resulting from fat embolism generally show perivascular hemorrhage and necrosis. Small purely ischemic lesions also occur but are found mainly in the gray matter. The lumina of the obstructed vessels may contain rounded clear spaces from which fat has been dissolved during tissue preparation. The diagnosis must be confirmed by performing fat stains on frozen sections.

Bone marrow embolism can also occur following skeletal trauma. As with fat embolism, most of the emboli are trapped in the lungs. Rarely, fragments of bone marrow may be seen in cerebral blood vessels (Fig. 3–13C). We have also encountered this in individuals who have had vigorous closed chest cardiac massage.

Most patients with cerebral metastases must have had embolism by neoplastic cells in order to give rise to the metastatic lesions. Figure 3–13D shows a mass of neoplastic cells in the lumen of a leptomeningeal blood vessel. Rarely, patients with various types of mucin-producing adenocarcinomas may develop hemorrhagic or nonhemorrhagic cerebral infarcts from mucin emboli. These may occur remote from or in the absence of cerebral metastases. An example of intravascular mucin adjacent to a cerebellar infarct is seen in Figure 3–13E. This rare phenomenon has been observed most often in women with mucin-producing carcinomas of the breast.

REFERENCES

Ghatak NR: Pathology of cerebral embolization caused by nonthrombotic agents. Hum Pathol 1975; 6:599-610.

Jacobson DM, Terrence CF, Reinmuth OM: The neurologic manifestations of fat embolism. Neurology 1986; 36: 847-851.

Kamenar E, Burger PC: Cerebral fat embolism: A neuropathological study of a microembolic state. Stroke 1980; 11:477–484.

Towfighi J, Simmonds MA, Davidson EA: Mucin and fat emboli in mucinous carcinomas. Arch Pathol Lab Med 1983; 107:646–649.

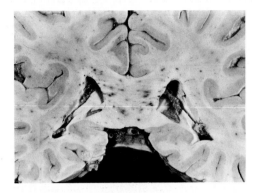

Figure 3–13A. Coronal section showing petechial hemorrhages in the splenium of the corpus callosum in a patient with fat embolism.

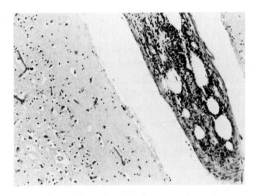

Figure 3–13C. Microscopic section showing a bone marrow embolus in a small leptomeningeal vessel.

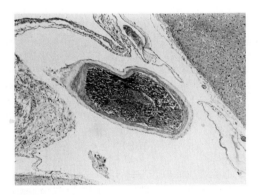

Figure 3–13E. Microscopic section, stained with mucicarmine, showing a mucin embolus adjacent to a cerebellar infarct in a woman with mucinous carcinoma of the breast.

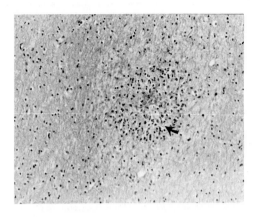

Figure 3–13B. Microscopic section showing foci of perivascular hemorrhage, necrosis and inflammation. Frozen sections demonstrated fat droplets in these lesions.

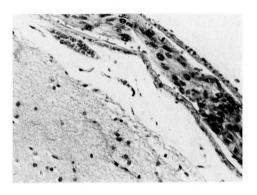

Figure 3–13D. Microscopic section showing a tumor embolus in a leptomeningeal blood vessel.

3.14   Temporal Arteritis

Giant Cell Arteritis

CLINICAL

This 89-year-old woman was in good health until she developed myalgias, headaches, scalp tenderness, and difficulty with chewing and swallowing. Shortly thereafter, she complained of double vision and awoke the next day, unable to see out of her left eye. On examination, she was found to have tortuous, firm superficial temporal arteries with prominent nodularity. An erythrocyte sedimentation rate was 105 mm/hr. A biopsy of the superficial temporal artery was performed.

PATHOLOGY

Histological examination of the biopsy specimen revealed a panarteritis (Fig. 3–14A). The vessel showed intimal proliferation with narrowing of the lumen, heavy mononuclear cell infiltrates in the media and adventitia, and fragmentation of the elastica with scattered giant cells (Fig. 3–14B).

COMMENT

Temporal arteritis is a systemic arteritis encountered predominantly in the elderly. Although any of the elastic arteries may be involved, the disease has a predilection for the superficial temporal, vertebral, ophthalmic, and posterior ciliary arteries. Common clinical manifestations include fever, headache, myalgia, tenderness of the temporal arteries, and monocular visual loss. The blindness is usually due to anterior ischemic optic neuropathy, reflecting involvement of the posterior ciliary arteries. Occasionally, visual loss may result from occlusion of the ophthalmic artery or even from occipital infarcts secondary to

vertebral artery disease. The intracranial arteries are usually spared, probably because of the paucity of elastica. About 50 percent of patients with temporal arteritis have pain and stiffness in proximal muscles, reflecting associated polymyalgia rheumatica. Laboratory studies may disclose mild anemia and leukocytosis; however, the most significant abnormality is a marked elevation of the erythrocyte sedimentation rate.

The diagnosis can often be confirmed by histological examination of a temporal artery biopsy specimen. All layers of the vessel wall are involved. The intima shows marked proliferation. This is the feature of the disease process that is mainly responsible for the vascular occlusion. The media and adventitia show infiltrates of inflammatory cells that are predominantly lymphocytes, plasma cells, and epithelioid cells. Occasional polymorphonuclear leukocytes and eosinophils also may be present. The internal elastic lamina becomes fragmented. Giant cells are an inconstant feature and are probably a response to the abnormal, fragmented elastica. The arteritis is segmental in distribution and multiple sections should be examined. Failure to demonstrate the characteristic histological features does not exclude the diagnosis.

REFERENCES

Bruetsch WL: Giant cell arteritis (Temporal arteritis, cranial arteritis, granulomatous angiitis). In Minckler J (ed): Pathology of the Nervous System. New York, McGraw-Hill, 1971, vol 2, chap 109, pp 1456-1468.

Dimant J, Grob D, Brunner NG: Ophthalmoplegia, ptosis, and miosis in temporal arteritis. Neurology 1980; 30:1054-1058.

Wilkinson IMS, Russell RWR: Arteries of the head and neck in giant cell arteritis. Arch Neurol 1972; 27:378-391.

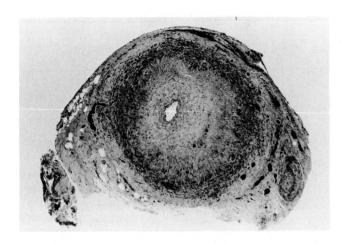

Figure 3–14A. Microscopic section of a temporal artery biopsy specimen showing panarteritis and narrowing of the lumen.

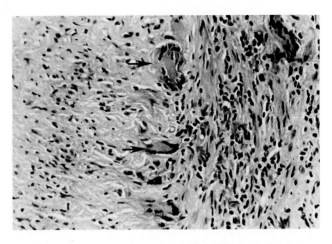

Figure 3–14B. Microscopic section at higher magnification showing multinucleated giant cells (arrow) near fragments of the disrupted elastica.

3.15 Granulomatous Angiitis

Polyarteritis
Other Vasculitides

CLINICAL

This 32-year-old man was evaluated following a seizure. The neurological examination was normal; however, a computerized tomogram of the head showed a wedge-shaped area of decreased attenuation in the right cerebral hemisphere. An angiogram demonstrated changes interpreted as vasculitis. Nine months later, the patient developed numbness and paresthesias of his left arm, right-sided headaches, and had another seizure. Repeat computerized tomography revealed a hypodense right fronto-temporal-parietal lesion with mild mass effect. Angiography again showed evidence of vasculitis. After further therapy with corticosteroids and anticonvulsants, a brain biopsy was performed.

PATHOLOGY

Histological examination of the biopsy specimen showed many of the intraparenchymal blood vessels to be surrounded by small mononuclear cells, epithelioid histiocytes and occasional giant cells (Fig. 3–15A). The intervening neural parenchyma was mildly gliotic.

COMMENT

The histological features encountered in this biopsy specimen were consistent with granulomatous angiitis. This condition is characterized by prominent histiocytic infiltrates and occasional giant cells involving predominantly the smaller intraparenchymal and meningeal blood vessels. Both arteries and veins are involved and the vasculitis is largely restricted to the central nervous system. The clinical manifestations are varied and reflect the multiple foci of vasculitis and resulting infarction. The cerebrospinal fluid often shows lymphocytic pleocytosis and elevated protein content. The etiology and pathogenesis of granulomatous angiitis are currently unknown. However, there is increasing evidence implicating the varicella zoster virus as the causative agent.

In contrast, polyarteritis nodosa is a systemic necrotizing vasculitis that typically affects small and medium sized arteries. During the active stages of the disease, the involved vessels show heavy inflammatory cell infiltrates with polymorphonuclear leukocytes and eosinophils. The vessel walls undergo fibrinoid necrosis and may become thrombosed. The healing stages are characterized by fibrosis and obliteration of the vessel lumina. Laboratory studies commonly show an elevated erythrocyte sedimentation rate, leukocytosis, and circulating immune complexes. About one third of the patients have hepatitis B antigenemia.

Patients with polyarteritis nodosa frequently have vasculitis in the vasa nervorum of peripheral nerves (Fig. 3–15B). As a result, peripheral neuropathies are commonly encountered in this disease and may even constitute the presenting complaints. By contrast, central nervous system involvement is seen in only about one third of the patients and usually occurs late in the course of the disease. The resulting lesions may appear as small infarcts (Fig. 3–15C) associated with mildly inflamed, scarred vessels (Fig. 3–15D). A vasculitis with morphologically similar lesions can be encountered in individuals who have abused amphetamines and amphetamine analogues.

Vasculitis is a prominent component of the pathological reaction to chronic infections with tuberculosis, syphilis, many fungi, and certain parasites. It also occurs in some patients with sarcoid. Recently, an acute necrotizing vasculitis has been described in a patient with ulcerative colitis (Fig. 3–15E).

REFERENCES

Blue MC, Rosenblum WI: Granulomatous angiitis of the brain with herpes zoster and varicella encephalitis. Arch Pathol Lab Med 1983; 107:126-128.

Moore PM, Cupps TR: Neurological complications of vasculitis. Ann Neurol 1983; 14:155-167.

Nelson J, Barron MM, Riggs JE, et al: Cerebral vasculitis and ulcerative colitis. Neurology 1986; 36:719-721.

Sigal LH: The neurologic presentation of vasculitis and rheumatologic syndromes. A review. Medicine 1987; 66:157-180.

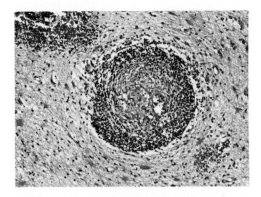

Figure 3–15A. Microscopic section showing granulomatous angiitis. The vessel lumen is surrounded by epithelioid cells and, more peripherally, lymphocytes.

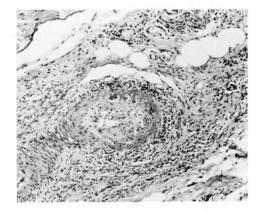

Figure 3–15B. Microscopic section of a sural nerve biopsy specimen from a patient with polyarteritis.

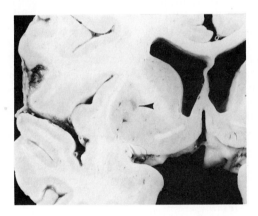

Figure 3–15C. Coronal section showing a small infarct (arrowhead) in the putamen of a patient with polyarteritis.

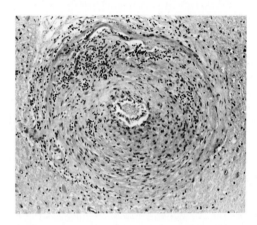

Figure 3–15D. Microscopic section showing a mildly inflamed, scarred vessel adjacent to the infarct shown in Figure 3–15C.

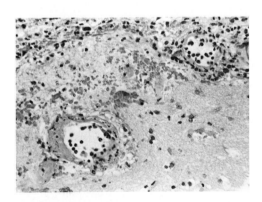

Figure 3–15E. Microscopic section showing necrotizing vasculitis in a patient with ulcerative colitis.

3.16   Lacunar Infarcts

CLINICAL

This 65-year-old man with a history of hypertension died from a myocardial infarct. No clinical neurological deficits had been documented.

PATHOLOGY

The brain was mildly swollen. The vessels at the base of the brain formed a normal circle of Willis and contained scattered atheromatous plaques. Horizontal sections of the cerebral hemispheres revealed lacunar infarcts in both caudate nuclei (Fig. 3–16A).

COMMENT

Lacunar infarcts are small cystic infarcts that result from occlusion of penetrating arteries. The infarcts generally measure 0.2 to 1.5 cm in diameter. Somewhat larger lesions are occasionally referred to as "super lacunes." Lacunar infarcts are found in the basal ganglia, internal capsules, thalami (Fig. 3–16B), and pons. These areas are perfused by vessels belonging to the lenticulostriate, thalamoperforating, and paramedian groups of arteries. The walls of the infarcts show reactive gliosis and the cavities may contain lipid- and pigment-laden macrophages. The walls of the vessels in and about the lacunar infarcts often show a waxy, eosinophilic degeneration described as lipohyalinosis (Fig. 3–16C). Vessels near some of the larger lacunar infarcts may show microatheromatous changes with intramural deposits of lipid-laden macrophages. Still other lacunar infarcts may be due to microemboli.

Lacunar infarcts are encountered predominantly in elderly individuals with hypertension and arteriosclerosis. The infarcts are frequently asymptomatic but may cause a wide variety of clinical manifestations including pure motor hemiparesis, pure sensory stroke, ataxic hemiparesis, and the dysarthria–clumsy hand syndrome.

Lacunar infarcts should be distinguished from the smooth-walled, enlarged perivascular spaces that also may be seen in the basal ganglia of older, hypertensive individuals. Fisher has designated the presence of these perivascular lesions as status cribrosus or etat crible. The literature is somewhat confusing since the same perivascular lesions have been designated as status lacunarus or etat lacunaire by some of the European authors. The clinical significance of these enlarged perivascular spaces is unclear.

REFERENCES

Fisher CM: Lacunar strokes and infarcts: A review. Neurology 1982; 32:871-876.
Miller VT: Lacunar stroke: A reassessment. Arch Neurol 1983; 40:129-134.
Mohr JP: Lacunes. In Barnett HJM, Mohr JP, Stein BM, Yatsu FM (eds): Stroke. Pathophysiology, Diagnosis, and Management. New York, Churchill Livingstone, 1986, vol 1, chap 26, pp 475-496.

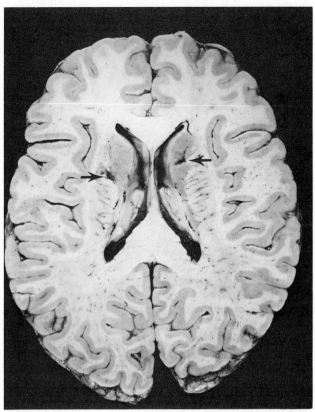

Figure 3–16A. Horizontal section showing bilateral lacunar infarcts (arrows) in the caudate nuclei.

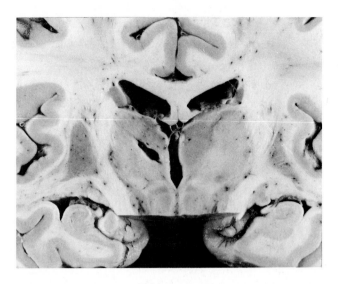

Figure 3–16B. Coronal section showing a lacunar infarct in the left thalamus.

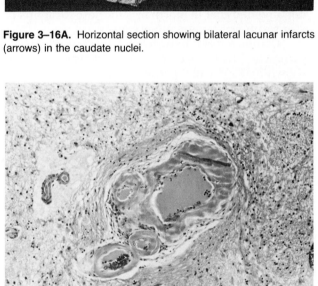

Figure 3–16C. Microscopic section showing lipohyalinosis of a small arteriole adjacent to a lacunar infarct.

3.17 Ganglionic Hemorrhage

Hypertensive Hemorrhage

CLINICAL

This 57-year-old woman with a history of hypertension, developed a headache and nausea, and subsequently collapsed. A computerized tomogram showed a large intraparenchymal hemorrhage involving the right basal ganglia with extension into the ventricular system (Fig. 3–17A). She died 1 day later.

PATHOLOGY

There was a small amount of blood in the subarachnoid space at the base of the brain and about the outlet foramina of the fourth ventricle. All gyri were swollen with correspondingly narrowed sulci. The right cingulate gyrus was displaced to the left. Both unci were grooved, the right more deeply than the left. Horizontal sections of the cerebral hemispheres, viewed from below upward, revealed a massive lateral ganglionic hemorrhage with dissection into the ventricular system (Fig. 3–17B). A thin rim of white matter dorsal and lateral to the hematoma was softened and contained petechial hemorrhages. Microscopic examination of the left basal ganglia and the pons revealed scattered arterioles that showed lipohyalinosis and/or aneurysmal dilatations (Fig. 3–17C).

COMMENT

Hemorrhages attributed to hypertension arise most often in the lateral portions of the basal ganglia. The hemorrhage often extends from the site of origin into the surrounding brain by dissecting along fiber tracts in the white matter. In doing so, the hematoma acts as a space-occupying mass and displaces surrounding structures. However, even when large, the hematoma usually destroys less neural parenchyma than a comparable sized infarct. In addition, the large hemorrhages often rupture into the ventricular system. Petechial hemorrhages are often encountered in the band of necrotic tissue surrounding the periphery of the hematoma. These lesions, so-called Staemmler's

marginal hemorrhages, are a secondary process and may be seen in association with hemorrhages from other causes. Vessels within the petechial hemorrhages may have necrotic walls (Fig. 3–17D).

The pathogenesis of hypertensive hemorrhages is controversial. Some authors attribute the hemorrhages to lipohyalinosis of penetrating arterioles in the basal ganglia, thalami, internal capsules, and pons. This is the same vascular alteration that has been implicated in the development of many lacunar infarcts. Other authors have attributed hypertensive hemorrhages to rupture of Charcot–Bouchard aneurysms, small aneurysmal dilatations that form on the penetrating arterioles with or without associated lipohyalinosis. Still others have concluded that the intraparenchymal hemorrhages are preceded by small infarcts. Finally, it must be emphasized that not all hemorrhages in the basal ganglia, thalami, internal capsules, and pons are necessarily due to hypertension. It has been well documented that hemorrhages in these locations can also result from many other causes.

Computerized tomography is very effective in demonstrating intracerebral hemorrhages. It has been shown that some of the lesions initially interpreted as infarcts are actually hemorrhages. Small hemorrhages, even with intraventricular extension, may have a favorable outcome.

REFERENCES

Drayer BP: Disease of the cerebral vascular system. In Rosenberg RN (ed): The Clinical Neurosciences. New York, Churchill Livingstone, 1983, vol 4, chap 3, pp IV:247–IV:360.

Fisher CM: Pathological observations in hypertensive cerebral hemorrhage. J Neuropathol Exp Neurol 1971; 30:536-550.

McCormick WF, Rosenfield DB: Massive brain hemorrhage: A review of 144 cases and an examination of their causes. Stroke 1973; 4:946-954.

Mohr JP, Kase CS: Cerebrovascular disease. In Rosenberg RN (ed): The Clinical Neurosciences. New York, Churchill Livingstone, 1983, vol 1, chap 3, pp I:167–I:231.

Zulch KJ: Hemorrhage, thrombosis, embolism. In Minckler J (ed): Pathology of the Nervous System. New York, McGraw-Hill, 1971, vol 2, chap 113, pp 1499-1536.

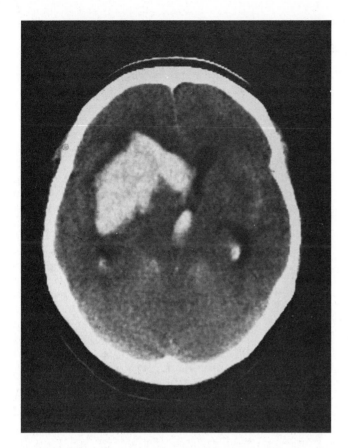

Figure 3–17A. Computerized tomogram showing a lateral ganglionic hemorrhage with extension into the ventricular system.

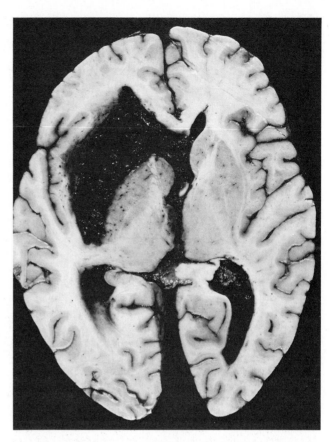

Figure 3–17B. Horizontal section showing a hypertensive lateral ganglionic hemorrhage with extension into the ventricular system.

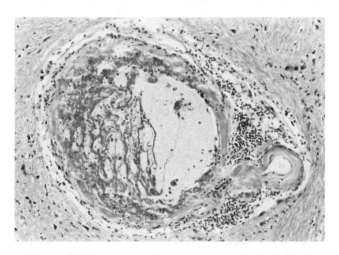

Figure 3–17C. Microscopic section showing lipohyalinosis and aneurysmal dilatation of a small arteriole.

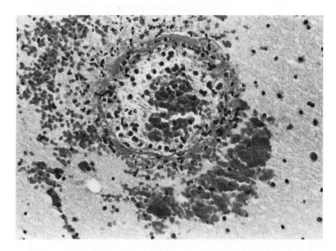

Figure 3–17D. Microscopic section showing necrosis of small vessels within the petechial hemorrhages at the margin of the hematoma.

3.18   Thalamic Hemorrhage

CLINICAL

This 63-year-old woman with a long history of hypertension had the acute onset of headache and right hemiparesis. Initially she was alert and communicative but soon became unresponsive and required intubation. A computerized tomogram revealed a large left thalamic hemorrhage. She died 3 weeks later.

PATHOLOGY

Horizontal sections of the cerebral hemispheres revealed a large hematoma involving predominantly the left thalamus (Fig. 3–18A). The hematoma had extended into the posterior limb of the left internal capsule and had dissected into the mesencephalon. The center of the hematoma had a reddish brown color while the periphery was reddish green.

COMMENT

The thalamus is one of the sites of predilection for hemorrhages attributed to hypertension. Another example is shown in Figure 3–18B. The thalamus was formerly thought to be the location of about 15 percent of hypertensive hemorrhages. Recent reports, based on computerized tomography, have suggested that the percentage in this location is even higher. Clinically, these patients often have small nonreactive pupils. They may also have restriction of upward gaze and downward ocular deviation when the hematoma extends into the mesencephalon.

Intracerebral hematomas undergo progressive changes with the passage of time. Within a few days, the hemorrhage elicits a prominent polymorphonuclear leukocyte response at its periphery. As the blood breaks down, the hematoma changes color. Macrophages invading the margins of the hematoma become laden with lipids and pigment granules. These pigments include hemosiderin, which is brown and contains iron, and hematoidin, which is yellow and derived from the non-heme portion of the hemoglobin. The surrounding neural parenchyma becomes gliotic but shows minimal fibrosis. If the patient survives, the hematoma is eventually resorbed and only a cavity with brown-stained walls remains.

REFERENCE

Weisberg LA: Thalamic hemorrhage: Clinical–CT correlations. Neurology 1986; 36:1382-1386.

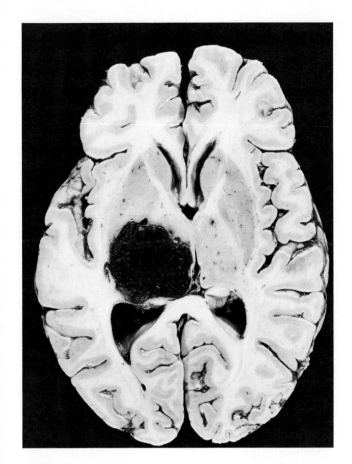

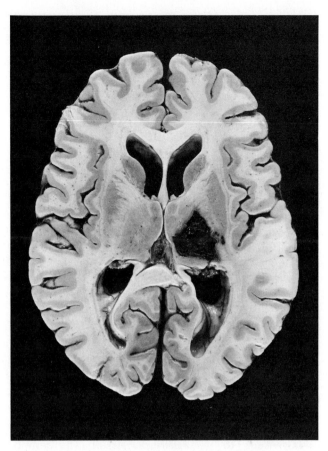

Figure 3–18A. Horizontal section showing a hypertensive hemorrhage in the left thalamus.

Figure 3–18B. Horizontal section showing a hypertensive hemorrhage in the right thalamus.

3.19   Pontine Hemorrhage

CLINICAL

This 70-year-old man, with a long history of hypertension, suddenly collapsed and developed respiratory difficulties. On examination, he was noted to be quadriplegic. His pupils were pinpoint but reactive to light. He died 1 day later.

PATHOLOGY

The vessels at the base of the brain showed severe atherosclerotic changes. The ventral surface of the pons was swollen and focally hemorrhagic (Fig. 3–19A). Sagittal section of the brain disclosed a large hematoma in the basis pontis (Fig. 3–19B).

COMMENT

The pons is the site of only 5 to 15 percent of hemorrhages attributed to hypertension. The hemorrhages usually arise from the midportion of the pons and involve the basis pontis and pontine tegmentum bilaterally. They often extend rostrally into the mesencephalon and occasionally extend caudally into the medulla. They are typically accompanied by quadriplegia, small but reactive pupils, and severe respiratory difficulties. Most pontine hemorrhages are rapidly lethal. Figure 3–19C is from a 47-year-old man with hypertension who was found dead in bed. In this case, the hemorrhage had ruptured into the fourth ventricle, filled the aqueduct and third ventricle, and entered the subarachnoid space through the outlet foramina of the fourth ventricle. Note the severe arteriosclerosis involving even distal portions of the cerebral arteries. Occasionally, computerized tomography has permitted identification of small unilateral pontine hemorrhages in patients who have survived.

REFERENCE

Kase CS, Caplan LR: Hemorrhage affecting the brain stem and cerebellum. In Barnett HJM, Mohr JP, Stein BM, Yatsu FM (eds): Stroke. Pathophysiology, Diagnosis, and Management. New York, Churchill Livingstone, 1986, vol 1, chap 30, pp 621-641.

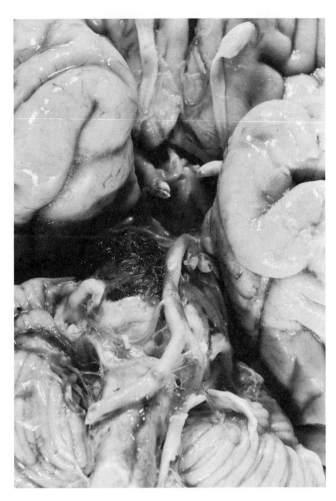

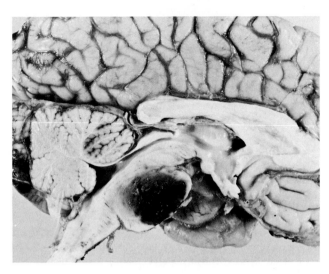

Figure 3–19B. Sagittal section of brain showing a pontine hemorrhage.

Figure 3–19A. Base of brain showing focal hemorrhage in left basis pontis. Note also, severe arteriosclerosis of basilar and vertebral arteries.

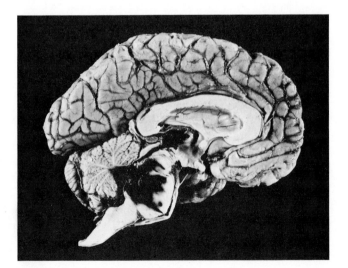

Figure 3–19C. Sagittal section of brain showing a pontine hemorrhage with rupture into the fourth ventricle. Note also the severe arteriosclerosis of basilar and anterior cerebral arteries.

3.20   Cerebellar Hemorrhage

CLINICAL

This 70-year-old man developed headache and nausea after climbing a flight of stairs. He subsequently became unresponsive. When seen in an emergency room the next day, he was comatose and had decerebrate posturing. A computerized tomogram showed a right cerebellar hemorrhage with obstructive hydrocephalus. A ventriculostomy was performed but the patient expired the following day.

PATHOLOGY

The vessels at the base of the brain contained numerous atherosclerotic plaques. The right cerebellar hemisphere was larger than the left and the cerebellar tonsils were displaced caudally. They were closely approximated in the midline and deeply grooved by the foramen magnum (Fig. 3–20A). Coronal sections of the cerebral hemispheres disclosed mildly enlarged ventricles. Sections of the cerebellum disclosed a large intraparenchymal hematoma arising from the central white matter of the right cerebellar hemisphere (Fig. 3–20B). The fourth ventricle and underlying brain stem were compressed.

COMMENT

The cerebellum is variously reported to be the site of 5 to 15 percent of hemorrhages attributed to hypertension. The hemorrhages generally arise from deep in the hemispheres near the central nuclei. The patients often experience an abrupt onset of nausea and vomiting, headache and ataxia. Loss of consciousness is less commonly an initial feature as compared with pontine hemorrhages. Early diagnosis is important since the outcome is variable and surgical intervention is indicated for some of these individuals. Death in patients with cerebellar hematomas is often the result of hydrocephalus and medullary compression.

REFERENCES

Melamed N, Satya-Murti S: Cerebellar hemorrhage: A review and reappraisal of benign cases. Arch Neurol 1984; 41:425-428.

Ott KH, Kase CS, Ojemann RG, Mohr JP: Cerebellar hemorrhage: Diagnosis and treatment. Arch Neurol 1974; 31:160-167.

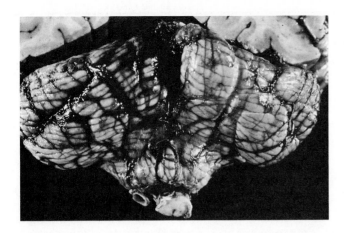

Figure 3–20A. Enlargement of the right cerebellar hemisphere and caudal displacement of the cerebellar tonsils due to a cerebellar hemorrhage.

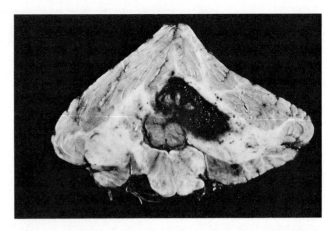

Figure 3–20B. Section of cerebellum and brain stem showing cerebellar hematoma.

3.21 Lobar Hemorrhage

Metastatic Carcinoma
Leukemia
Thrombocytopaenia

CLINICAL

This 73-year-old man was admitted to the hospital with a 2-week history of back pain. He was found to have a pulmonary infiltrate in the posterior segment of the left upper lobe. Shortly after admission, the patient became obtunded and developed a left hemiparesis. A computerized tomogram revealed a hematoma in the right frontal lobe. The patient died a few days later.

PATHOLOGY

The brain was mildly asymmetrical due to fullness of the right cerebral hemisphere. There was a small amount of blood in the subarachnoid space over the lateral surface of the left hemisphere and in the interhemispheric fissure. Horizontal sections of the cerebral hemispheres revealed a large hematoma in the white matter of the right hemisphere (Fig. 3–21A) and small hemorrhagic and nonhemorrhagic metastases in the left hemisphere and cerebellum.

COMMENT

Although some lobar hemorrhages can be attributed to hypertension, these hemorrhages are more likely to be the result of other disease processes, including neoplasms. Among the primary neoplasms, oligo-dendrogliomas, glioblastomas, and hemangioblast-omas of the cerebellum are well known for producing hemorrhages. Metastatic lesions may also become hemorrhagic and even may present clinically as an acute cerebrovascular accident. Among metastases, carcinoma of the lung, melanoma, choriocarcinoma, and Kaposi's sarcoma are especially prone to be hemorrhagic.

In the past, many patients dying with leukemia had multiple intracerebral hemorrhages (Fig. 3–21B). These were variously attributed to obstruction of blood vessels by the large numbers of leukemic cells or the associated thrombocytopaenia. Figure 3–21C illustrates an intraparenchymal hemorrhage secondary to thrombocytopaenia in a young man with aplastic anemia. Other important causes of massive lobar hemorrhage include various abnormal coagulation states, venous thrombosis, ruptured vascular malformations, and ruptured saccular aneurysms.

REFERENCES

Kase CS, Williams JP, Wyatt DA, Mohr JP: Lobar intracerebral hematomas: Clinical and CT analysis of 22 cases. Neurology 1982; 32:1146-1150.

Ropper AH, Davis KR: Lobar cerebral hemorrhages: Acute clinical syndromes in 26 cases. Ann Neurol 1980; 8:141-147.

Schwartzman RJ, Hill JB: Neurologic complications of disseminated intravascular coagulation. Neurology 1982; 32:791-797.

Toffol GJ, Biller J, Adams HA Jr: Nontraumatic intracerebral hemorrhage in young adults. Arch Neurol 1987; 44:483-485.

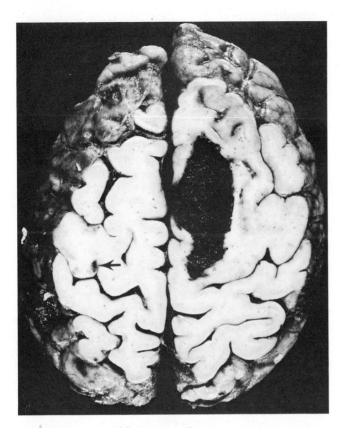

Figure 3–21A. Horizontal section showing a lobar hemorrhage secondary to metastatic carcinoma from the lung. Note also the small hemorrhagic metastasis in the left hemisphere (arrow).

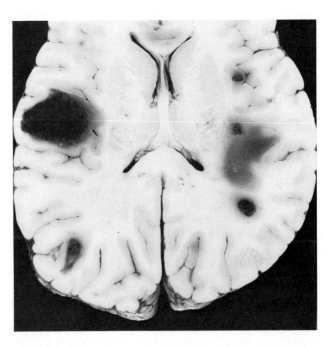

Figure 3–21B. Horizontal section showing multiple lobar hemorrhages secondary to leukemia.

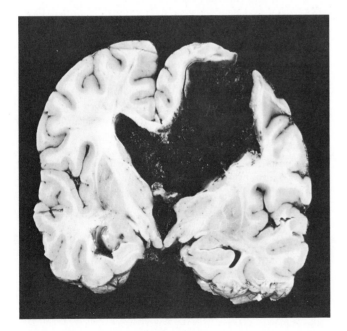

Figure 3–21C. Coronal section showing a massive lobar hemorrhage with rupture into the ventricular system in a man with thrombocytopenia secondary to aplastic anemia.

3.22 Amyloid Angiopathy

CLINICAL

This 73-year-old man was brought to the emergency room in cardiopulmonary arrest. Resuscitative measures were unsuccessful. The patient had a long history of cardiac disease but no clinically documented cerebrovascular accidents.

PATHOLOGY

Death was attributed to a recent posterior myocardial infarct. The patient had advanced systemic arteriosclerosis but the vessels at the base of the brain contained only scattered atheromatous plaques. Coronal sections of the cerebral hemispheres revealed a thin, slit-like cavity in the convolutional white matter underlying the left superior frontal gyrus (Fig. 3–22A). The walls of this lesion were stained faintly brown. Histological examination of the brain showed numerous intracortical (Fig. 3–22B) and occasional leptomeningeal blood vessels that had thickened, hyalinized walls. The abnormal vessels were stained deep orange with Congo red (Fig. 3–22C) and showed a yellow-green birefringence color when viewed with polarized light (Fig. 3–22D). Some of the smaller vessels showed "brush-like" perivascular deposits of amyloid that extended into the surrounding neural parenchyma. The brain also contained scattered senile plaques and occasional neurofibrillary tangles.

COMMENT

Brains of patients with Alzheimer's disease and occasionally from nondemented elderly individuals contain amyloid in the cores of senile (neuritic) plaques and in the walls of blood vessels. In some brains, the vascular deposits are especially prominent and have been designated as congophilic angiopathy or cerebral amyloid angiopathy. The amyloid deposition is found in small leptomeningeal and intraparenchymal blood vessels throughout the brain but tends to be most severe in the occipital and parietal lobes. The distinctive staining properties of amyloid are the result of the structure of the amyloid fibrils rather than their composition. There are several different types of amyloid, each derived from different proteins. The composition and derivation of cerebral amyloid is unsettled.

Cerebral amyloid angiopathy occurs independently of primary or secondary systemic amyloidosis. It becomes more prevalent with increasing age and is a common accompaniment of Alzheimer's disease. In recent years, cerebral amyloid angiopathy has been implicated as an important cause of intracerebral hemorrhage in the elderly. The hemorrhages attributed to this condition are usually lobar and may be multiple. They may be in unusual locations such as the frontal lobe (as in the present case) or in the occipital lobe, as seen in Figure 3–22E. In contrast to hypertension, hemorrhages associated with cerebral amyloid angiopathy rarely involve the basal ganglia, brain stem, or cerebellum. The mechanisms by which the cerebral amyloid angiopathy precipitate intraparenchymal bleeding are unclear.

REFERENCES

Cosgrove GR, Leblanc R, Meagher-Villemure K, Ethier R: Cerebral amyloid angiopathy. Neurology 1985; 35:625-631.

Drury I, Whisnant JP, Garraway WM: Primary intracerebral hemorrhage: Impact of CT on incidence. Neurology 1984; 34:653-657.

Gilles C, Brucher JM, Khoubesserian P, Vanderhaeghen JJ: Cerebral amyloid angiopathy as a cause of multiple intracerebral hemorrhages. Neurology 1984; 34:730-735.

Mandybur TI: Cerebral amyloid angiopathy: The vascular pathology and complications. J Neuropathol Exp Neurol 1986; 45:79-90.

Vinters HV: Cerebral amyloid angiopathy: A critical review. Stroke 1987; 18:311-324.

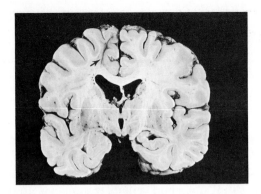

Figure 3–22A. Coronal section showing a slit-like hematoma cavity in the white matter of the left superior frontal gyrus (arrow). Note the brown, hemosiderin-stained walls.

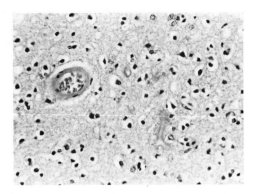

Figure 3–22B. Microscopic section showing thickened, hyalinized intracortical blood vessels.

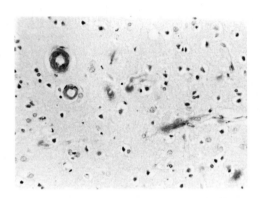

Figure 3–22C. Microscopic section, stained with Congo red, showing amyloid deposition in the vessel walls.

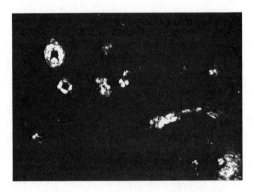

Figure 3–22D. Identification of the amyloid was further established by the yellow-green birefringence color when viewed with polarized light.

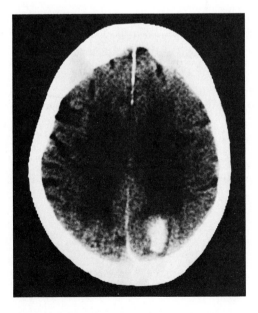

Figure 3–22E. Computerized tomogram showing an occipital hemorrhage due to amyloid angiopathy.

3.23 Venous Thrombosis

Congenital Heart Disease

CLINICAL

This female infant was evaluated at 13 days of age because of tachypnea, cyanosis, and difficulty feeding. She was found to have a heart murmur and an enlarged right ventricle. Cardiac catheterization confirmed a diagnosis of Ebstein's anomaly. The child had multiple hospitalizations for respiratory distress and pneumonia and died at 7 months of age.

PATHOLOGY

At the time of autopsy, the sagittal sinus was noted to contain thrombus. The brain was swollen but the cerebral hemispheres were symmetrical. Blood was present in the subarachnoid space over the dorsal surface of the cerebral hemispheres but not at the base of the brain. The cortical veins were markedly congested and some were thrombosed. Multiple coronal sections of the cerebral hemispheres revealed extensive areas of hemorrhagic necrosis involving the cortex and convolutional white matter (Figs. 3–23A and 3–23B). In addition, there were small foci of hemorrhagic necrosis in the left putamen and caudate nucleus.

COMMENT

There are many conditions that predispose individuals to dural sinus and venous thrombosis. In the past, infants with this condition often had dehydration from vomiting and diarrhea. In this case, congenital heart disease and dehydration associated with a febrile illness were the major contributory factors. Either the deep or superficial venous system alone, or both, may be involved. Among the dural sinuses, the superior sagittal and lateral sinuses are the most commonly occluded. Cortical infarcts are more extensive when there is concomitant thrombosis of the cortical veins. The resulting infarcts may be unilateral or bilateral. However, even when bilateral, they may be markedly asymmetrical. The infarcts are typically hemorrhagic and quite irregular in shape. Thrombosis of the vein of Galen and internal cerebral veins produces necrosis in the basal ganglia, thalamus, and central white matter. Cortical vein thrombosis is often accompanied by subarachnoid hemorrhage while deep venous thrombosis often produces intraventricular hemorrhage.

REFERENCE

Friede RL: Developmental Neuropathology. New York, Springer Verlag, 1975, pp 135-144.

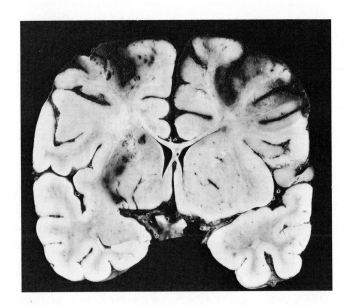

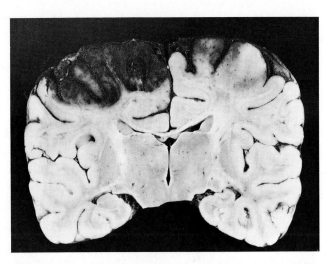

Figure 3–23B. Coronal section, at a more caudal level, showing bilateral but asymmetrical hemorrhagic infarcts.

Figure 3–23A. Coronal section showing bilateral hemorrhagic infarcts due to sagittal sinus and cortical vein thrombosis. Note also the small foci of hemorrhagic necrosis in the left putamen and caudate nucleus.

3.24 Venous Thrombosis

Meningitis
Trauma
Associated with Malignancy

CLINICAL

This 60-year-old man was hospitalized with lethargy, headaches, and neck pain. A lumbar puncture was performed and the cerebrospinal fluid was consistent with pneumococcal meningitis. He was treated with antibiotics but developed focal seizures 10 days later. A computerized tomogram showed a right fronto-parietal mass lesion and an angiogram demonstrated thrombosis of the sagittal sinus. The patient died 1 month later from aspiration pneumonia.

PATHOLOGY

The sagittal and sigmoid sinuses were thrombosed. On transverse sections, the thrombus had a mottled gray-brown color (Fig. 3–24A). The cerebral hemispheres were symmetrical. The leptomeninges were focally opacified and hemorrhagic over the posterior portion of the frontal lobe and the parietal lobe on the right. Cortical veins in this area were thrombosed. Horizontal sections of the cerebral hemispheres revealed a large area of partially hemorrhagic encephalomalacia in the right parietal lobe and another smaller area of focally hemorrhagic encephalomalacia in the left frontal lobe (Fig. 3–24B).

COMMENT

Meningitis is one of the many diseases that predispose patients to dural sinus and cortical vein thrombosis. Seizures are a common manifestation and probably reflected the onset of the process in this patient. Although computerized tomography showed a mass lesion, the definitive diagnosis was derived from angiography.

Head trauma, even relatively mild trauma, is another widely recognized antecedent event. Figures 3–24C and 3–24D show cortical vein thrombosis and venous infarction in a young man who developed right sided weakness and multiple seizures following a fall. He had thrombosed cortical veins and a hemorrhagic infarct in the left frontal region.

Dural sinus and cortical vein thrombosis may be encountered in patients with various neoplasms even when the neoplasm does not directly involve the brain. Figure 3–24E shows hemorrhagic infarcts in a patient with carcinoma of the lung and a superior vena cava syndrome, but no cerebral metastases. Note the overlying distended, thrombosed cortical veins. Formerly, childbirth was another important predisposing condition.

REFERENCES

Bousser M-G, Chiras J, Bories J, Castaigne P: Cerebral venous thrombosis—A review of 38 cases. Stroke 1985; 16:199-213.

Sigsbee B, Deck MDF, Posner JB: Nonmetastatic superior sagittal sinus thrombosis complicating systemic cancer. Neurology 1979; 29:139-146.

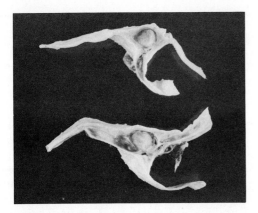

Figure 3–24A. Transverse sections of the sagittal sinus showing mottled intralumenal thrombus.

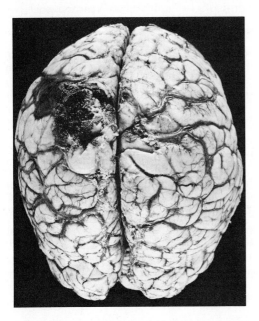

Figure 3–24C. Dorsal surface of the brain showing cortical vein thrombosis and a venous infarct in a man who suffered a fall.

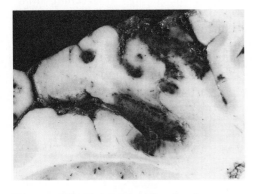

Figure 3–24E. Horizontal section showing venous thrombosis and hemorrhagic infarction in a man with carcinoma of the lung and superior vena cava syndrome.

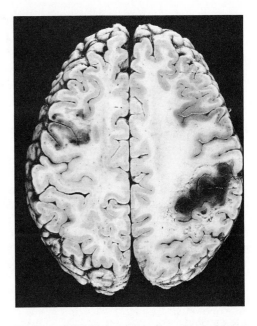

Figure 3–24B. Horizontal section showing large hemorrhagic infarct in right parietal lobe and smaller hemorrhagic infarct in the left frontal lobe due to venous thrombosis. Note the distended cortical veins.

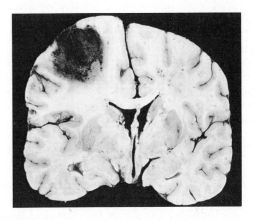

Figure 3–24D. Coronal section showing the hemorrhagic infarct due to venous thrombosis.

3.25 Arteriovenous Malformation

CLINICAL

This 73-year-old woman complained of a headache and called the emergency medical services. When they arrived, the patient was lethargic and unable to communicate. She was taken to a hospital, where she lapsed into coma with fixed and dilated pupils. A computerized tomogram revealed a massive left intracerebral hematoma. The patient died the following day. Further history revealed that she had had focal seizures for the past 40 years.

PATHOLOGY

Examination of the brain revealed numerous abnormal blood vessels on the dorsolateral aspect of the left frontal lobe (Fig. 3–25A). The meninges overlying these vessels were mildly thickened and opacified. Coronal sections through this area revealed a wedge-shaped collection of abnormal vascular channels (Fig. 3–25B). There was a large intracerebral hematoma ventromedial to the vascular malformation. Histological examination demonstrated the lesion to be an arteriovenous vascular malformation composed of congeries of thick-walled arteries, veins, and arterialized veins (Fig. 3–25C). Gliotic neural parenchyma was interposed between some of the anomalous vascular channels.

COMMENT

Vascular malformations are collections of aberrant vascular channels. They can be classified into four categories — arteriovenous malformations, cavernous angiomas, venous angiomas, and telangiectases. Vascular malformations of one type or another are encountered in about 5 percent of brains examined at autopsy. The venous angiomas and telangiectases are the more common types but are usually asymptomatic. Arteriovenous malformations and cavernous angiomas are less common but are more likely to produce symptoms in the form of headaches, seizures, focal neurological deficits, or hemorrhage.

The arteriovenous malformations comprise about 12 percent of cerebral vascular malformations encountered at autopsy but are more heavily represented in clinically ascertained series. They occur in all portions of the brain without predilection for specific locations. They are also found in the spinal cord. Large arteriovenous malformations in the cerebral hemispheres are often cone shaped, with their base at the pial surface. As in the present case, they are characterized by an admixture of arteries, veins, and arterialized veins. The walls of the component vessels vary in thickness and the lumina are often irregular. The interposed neural parenchyma is usually gliotic. Occasionally, some of the vascular channels undergo thrombosis. When this occurs, the occluded vessels may be surrounded by inflammatory cells. Some of the vessels and surrounding neural tissue may become mineralized. Focal deposits of lipid- and hemosiderin-laden macrophages, from prior bleeding, are often encountered, even when there is no previous history of hemorrhage. Massive intraparenchymal hemorrhages are the most devastating complications of these lesions. The hemorrhages may extend into the subarachnoid space or ventricular system. The initial hemorrhages often occur during late adolescence or early adult life and may recur subsequently. The circumstances that precipitate bleeding from these lesions are unclear.

REFERENCES

Graf CJ, Perret GE, Torner JC: Bleeding from cerebral arteriovenous malformations as part of their natural history. J Neurosurg 1983; 58:331-337.

McCormick WF: Vascular diseases. In Rosenberg RN (ed): The Clinical Neurosciences. New York, Churchill Livingstone, 1983, vol 3, chap 2, pp III:35–III:83.

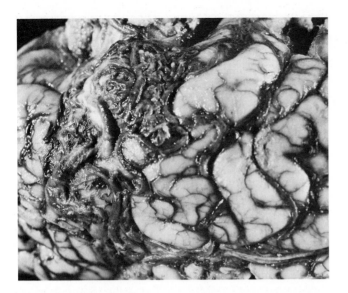

Figure 3–25A. Arteriovenous malformation on the dorsolateral aspect of the left frontal lobe.

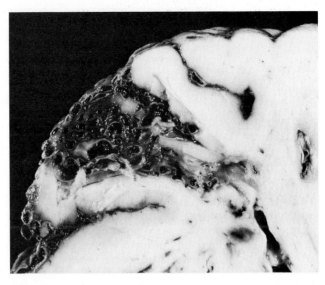

Figure 3–25B. Coronal section showing the arteriovenous malformation.

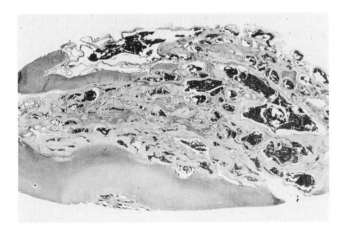

Figure 3–25C. Macrosection of the arteriovenous malformation showing the admixture of thick-walled arteries, veins, and arterialized veins.

3.26 Arteriovenous Malformation

Delayed Hemorrhage Following Proton-Beam Radiation

CLINICAL

This 44-year-old man had a long history of alcoholism and seizures. An orbital bruit was detected during an examination following a brief episode of unconsciousness and headache. Computerized tomography and arteriography disclosed a large left posterior temporal-parietal arteriovenous malformation (Fig. 3–26A). The patient died from an intracranial hemorrhage approximately 1 month following Bragg-peak proton-beam radiation.

PATHOLOGY

There was an abundant amount of fresh blood in the subarachnoid space at the base of the brain and on the lateral aspect of the left cerebral hemisphere (Fig. 3–26B). The leptomeninges over the left posterior temporal and parietal lobes were focally thickened and covered a congeries of abnormal, tortuous blood vessels. Coronal sections revealed a large arteriovenous vascular malformation (Fig. 3–26C). The white matter immediately surrounding the left occipital horn was focally softened and a small amount of blood was present within the ventricular system.

COMMENT

The risk of hemorrhage from arteriovenous vascular malformations has been variously reported to be between 1 and 3 percent per year. Some authors regard the risk of hemorrhage to be greater in individuals with small arteriovenous malformations than in individuals with large malformations. Although surgery remains the mainstay of definitive therapy, alternative regimens have included embolization and proton beam irradiation.

REFERENCES

Aminoff MJ: Treatment of unruptured cerebral arteriovenous malformations. Neurology 1987; 37:815-819.

Heros RC, Tu Y-K: Is surgical therapy needed for unruptured arteriovenous malformations? Neurology 1987; 37:279-286.

Kjellberg RN, Hanamura T, Davis KR, et al: Bragg-peak proton - beam therapy for arteriovenous malformations of the brain. N Engl J Med 1983; 309:269-274.

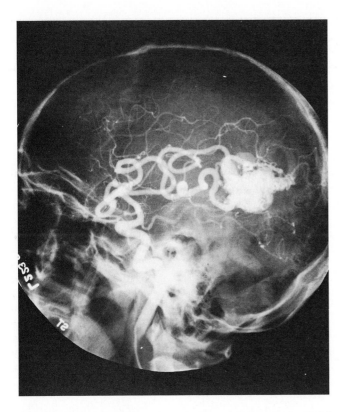

Figure 3–26A. Angiogram showing large left temporal–parietal arteriovenous malformation.

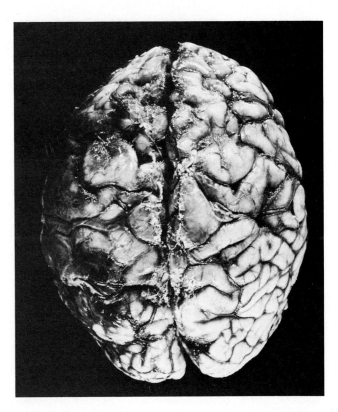

Figure 3–26B. Dorsal view of brain showing subarachnoid blood on the left cerebral hemisphere.

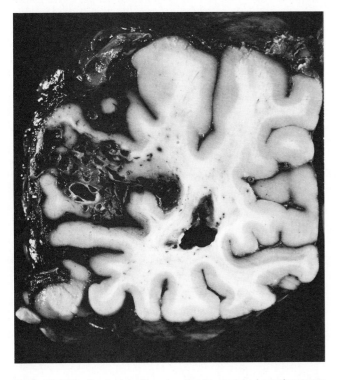

Figure 3–26C. Coronal section showing the ruptured arteriovenous malformation.

3.27 Vein of Galen Aneurysm

CLINICAL

This female infant was the product of a normal gestation and delivery. She was noted to be in congestive heart failure and on examination had a systolic murmur that radiated to the right axilla. An echocardiogram and cardiac catheterization revealed an atrial septal defect, right ventricular dilatation, and pulmonary hypertension. A computerized tomogram of the head disclosed an arteriovenous malformation and arteriography demonstrated a vein of Galen aneurysm. The child died during surgery.

PATHOLOGY

The brain was abnormally small and the right cerebral hemisphere was more atrophic than the left (Fig. 3–27A). Many of the gyri were severely shrunken (ulegyric) and abnormally firm. The vein of Galen was markedly dilated (Figs. 3–27B and 3–27C) and in continuity with abnormally enlarged dural sinuses. Histological examination of sections from the medial aspects of the cerebral hemispheres revealed numerous abnormal thick walled vessels on the pial surface and within the underlying neural parenchyma. The remaining cortex and white matter showed widespread partially cystic encephalomalacia, gliosis, and foci of mineralization.

COMMENT

The aneurysmal dilatation of the vein of Galen results from the abnormal shunting of arterial blood through an arteriovenous malformation or arteriovenous fistula into the normally low pressure Galenic system. The clinical manifestations vary with the age of the patient. Neonates usually display congestive heart failure from the abnormal shunting of blood. Older infants may present with seizures or hydrocephalus from compression of the aqueduct by the enlarged vein of Galen and increased venous pressure. Older children and adults may have headaches, mental retardation, and evidence of intracranial bleeding. Other neurological deficits can be attributed to the cerebral ischemia (the "steal" phenomena) that results from the abnormal perfusion of the neural parenchyma.

REFERENCES

Hoffman HJ, Chuang S, Hendrick EB, Humphreys RP: Aneurysms of the vein of Galen. J Neurosurg 1982; 57:316-322.

Montoya G, Dohn DF, Mercer RD: Arteriovenous malformation of the vein of Galen as a cause of heart failure and hydrocephalus in infants. Neurology 1971; 21:1054-1058.

Stehbens WE: Pathology of the Cerebral Blood Vessels. St. Louis, Mosby, 1972, pp 493-495.

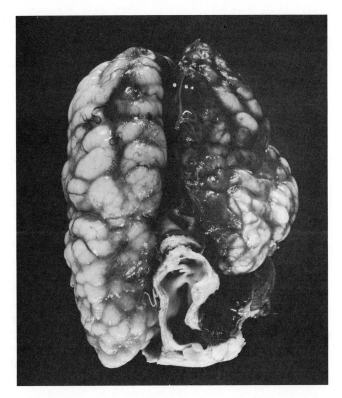

Figure 3–27A. Dorsal surface of a brain with a vein of Galen aneurysm. Note the cerebral atrophy, ulegyria, and enlargement of torcula and sigmoid sinuses.

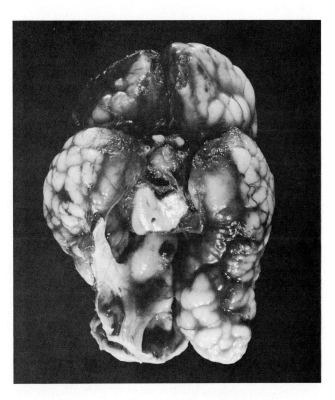

Figure 3–27B. Ventral surface of the brain with brain stem and cerebellum removed. Note the enlargement of the vein of Galen.

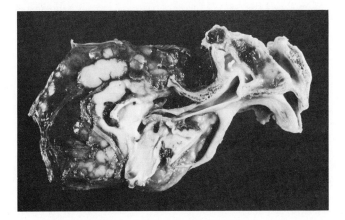

Figure 3–27C. Sagittal section showing part of the enlarged vein of Galen and enlarged dural sinuses.

3.28 Cavernous Angioma

CLINICAL

This 17-year-old boy had a history of headaches and recently developed seizures. Computerized tomography revealed a partially calcified, minimally enhancing lesion without significant mass effect in the right frontal lobe. Angiography showed minimal vascularity. The lesion was surgically resected.

PATHOLOGY

The lesion involved both cortex and underlying white matter and was composed of numerous compactly aggregated vascular channels (Fig. 3–28A). Some of the component vessels were thrombosed while others contained deposits of mineral (Fig. 3–28B). The surrounding neural parenchyma at the periphery of the lesion was focally discolored brown and yellow, reflecting prior bleeding. Histological examination revealed thick-walled sinusoidal vascular channels without intervening neuroglial tissue. There were small numbers of macrophages containing lipid and hemosiderin in the discolored gliotic tissue at the periphery of the lesion.

COMMENT

Cavernous angiomas are the least common type of vascular malformation, as judged from autopsy series. Many are asymptomatic and encountered as an incidental finding at the time of autopsy (Figs. 3–28C and 3–28D). When symptomatic, they are more apt to cause seizures than massive hemorrhage. Nevertheless, they are often accompanied by small numbers of pigment- and lipid - laden macrophages, reflecting minor bleeding. Histologically, they appear as compact aggregates of sinusoidal vessels without significant interposed neural parenchyma (Fig. 3–28D). The neural parenchyma immediately surrounding the angioma is usually gliotic. As in the present case, they often become partially mineralized. Some may be demonstrated by computerized tomography or even plain skull x-ray. However, because of their lack of major arterial supply, they are rarely visualized by angiography. Recently, it has been suggested that magnetic resonance imaging may be especially effective for demonstrating these lesions.

REFERENCES

McCormick WF: Vascular diseases. In Rosenberg RN (ed): The Clinical Neurosciences. New York, Churchill Livingstone, 1983, vol 3, chap 2, pp III:35–III:83.

Rigamonti D, Drayer BP, Johnson PC, et al: The MRI appearance of cavernous malformations (angiomas). J Neurosurg 1987; 67:518-524.

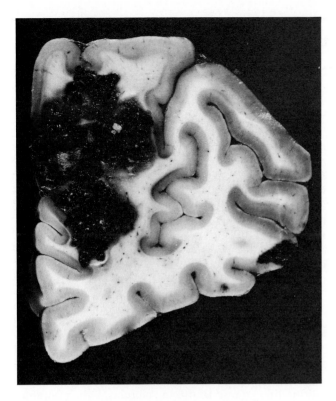

Figure 3–28A. Cavernous angioma of the right frontal lobe.

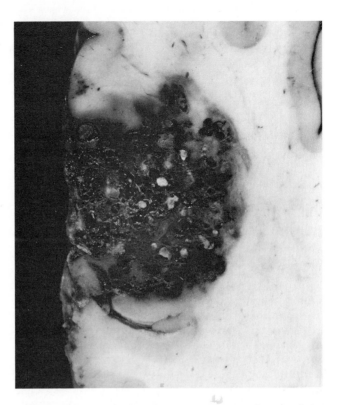

Figure 3–28B. Cavernous angioma with yellow-gray deposits of mineral in some of the vascular channels.

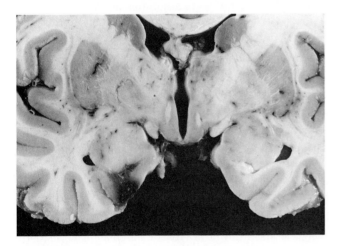

Figure 3–28C. Incidental cavernous angioma of left temporal lobe.

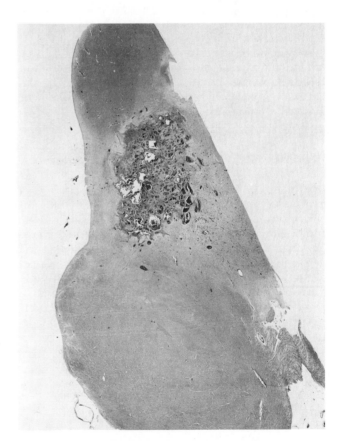

Figure 3–28D. Macrosection showing an incidental cavernous angioma of the mesencephalon.

3.29　Cavernous Angiomas

Multiple

CLINICAL

This 59-year-old man had a long complicated neurological history. Sixteen years previously he had presented with ataxia, decreased right facial sensation, decreased hearing, dysphagia, and right hemiparesis. He regained full use of his extremities and did well for the following 5 years. At that time, he had the acute onset of impaired balance, decreased vision on the right, facial weakness, and dysphagia. Three weeks later, he developed tinnitus and loss of hearing on the right. Within 1 month all of these symptoms cleared except for ataxia. His condition was stable for the next 4 years and then he again developed right hemiparesis and a right peripheral facial palsy. Subsequently, a computerized tomogram showed an area of increased attenuation in the right cerebral peduncle displacing the fourth ventricle to the left and foci of decreased attenuation in the left parieto-occipital area.

His final admission was prompted by the development of increased weakness and impairment of speech. While being evaluated, he suffered a cardiac arrest from which he was successfully resuscitated. At that time, a computerized tomogram disclosed three moderately dense lesions in the brain stem and cerebellum. Angiography was unremarkable. The patient developed renal failure and died 3 weeks after his final admission.

PATHOLOGY

Examination of the brain revealed a small amount of fresh blood in the subarachnoid space near the right cerebellopontine angle. Horizontal sections of the cerebral hemispheres revealed multiple small cavernous angiomas in the white matter of the right cerebral hemisphere (Fig. 3–29A). The right ventrolateral aspect of the medulla was swollen and discolored. Multiple transverse sections of the brain stem revealed a large cavernous angioma in the right half of the dorsal pons (Fig. 3–29B). This lesion partially filled the fourth ventricle and extended caudally into the right dorsolateral quadrant of the medulla (Fig. 3–29C). Histologically, the lesions were typical cavernous angiomas (Fig. 3–29D). Some of the vascular channels were thrombosed while others contained mineralized concretions. The adjacent neural parenchyma was gliotic and contained macrophages that were laden with lipid and hemosiderin as the result of remote hemorrhages.

COMMENT

Patients with vascular malformations of the brain stem may have complex fluctuating clinical manifestations that mimic multiple sclerosis. Other patients with multiple cavernous angiomas may have symptoms that resemble pseudotumor cerebri. Occasionally, multiple cavernous angiomas are familial.

REFERENCES

Britt RH, Connor WS, Enzmann DR: Occult arteriovenous malformation of the brain stem simulating multiple sclerosis. Neurology 1981; 31:901-903.

DeJong RN, Hicks SP: Vascular malformation of the brainstem: Report of a case with long duration and fluctuating course. Neurology 1980; 30:995-997.

Dobyns WB, Michels VV, Groover RV, et al: Familial cavernous malformations of the central nervous system and retina. Ann Neurol 1987; 21:578-583.

Stahl SM, Johnson KP, Malamud N: The clinical and pathological spectrum of brain-stem vascular malformations: Long-term course simulates multiple sclerosis. Arch Neurol 1980; 37:25-29.

Tindall RSA, Kirkpatrick JB, Sklar F: Multiple small cavernous angiomas of the brain with increased intracranial pressure. Ann Neurol 1978; 4:376-378.

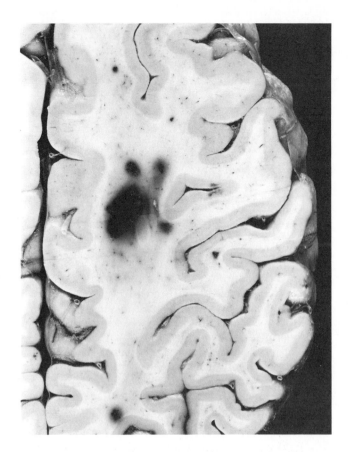

Figure 3–29A. Horizontal section showing multiple cavernous angiomas in the white matter of the right cerebral hemisphere.

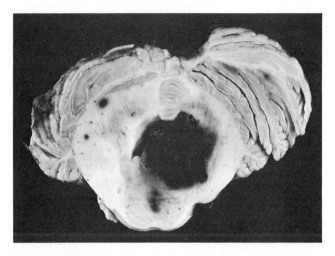

Figure 3–29B. Section of pons and cerebellum showing a cavernous angioma of the pons.

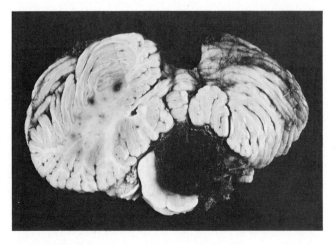

Figure 3–29C. Section of the medulla and cerebellum showing a cavernous angioma.

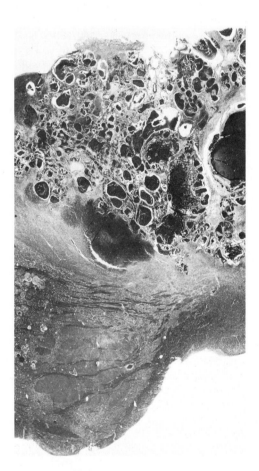

Figure 3–29D. Microscopic section showing compactly aggregated vessels consistent with cavernous angioma.

3.30 Other Vascular Malformations

Venous Angiomas
Capillary Telangiectases
Sturge–Weber Syndrome

Venous angiomas are the most common type of vascular malformation, comprising about 67 percent of vascular malformations, as judged from autopsy series. They are rarely detected angiographically and are rarely clinically significant. They appear as a loose aggregate of various sized veins separated from one another by intact neural parenchyma (Fig. 3–30A). Occasionally, a large draining vein can be demonstrated extending to the meningeal veins or, less commonly, to the deep venous system. They occur in all parts of the brain but are recognized more commonly in the cerebrum and cerebellum.

Capillary telangiectases comprise about 11 percent of all vascular malformations as judged from autopsy series. They are rarely symptomatic. They appear as compact congeries of small vessels (Figs. 3–30B and 3–30C). Histologically, the component vessels are like capillaries with thin walls but have variable sized lumina (Fig. 3–30D). The intervening neural parenchyma is generally relatively normal. Some of these lesions show transitions to cavernous angiomas.

The Sturge–Weber syndrome is a neurocutaneous syndrome characterized by a cutaneous vascular nevus on the face in the distribution of one or more divisions of the trigeminal nerve and an ipsilateral meningeal angioma. The parietal and occipital regions are the most common sites of the meningeal angioma. The leptomeninges harboring the angioma often contain unusually prominent melanocytes. The neural parenchyma underlying the meningeal angioma usually becomes mineralized (Fig. 3–30E). The mineral deposits in adjacent gyri produce the characteristic "tram-track" appearance seen radiologically. These lesions cause seizures and mental deterioration but rarely significant intracranial hemorrhage. There also may be an angioma of the choroid of the ipsilateral eye. This can lead to blindness.

REFERENCES

Alexander GL: Sturge—Weber syndrome. In Vinken PJ, Bruyn GW (eds): Handbook of Clinical Neurology. Amsterdam, Elsevier, 1972, vol 14, chap 7, pp 223-240.

McCormick WF: Vascular diseases. In Rosenberg RN (ed): The Clinical Neurosciences. New York, Churchill Livingstone, 1983, vol 3, chap 2, pp III:35–III:83.

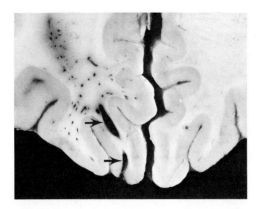

Figure 3–30A. Incidental venous angioma in left frontal lobe. Note the large draining vein (arrows).

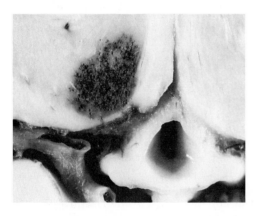

Figure 3–30C. Capillary telangiectasis of frontal lobe.

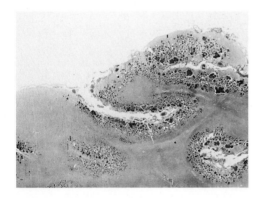

Figure 3–30E. Macroscopic section from patient with Sturge–Weber syndrome. Note the mineral is in the cerebral cortex.

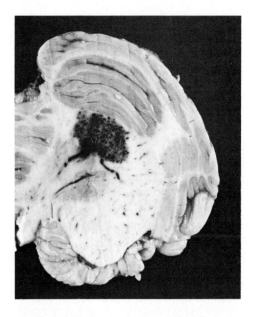

Figure 3–30B. Capillary telangiectasis in cerebellar hemisphere.

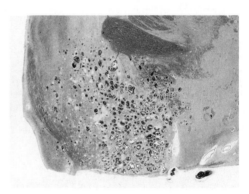

Figure 3–30D. Macroscopic section of telangiectasis showing thin-walled vessels.

3.31 Saccular Aneurysm

Unruptured

CLINICAL

This 64 year-old-woman died from metastatic lung carcinoma.

PATHOLOGY

Examination of the brain revealed an unruptured saccular aneurysm at the bifurcation of the right middle cerebral artery (Fig. 3–31A). The aneurysm measured approximately 0.5 × 0.5 × 0.5 cm after formalin fixation. The dome of the aneurysm contained atherosclerotic plaques.

COMMENT

Saccular or "berry" aneurysms are encountered at autopsy in about 5 percent of all patients over the age of 20 years. They are more common in women than men. An increased prevalence has been reported in individuals with adult polycystic kidney disease. In addition, there are rare familial cases. About 85 percent of the aneurysms arise from bifurcations of the proximal vessels of the anterior circulation. Among individuals with saccular aneurysms, about 25 percent will have multiple lesions and about 15 percent will have bilateral, "mirror image," aneurysms (Fig. 3–31B).

As determined by autopsy series, saccular aneurysms occur most commonly on the middle cerebral arteries. This is in contrast to clinical series in which the aneurysms arising from the junction of the anterior cerebral and anterior communicating arteries (Fig. 3–31C) and the junction of the internal carotid and posterior communicating arteries are more heavily represented. This discrepancy reflects the greater risk of hemorrhage from aneurysms in the latter two sites as well as the tendency for internal carotid–posterior communicating aneurysms to produce third nerve compression rather than hemorrhage. Only about 15 percent of saccular aneurysms arise from vessels of the posterior circulation. Figures 3–31D and 3–31E illustrate an unruptured aneurysm arising from the bifurcation of the basilar artery.

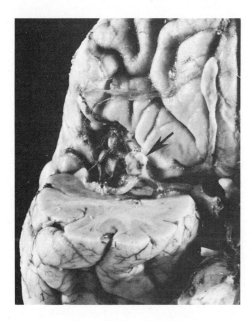

Figure 3–31A. Unruptured saccular aneursym (arrow) at bifurcation of right middle cerebral artery.

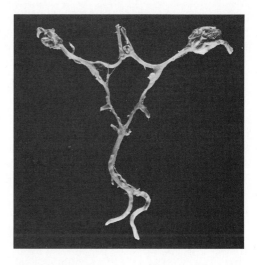

Figure 3–31B. Multiple saccular aneurysms (left and right middle cerebral arteries and anterior communicating artery).

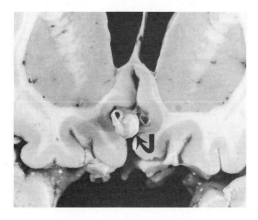

Figure 3–31C. Anterior communicating artery aneurysm (curved arrow).

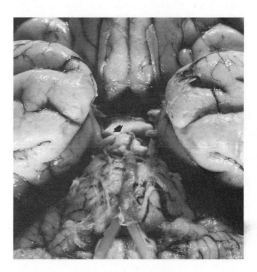

Figure 3–31D. Unruptured, bilobed basilar tip aneurysm (arrow).

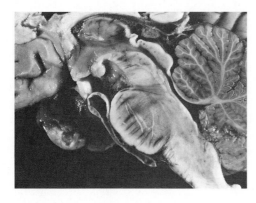

Figure 3–31E. Sagittal section showing unruptured basilar tip aneurysm.

Occasionally, the lumen of an aneurysm will contain laminated thrombus, making angiographic evaluation of its size or even detection difficult (Fig. 3–31F). Conversely, some aneurysms are deeply embedded in the adjacent neural parenchyma and are not readily evident from external examination of the brain (Fig. 3–31G). Aneurysms appear smaller at the time of autopsy since they are not distended by the pressure of the circulating blood and even smaller at brain cutting since they shrink significantly following formalin fixation. As shown in these examples, the majority of the small saccular aneurysms remain asymptomatic.

REFERENCES

McCormick WF: Vascular diseases. In Rosenberg RN (ed): The Clinical Neurosciences. New York, Churchill Livingstone, 1983, vol 3, chap 2, pp III:35–III:83.

Stehbens WE: Pathology of the Cerebral Blood Vessels. St Louis, Mosby, 1972, pp 351-470.

Wiebers DO, Whisnant JP, Sundt TM Jr, O'Fallon WM: The significance of unruptured intracranial saccular aneurysms. J Neurosurg 1987; 66:23-29.

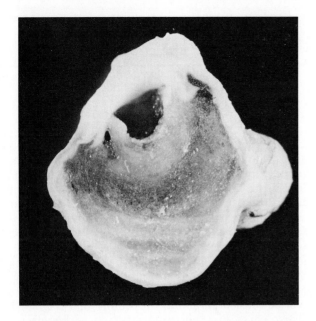

Figure 3–31F. Saccular aneurysm partially filled with laminated thrombus.

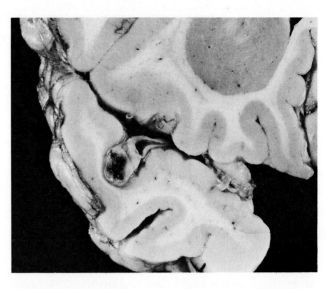

Figure 3–31G. Unruptured saccular aneurysm deeply embedded in temporal lobe.

3.32 Saccular Aneurysm

Ruptured

CLINICAL

This 44-year-old man with a history of hypertension was found dead in his apartment.

PATHOLOGY

There was abundant blood in the subarachnoid space at the base of the brain. The hemorrhage originated from a ruptured saccular aneurysm located at the junction between the left internal carotid and posterior communicating arteries (Fig. 3–32A). The aneurysm measured approximately 2.5 × 1.5 × 1.5 cm. The dome contained atherosclerotic plaques.

COMMENT

Ruptured saccular aneurysms are usually greater than 0.7 cm in maximal diameter. The immediate cause of the rupture is controversial although many authors have implicated a sudden, acute rise in blood pressure. The rupture generally leads to subarachnoid hemorrhage with varying degrees of intracerebral and intraventricular extension. As in the present case, the hemorrhage is usually most abundant at the base of the brain in the vicinity of the ruptured aneurysm. Occasionally, following the rupture of a middle cerebral artery aneurysm, much of the blood will be largely confined to the Sylvian fissure producing a Sylvian hematoma. When the aneurysm has been largely buried in the brain, most of the hemorrhage will be intracerebral and intraventricular (Fig. 3–32B). These cases may be misinterpreted as hypertensive hemorrhages until the aneurysm is discovered.

Aneurysms arising from the junction of the anterior cerebral and anterior communicating arteries (Fig. 3–32C) are especially prone to rupture. Often part of the hemorrhage will extend onto the dorsal surface of the corpus callosum (Fig. 3–32D). In these cases, vasospasm often leads to necrosis of the underlying corpus callosum and to infarcts in the perfusion bed of the distal branches of the anterior cerebral arteries (Fig. 3–32E).

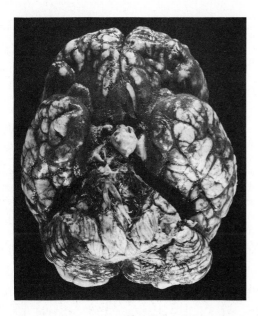

Figure 3–32A. Subarachnoid hemorrhage from ruptured saccular aneurysm located at junction between left internal carotid and posterior communicating arteries.

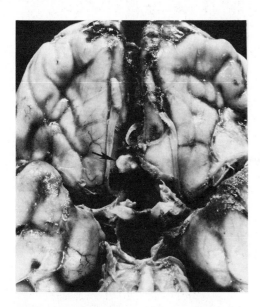

Figure 3–32C. Ruptured aneurysm arising from junction between anterior cerebral and anterior communicating arteries.

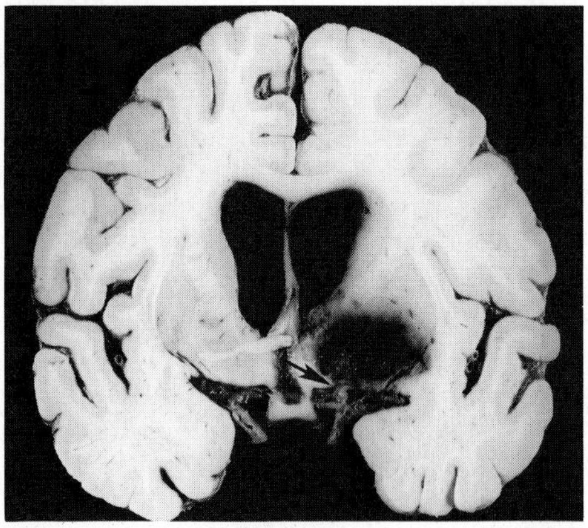

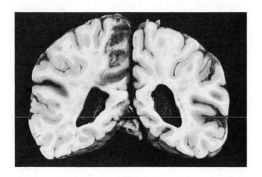

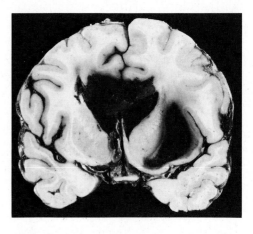

Figure 3–32B. Intraparenchymal and intraventricular hemorrhage secondary to ruptured aneurysm (arrow).

Figure 3–32D. The subarachnoid hemorrhage from the ruptured aneurysm extended onto the dorsal surface of the corpus callosum causing extensive necrosis of the corpus callosum.

Figure 3–32E. Infarct of the medial aspect of the left posterior frontal and parietal lobe secondary to vasospasm.

Although less common, aneurysms on posterior circulation vessels are similarly subject to rupture. Figure 3–32F illustrates a large ruptured basilar tip aneurysm. Other, even less common sites may harbor aneurysms that are responsible for otherwise unexplained, nontraumatic subarachnoid hemorrhages. This is illustrated in Figure 3–32G, which shows a subarachnoid hemorrhage due to a ruptured aneurysm arising from a branch of the right vertebral artery.

The blood from ruptured aneurysms often impairs the function of the pacchionian granulations and impedes egress of cerebrospinal fluid. This in turn, can lead to acute hydrocephalus. Large supratentorial hematomas from ruptured aneurysms may cause cerebral herniation. Figure 3–32H shows hemorrhagic infarction in the posterior temporal and occipital cortex in a patient with a ruptured anterior communicating artery aneurysm. The infarcts resulted from transient kinking of the posterior cerebral arteries as the brain stem moved caudally during the course of the cerebral herniation.

REFERENCES

Heros RC, Zervas NT, Varso V: Cerebral vasospasm after subarachnoid hemorrhage: An update. Ann Neurol 1983; 14:599-608.

Hijdra A, Van Gijn J, Stefanko S, et al: Delayed cerebral ischemia after aneurysmal subarachnoid hemorrhage: Clinicoanatomic correlations. Neurology 1986; 36:329-333.

Sacco RL, Wolf PA, Bharucha NE, et al: Subarachnoid and intracerebral hemorrhage: Natural history, prognosis, and precursive factors in the Framingham Study. Neurology 1984; 34:847-854.

Weisberg LA: Ruptured aneurysms of anterior cerebral or anterior communicating arteries: CT patterns. Neurology 1985; 35:1562-1566.

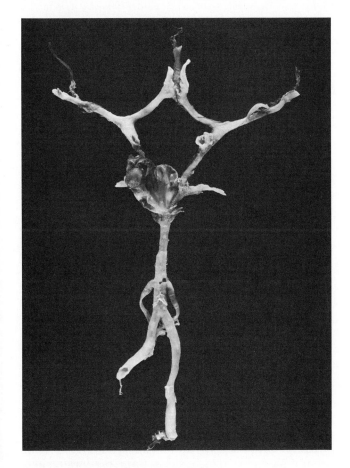

Figure 3–32F. Ruptured basilar tip aneurysm.

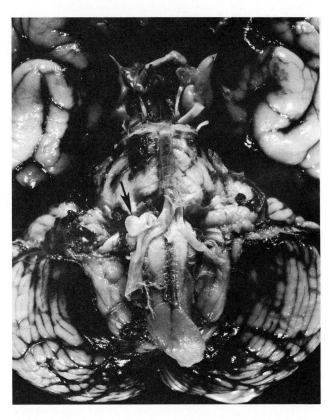

Figure 3–32G. Ruptured aneurysm (arrow) arising from a branch of the right vertebral artery.

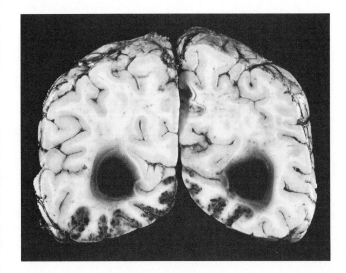

Figure 3–32H. Hemorrhagic infarction of posterior temporal and occipital cortices secondary to herniation and kinking of the posterior cerebral arteries.

3.33   Other Aneurysms

"Mycotic" Aneurysms
Arteriosclerotic Aneurysm

CLINICAL

This 43-year-old woman, a known intravenous drug user, developed headaches. When hospitalized she was febrile and had a heart murmur consistent with aortic insufficiency. She died shortly thereafter.

PATHOLOGY

Examination of the heart revealed acute bacterial endocarditis affecting the aortic and mitral valves. The dura was focally adherent to the lateral aspect of the left frontal lobe. At the site of adhesion, there was a hemorrhagic lesion measuring approximately 1 cm in diameter (Fig. 3–33A). Coronal sections of the cerebral hemispheres disclosed a small area of hemorrhage and necrosis in the cortex and subcortical white matter (Fig. 3–33B). Histological examination revealed the inner part of an inflamed wall of a mycotic aneurysm (Fig. 3–33C). The outer part of the aneurysm had remained attached to the overlying dura.

COMMENT

Inflammatory aneurysms, commonly referred to as "mycotic" aneurysms, result from focal weakening and subsequent aneurysmal dilatation of intracranial blood vessels. In contrast to saccular aneurysms, they are generally found on peripheral branches of the cerebral arteries and may be multiple. They are relatively uncommon and found predominantly in individuals with endocarditis, especially acute bacterial endocarditis. The causative organisms are usually streptococci or staphylococci. Experimental studies have shown that the lesions develop rapidly after septic embolization. In addition, these studies have shown that the inflammatory process begins in the adventitia and progresses centripetally toward the intima. Inflammatory aneurysms have also been encountered in patients with meningitis. In rare instances, inflammatory aneurysms have been caused by fungal infections or various forms of vasculitis.

Another uncommon type of intracranial aneurysm is the arteriosclerotic aneurysm. These are found predominantly in elderly individuals with advanced cerebral arteriosclerosis. Unlike saccular aneurysms, they do not arise from arterial bifurcations. They are generally fusiform with focal sacculations and may become quite large. They most often involve the basilar artery (Fig. 3–33D). Large symptomatic arteriosclerotic aneurysms usually produce brain stem compression or undergo thrombosis resulting in brain stem infarction. Hemorrhage from rupture is less common.

REFERENCES

Bohmfalk GL, Story JL, Wissinger JP, Brown WE Jr: Bacterial intracranial aneurysm. J Neurosurg 1978; 48:369-382.

Molinari GF, Smith L, Goldstein MN, Satran R: Pathogenesis of cerebral mycotic aneurysms. Neurology 1973; 23:325-332.

Nijensohn DE, Saez RJ, Reagan TJ: Clinical significance of basilar artery aneurysms. Neurology 1974; 24:301-305.

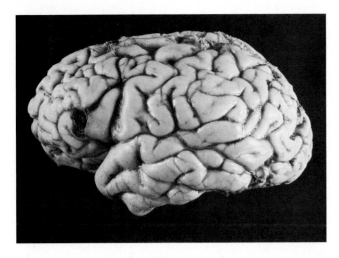

Figure 3–33A. Mycotic aneurysm in a drug user with endocarditis.

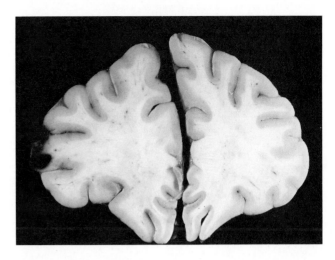

Figure 3–33B. Coronal section showing the mycotic aneurysm.

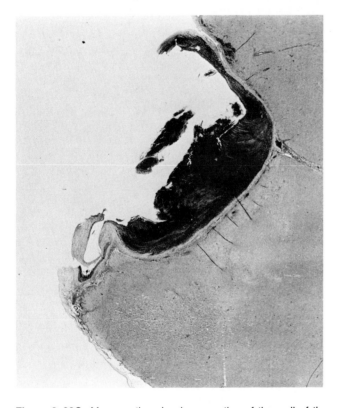

Figure 3–33C. Macrosection showing a portion of the wall of the mycotic aneurysm.

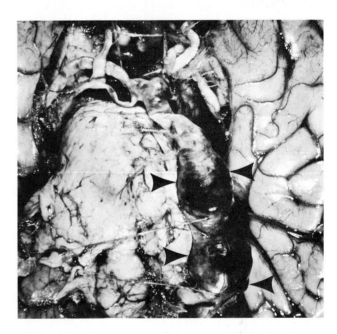

Figure 3–33D. Arteriosclerotic aneurysm of basilar artery (arrowheads).

4

Trauma

4.1   Epidural Hematoma

CLINICAL

This 32-year-old man had been struck on the side of the head. When seen, 36 hours later, at a referral hospital, he was comatose and decerebrate. The scalp on the right side of his head was swollen and faintly discolored. His tympanic membranes were intact. Computerized tomography disclosed a right-sided epidural hematoma. The patient's condition did not improve significantly following evacuation of the hematoma and he died on the second hospital day.

PATHOLOGY

Examination of the skull revealed fractures extending from the surgical defect dorsally to the sagittal suture and inferiorly into the middle fossa. There was residual epidural hematoma on the outer surface of the right dural leaf (Fig. 4–1A). The brain showed a large contusion involving the posterior portion of the right parietal lobe and the right occipital lobe (Fig. 4–1B). There was a small amount of subdural blood in the interhemispheric fissure and a small amount of subarachnoid blood, especially at the base of the brain.

COMMENT

As in this case, epidural hematomas are generally the result of head trauma. In adults, they are most fre-quently located in the temporoparietal area and are usually caused by skull fractures that lacerate branches of the middle meningeal artery. Some are found in other locations and may be venous in nature. This generally results from tears in the dural sinuses. Children occasionally have epidural hematomas without an associated skull fracture.

Traditionally, epidural hematomas are thought to produce rapidly evolving neurological deficits without being accompanied by other traumatic lesions. More recently, largely as the result of computerized tomography, it has become apparent that some patients may have a delayed onset of symptoms. In addition, nearly one third of the patients have been found to have significant intradural injuries. Since epidural hematomas press the dura against the underlying brain, the apices of the compressed gyri tend to be more severely flattened than when the deformity is produced by a subdural hematoma.

REFERENCES

Jamieson KG, Yelland JDN: Extradural hematoma: Report of 167 cases. J Neurosurg 1968; 29:13-23.

Borovich B, Braun J, Guilburd JN, et al: Delayed onset of traumatic extradural hematoma. J Neurosurg 1985; 63:30-34.

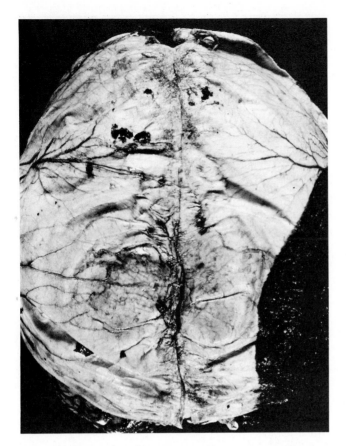

Figure 4–1A. Outer surface of dura with an epidural hematoma overlying the right parietal and occipital lobes.

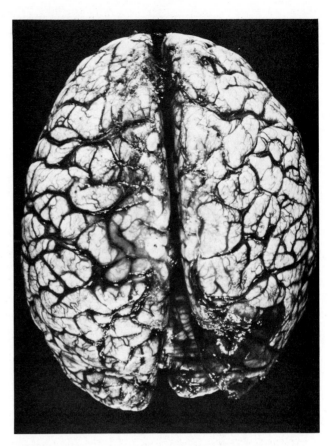

Figure 4–1B. Contusion of right parietal and occipital lobes underlying the epidural hematoma.

4.2 Acute Subdural Hematoma

"Burst lobe"

CLINICAL

This 31-year-old woman fell from a moving truck. She was unconscious at the scene of the accident. She was found to have abrasions and lacerations of the scalp, a left parietal skull fracture, and an acute subdural hematoma. Although the hematoma was evacuated surgically, she never regained consciousness and died 1½ days later.

PATHOLOGY

Residual clotted subdural blood was present beneath the surgical defect over the lateral surface of the right temporal lobe (Fig. 4–2A). There were contusions on the lateral aspect of the right temporal lobe and inferior surface of the right frontal lobe. Coronal sections revealed extensive cortical contusions and lacerations beneath the subdural hematoma (Fig. 4–2B). The right cerebral hemisphere was severely swollen. As a result, there was herniation of the right cingulate gyrus beneath the falx, compression of right lateral ventricle, bowing of the third ventricle to the left, central herniation, and bilateral uncal herniation. The herniated unci also were contused.

COMMENT

Subdural hematomas have been classified according to the nature of their contents into acute, subacute, and chronic. Acute subdural hematomas contain clotted blood, subacute hematomas contain a mixture of clotted and liquefied blood, and chronic hematomas contain predominantly liquefied blood. Acute subdural hematomas can arise from either venous or arterial bleeding. Torn meningeal vessels at the site of cortical contusions have been implicated in the majority of these cases. In some patients, intraparenchymal hematomas are in continuity with the overlying acute subdural hematomas. These lesions have been designated as "burst lobes." The frontal and temporal lobes are most commonly involved. Acute subdural hematomas are common traumatic lesions and have a high mortality of 30 to 90 percent. They may result from falls and blows, as well as vehicular accidents.

REFERENCES

Lindenberg R: Trauma of meninges and brain. In: Minckler J (ed): Pathology of the Nervous System. New York, McGraw-Hill, 1971, vol 2, chap 133, pp 1705-1765.

Seeling JM, Becker DP, Miller JD, et al: Traumatic acute subdural hematoma: Major mortality reduction in comatose patients treated within four hours. N Engl J Med 1981; 304:1511-1518.

Shenkin HA: Acute subdural hematoma: Review of 39 consecutive cases with high incidence of cortical artery rupture. J Neurosurg 1982; 57:254-257.

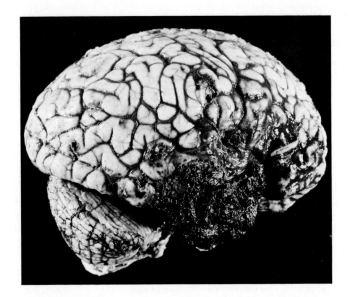

Figure 4–2A. Lateral surface of brain showing an acute subdural hematoma.

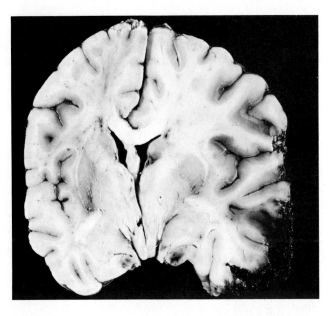

Figure 4–2B. Coronal sections showing the cortical contusions and lacerations underlying the acute subdural hematoma. Note also herniation of the right cingulate gyrus, the shift of the right lateral and third ventricles, herniation contusions on both unci, and central herination.

4.3 Chronic Subdural Hematoma

CLINICAL

This 62-year-old man, a known alcohol abuser, died from carbon monoxide poisoning in a house that was partially destroyed by fire.

PATHOLOGY

Postmortem toxicology revealed a carbon monoxide saturation level of 80 percent and a blood alcohol level of 0.27 g/dL. Examination of the brain disclosed thick brown-stained subdural membranes on the undersurface of the left dural leaf (Figs. 4–3A and 4–3B). In areas, these membranes measured up to 0.5 cm in thickness. The membranes could be separated easily from the overlying dura and underlying arachnoid. Soft tan material occupied the space between the inner and outer membranes. Macrosections (Fig. 4–3C) through the membranes showed the outer membrane (arrows) to be thicker than the inner membrane. The leptomeningeal blood vessels were congested and abnormally red from the presence of carboxyhemoglobin. No contusions were evident.

COMMENT

Chronic subdural hematomas are generally the result of bleeding from bridging veins torn by trauma. The trauma may be minimal or even forgotten by the patient. Furthermore, the trauma need not be directly to the head. Falls on the buttocks have been implicated in many cases. Individuals who are at special risk for chronic subdural hematomas include the elderly with cerebral atrophy, and alcohol abusers and epileptics who are subject to falls. In addition, individuals with clotting abnormalities are at increased risk. This group includes patients with clotting disorders such as hemophilia, alcohol abusers with liver disease and abnormal platelet function, and patients who are therapeutically anticoagulated. Figures 4–3D and 4–3E illustrate the undersurface of the dura and cross sections of a chronic subdural hematoma in a patient who was anticoagulated for long-term hemodialysis.

Chronic subdural hematomas are most commonly encountered over the frontal, parietal, and temporal convexities. In about 20 percent of cases, the hematomas are bilateral. On rare occasions, they may be located at the base of the brain, in the interhemispheric fissure, or in the posterior fossa. Although chronic subdural hematomas are generally described as being in the subdural space, studies by Schachenmayr and Friede have suggested that the blood is actually located in a cleavage plane within the inner layers of the dura, at the dura-arachnoid interface. Furthermore, they suggest that under normal circumstances, there is no subdural space.

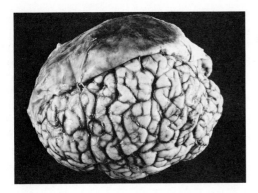

Figure 4–3A. Dorsolateral view of brain with partially reflected left dural leaf showing the thick brownstained membranes from a chronic subdural hematoma.

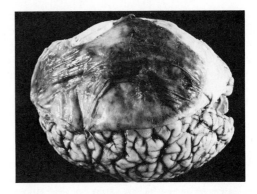

Figure 4–3B. Dorsal view of brain with reflected left dural leaf. The subdural membranes were easily separated from the overlying dura and underlying arachnoid.

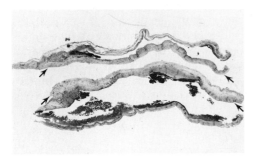

Figure 4–3C. Macrosections of the subdural membranes showing the outer membranes (arrows) to be thicker than the inner membranes. Only a small amount of blood is enclosed between the membranes.

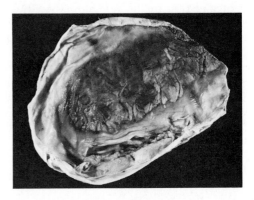

Figure 4–3D. Undersurface of dura with a large chronic subdural hematoma from a patient who was anticoagulated for hemodialysis.

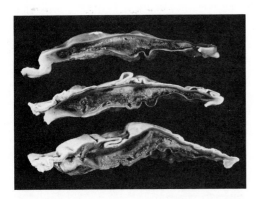

Figure 4–3E. Cross sections of the chronic subdural hematoma shown in Figure 4–3D.

Symptoms from chronic subdural hematomas are usually a result of mass effects and may be accompanied by herniation. Figures 4–3F and 4-3G illustrate a case with bilateral hematomas that resulted in central and uncal herniation. Progressive enlargement of chronic subdural hematomas may occur and has been the subject of extensive investigations. Formerly, it was thought that the membranes surrounding the partially lysed blood acted as a semipermeable membrane and that the enlargement was the result of oncotic pressure. More recently, the enlargement has been attributed to recurrent bleeding from abnormally large, thin-walled vessels in the outer membrane. These so-called giant capillaries are unusually permeable, and the endothelial cells are joined by gap junctions.

The outer membrane is generally thicker and more vascular than the inner membrane. Because of recurrent bleeding in the hematoma cavity and the coexistence of highly vascularized and densely organized fibrous areas in the membranes, accurate determination of the age of a subdural hematoma by histological examination is often difficult or even impossible. Eventually, both membranes become densely fibrotic and the inner and outer membranes may become adherent to one another. Occasionally, the residual lesion becomes mineralized.

Typically, chronic subdural hematomas appear as relatively low-density lesions by computerized tomography. Because of the high protein content, they are somewhat more dense than cerebrospinal fluid. After recurrent bleeds, they may acquire the same density as the adjacent brain, that is, become isodense, making radiographic diagnosis somewhat difficult. Under these circumstances, displacement of the white matter and ventricular system may be significant features.

REFERENCES

Markwalder T-M: Chronic subdural hematomas: A review. J Neurosurgery 1981; 54:637-645.

Schachenmayr W, Friede RL: The origin of subdural neomembranes. I. Fine structure of the dura-arachnoid interface in man. Am J Pathol 1978; 92:53-68.

Yamashima T, Yamamoto S, Friede RL: The role of endothelial gap junctions in the enlargement of chronic subdural hematomas. J Neurosurg 1983; 59:298-303.

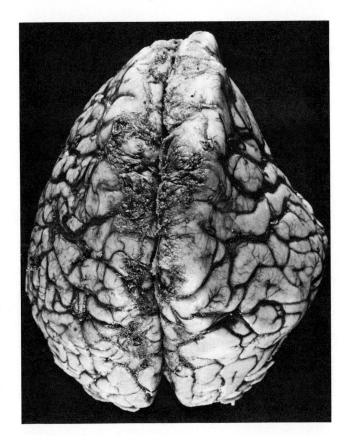

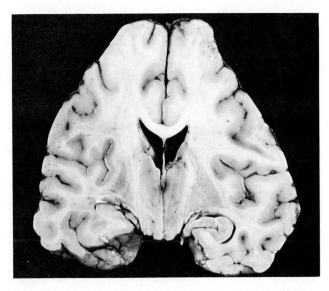

Figure 4–3G. Coronal section showing the deformations caused by the bilateral subdural hematomas. Note also the compression of the third ventricle, central herniation, and bilateral uncal herniation.

Figure 4–3F. Dorsal surface of brain from a patient with bilateral chronic subdural hematomas. The hematoma over the right hemisphere was much larger than the hematoma on the left.

4.4 Contusions

Old and Recent

CLINICAL

This 74-year-old man was involved in a vehicular accident. After being removed from his automobile, he was moving spontaneously but not following commands. He had multiple fractures of both legs. His left pupil dilated while he was being taken to the emergency room. Examination revealed a large left frontal scalp laceration with an underlying linear skull fracture. Computerized tomography revealed no intracranial blood. He died shortly after admission to the hospital.

PATHOLOGY

Examination of the brain revealed fresh blood in the subarachnoid space. There were multiple recent contusions on the lateral surface of the left frontal lobe and inferior surface of both frontal and the right temporal lobes (Fig. 4–4A). The acute contusions appeared as hemorrhagic areas in the apices of gyri. There were also remote contusions on the orbital surface of the right frontal lobe and on the inferior and lateral surfaces of the right temporal lobe (Fig. 4–4A, curved arrow). The remote contusions were excavated areas and had a yellow-brown color. In a coronal section, the recent contusions appeared as hemorrhages oriented perpendicular to the pial surface (Fig. 4–4B). By contrast, the remote contusions appeared as wedge-shaped areas from which cortex and white matter had been excavated (Fig. 4–4C).

COMMENT

This case illustrates the common occurrence of subarachnoid hemorrhage in individuals with head trauma. The case also contrasts the appearance of contusions suffered during the recent accident with contusions sustained in the remote past. Contusions are typically wedge-shaped and preferentially affect the apices of gyri. Recent contusions consist of necrotic neural parenchyma in which there are usually streak-like hemorrhages. The hemorrhages are generally oriented perpendicular to the overlying pial surface (Fig. 4–4D). With the passage of time, the necrotic tissue is removed and remote contusions generally appear as excavated, wedge-shaped lesions on the apices of gyri (Fig. 4–4E). The surface is typically disrupted, in contrast to infarcts, where the molecular layer may remain intact as the result of perfusion from meningeal vessels.

As in the present case, the site of impact is best determined from the location of the scalp injuries and skull fractures. Contusions located beneath the site of impact are often designated as coup lesions. Blows to an unsupported, movable head often result in contusions that are confined to the area beneath the site of impact. Lesions that are away from the site of impact, often on the opposite side of the brain, are usually designated as contrecoup lesions. A combination of coup and contrecoup lesions is best seen in low velocity decelerative injuries such as falls. However, the same combination can also result from accelerative injuries such as blows to the head when the forces are especially great. Contrecoup contusions are especially prominent following falls with impact on the occiput. In such cases, there are often extensive contusions on the inferior surfaces of the frontal and temporal lobes with minimal or no contusions beneath the site of impact. The exact mechanisms responsible for producing the more prominent

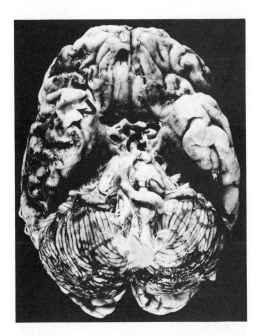

Figure 4–4A. Base of brain showing both recent and old contusions. Recent contusions can be seen on the inferior surface of both frontal lobes and the right temporal lobe. They appear as hemorrhagic, discolored areas. Remote contusions can be seen on the inferior surface of the right frontal and temporal lobe (curved arrow). They appear as shallow excavations on the apices of gyri.

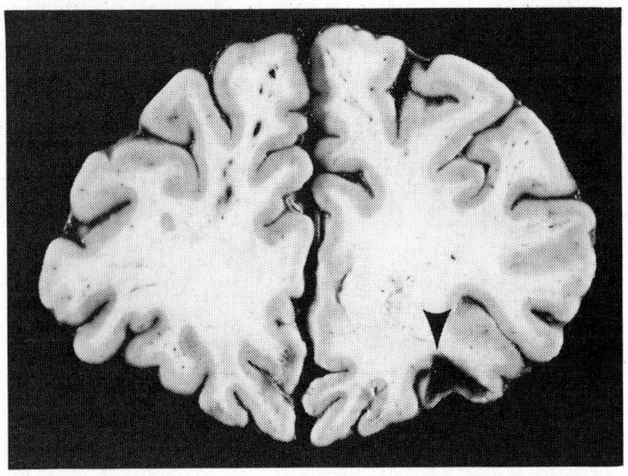

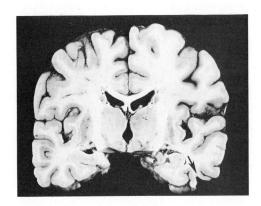

Figure 4–4C. Coronal section showing a wedge-shaped remote contusion in the right inferior temporal convolution (arrow).

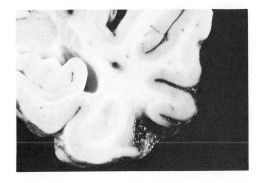

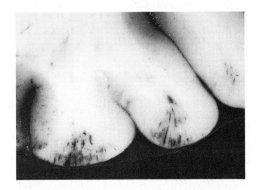

Figure 4–4B. Coronal section showing an acute contusion on the orbital surface of the right frontal lobe (arrowhead) and a gliding contusion in the white matter of the left superior frontal convolution.

Figure 4–4D. Recent contusions typically involving the apices of gyri and containing streak-like hemorrhages oriented perpendicular to the pial surface.

Figure 4–4E. A remote contusion represented by a wedge-shaped excavation involving the apex of a gyrus.

contrecoup lesions are unclear. It is in part due to the greater irregularity of the base of the skull at these sites. Occasionally, contusions are encountered on the dorso-medial surface of the temporal lobe adjacent to the Sylvian fissure (Fig. 4–4F). The occurrence of the lesions in this location is more difficult to explain.

Special terms have been applied to contusions and related lesions encountered in certain specific locations. Contusions on the unci (Fig. 4-4G) and on the cerebellar tonsils (Fig. 4–4H) may be designated as herniation contusions when they result from herniation of these structures. Contusions beneath fracture lines may be characterized by the term fracture contusions. The term gliding contusions has been applied to hemorrhagic lesions in the cortex and subcortical white matter of the superior frontal convolutions (Fig. 4–4B). The lesions have been attributed to the injurious effects of the brain shifting back and forth following impact.

Intraparenchymal hemorrhages located between the coup and contrecoup lesions have been described by Lindenberg as intermediary coup contusions. The use of this designation has been challenged in recent years. It may be more appropriate to consider intermediary contusions and gliding contusions in the context of diffuse brain injury. Parenthetically, it should be noted that several authors have emphasized the inhibitory role of alcohol on platelet function in promoting the development of acute intraparenchymal hematomas. Disseminated intravascular coagulation, initiated by disrupted neural parenchyma, probably plays a similar role in the delayed development of these hematomas.

REFERENCES

Adams JH, Doyle D, Graham DI, et al: Gliding contusions in nonmissile head injury in humans. Arch Pathol Lab Med 1986; 110:485-488.

Lindenberg R: Trauma of meninges and brain. In Minckler J (ed): Pathology of the Nervous System, New York, McGraw-Hill, 1971, vol 2, chap 133, pp 1705-1765.

McCormick WF: Trauma. In Rosenberg RN (ed): The Clinical Neurosciences. New York, Churchill Livingstone, 1983, vol 3, chap 6, pp III:241–III:283.

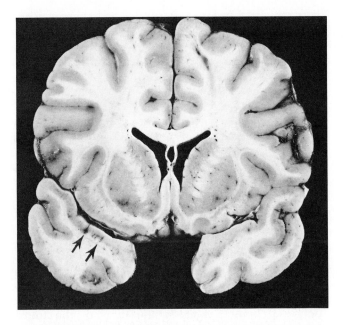

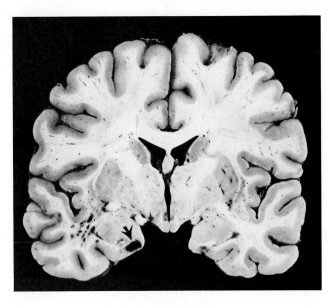

Figure 4–4F. Recent contusions represented by streak-like hemorrhages (arrows) involving the dorso-medial aspect of the temporal lobe adjacent to the sylvian fissure.

Figure 4–4G. Recent herniation contusion involving the left uncus (arrow).

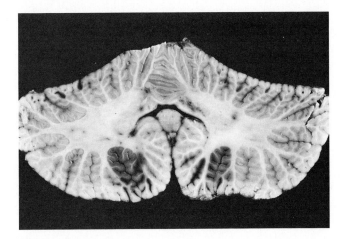

Figure 4–4H. Recent contusions from herniation of cerebellar tonsils, secondary to gunshot wound of cerebrum.

4.5   Ponto-Medullary Laceration

CLINICAL

This 30-year-old man died following a head-on vehicular accident.

PATHOLOGY

Autopsy revealed an ecchymotic area on the undersurface of the mandible and parieto-occipital and basilar skull fractures. Contusions were noted on the frontal and temporal lobes (Fig. 4–5A). In addition, there was partial disruption of the ponto-medullary junction. Sagittal sections of the brain stem disclosed partial laceration of the ponto-medullary junction with small numbers of petechial hemorrhages in the surrounding neural parenchyma (Fig. 4–5B). More numerous hemorrhages were evident microscopically (Fig. 4–5C).

COMMENT

Ponto-medullary lacerations have been documented with increased frequency in recent years. They generally result from traumatic hyperextension of the head and are commonly accompanied by fractures of the skull and/or cervical spine. Ponto-medullary lacerations are usually rapidly fatal, although some patients with this lesion have lived for a few days.

As in the present case, there is often relatively little subarachnoid hemorrhage around the laceration. Since this area may be disrupted artifactually at the time of brain removal, it is imperative to demonstrate intraparenchymal hemorrhages around the laceration by gross and histological examination. Figure 4–5D shows a parasagittal section from another case with a smaller laceration. In this case there were also petechial hemorrhages in the floor of the fourth ventricle.

REFERENCES

Hardman JM: Cerebrospinal trauma. In Davis RL, Robertson DM (ed): Textbook of Neuropathology. Baltimore, Williams & Wilkins, 1985, chap 17, pp 842-882.

Lindenberg R, Freytag E: Brainstem lesions characteristic of traumatic hyperextension of the head. Arch Pathol 1970; 90:509-515.

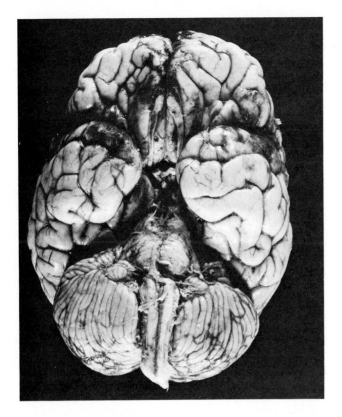

Figure 4–5A. Base of brain showing acute contusions on frontal and temporal lobes and partial laceration of the ponto-medullary junction.

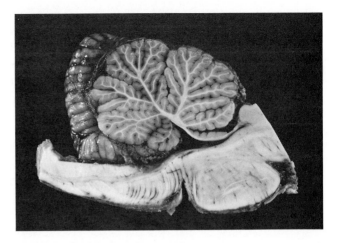

Figure 4–5B. Sagittal section of brain stem showing wedge-shaped laceration of ponto-medullary junction.

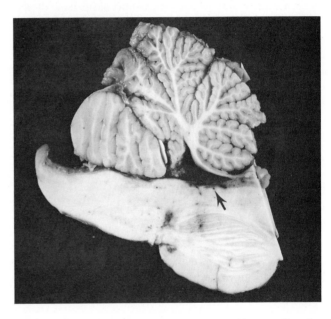

Figure 4–5D. Sagittal section of a brain stem with a small ponto-medullary laceration and petechial hemorrhages in the floor of the fourth ventricle (arrow).

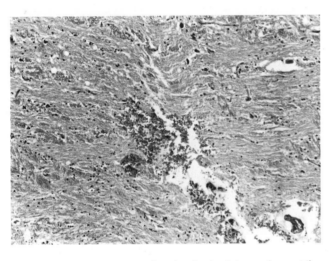

Figure 4–5C. Microscopic section showing fresh hemorrhage at the apex of the ponto-medullary laceration.

4.6   Diffuse Brain Injury

Diffuse Axonal Injury

CLINICAL

This 28-year-old man was struck in the head by a snapped cable. He was unconscious from the time of the accident until his death a few hours later.

PATHOLOGY

There were scalp contusions in the occipital region and fractures of the calvarium and skull base. There was a thin film of subarachnoid blood that was maximal over the right frontal lobe. Contusions were present on the lateral and inferior surfaces of both frontal and temporal lobes (Fig. 4–6A). Coronal sections of the cerebral hemispheres disclosed a small number of petechial hemorrhages in the corpus callosum, in addition to the contusions noted externally. Sections of the brain stem revealed small hemorrhages in the tegmentum of the mesencephalon (Fig. 4–6B) and pons (Fig. 4–6C). Histological examination revealed petechial hemorrhages but no reactive axons.

COMMENT

Despite numerous pathological studies of head trauma, there has been relatively poor correlation between the various focal lesions and clinical outcome. Many individuals died despite an apparent paucity of grossly discernible lesions. In recent years, there has been a shift in emphasis from the obvious focal lesions to the more subtle, diffuse brain injuries. The newer interpretations regarding the lesions observed in human material have been corroborated in part by experimental studies in primates. These studies have shown that death from severe diffuse brain injury may occur in the absence of extensive focal lesions. Several types of diffuse brain injury have been delineated by Adams and his co-workers. These include diffuse axonal injury, hypoxic brain damage, brain swelling, and multiple large or small intraparenchymal hemorrhages.

Diffuse axonal injury is the result of shearing of axons at the moment of impact. The damage is widespread in the brain and the individuals generally remain unconscious from the time of the accident until their death. When death is instantaneous or very rapid, there may be no grossly discernible lesions or only scattered petechial hemorrhages. When survival is somewhat longer, petechial and other small hemorrhages may be evident in certain areas. These areas of predilection include the dorsolateral quadrants of the rostral brain stem and the corpus callosum (Fig. 4–6D). In some cases, the fornices and leaves of the septum pellucidum also may be disrupted (Fig. 4–6E).

The rostral brain stem hemorrhages associated with diffuse axonal injury typically occur in the tectum and tegmentum of the mesencephalon and the tegmentum of the pons, adjacent to the superior cerebellar peduncles. These hemorrhages must be

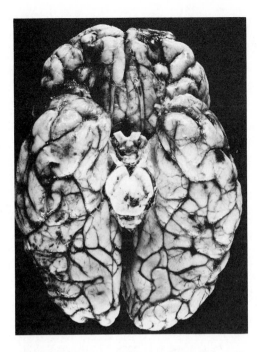

Figure 4–6A. Base of brain showing multiple acute contusions on frontal and temporal lobes and small hemorrahges in mesencephalic tegmentum.

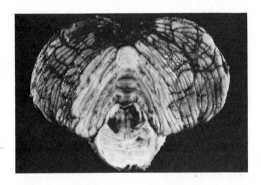

Figure 4–6C. Section of cerebellum and pons showing multiple small hemorrhages in pontine tegmentum and superior cerebellar peduncles. This is a typical location for hemorrhages associated with diffuse axonal injury.

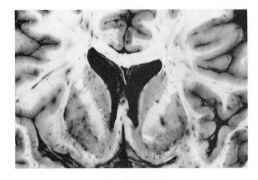

Figure 4–6E. Coronal section showing traumatic disruption of the leaves of a cavum septi pellucidi.

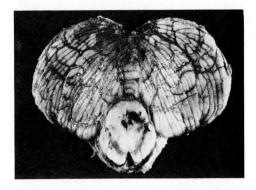

Figure 4–6B. Brain stem and cerebellum showing multiple small hemorrhages in mesencephalic tegmentum.

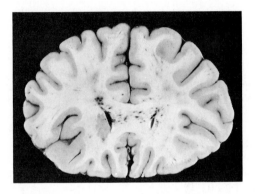

Figure 4–6D. Petechial hemorrhages in corpus callosum from another case with diffuse axonal injury.

distinguished from the so-called Duret hemorrhages or secondary brain stem hemorrhages that result from downward displacement of the brain stem in association with expanding supratentorial mass lesions. Duret hemorrhages typically involve the basis pontis rostral to the level of the trigeminal nerve roots (Figs. 4–6F and 4–6G). The Duret hemorrhages arise from vessels entering the brain stem from the basilar artery. These penetrating vessels are kinked and torn when the brain stem moves caudally in relation to the basilar artery.

REFERENCES

Adams JH: Head Injury. In Adams JH, Corsellis JAN, Duchen LW (eds): Greenfield's Neuropathology, 4th ed. New York, Wiley, 1984, chap 3, pp 85-124.

Adams JH, Graham DI, Murray LS, Scott G: Diffuse axonal injury due to nonmissile head injury in humans: An analysis of 45 cases. Ann Neurol 1982; 12:557-563.

Gennarelli TA, Thibault LE, Adams JH, et al: Diffuse axonal injury and traumatic coma in the primate. Ann Neurol 1982; 12:564-574.

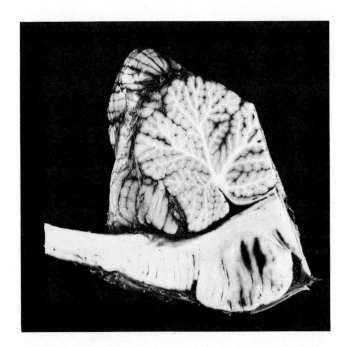

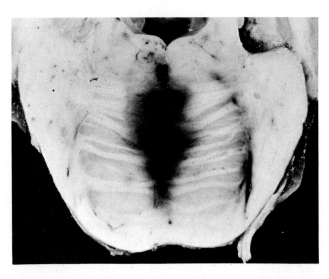

Figure 4–6G. Transverse section of brain stem showing a Duret hemorrhage in the basis pontis secondary to expanding supratentorial mass lesion.

Figure 4–6F. Sagittal section of brain stem showing brain stem hemorrhages secondary to an expanding supratentorial mass lesion (so-called Duret hemorrhages).

4.7 Diffuse Axonal Injury

Delayed Death

CLINICAL

This 18-year-old woman was involved in a motor vehicle accident and was unconscious at the scene. Her left pupil measured 6 mm and was nonreactive while the right pupil measured 4 mm and was reactive to light. Bilateral temporal burr holes were performed but no epidural hematomas were encountered. Computerized tomography disclosed subarachnoid and intraventricular blood but no intraparenchymal hematomas. The patient remained in a vegetative state until her death 10 days later.

PATHOLOGY

Examination of the brain revealed a small amount of subarachnoid blood, maximal over the right posterior frontal and parietal lobes (Fig. 4-7A). There were small cortical contusions in the left temporal pole (Fig. 4–7B). Coronal sections of the cerebral hemispheres revealed foci of hemorrhagic necrosis in the corpus callosum and leaves of the septum pellucidum and right fornix (Figs. 4–7C and 4–7D). Sections through the brain stem disclosed additional areas of hemorrhagic necrosis in the mesencephalic tectum and tegmentum (Fig. 4–7B) and in the superior cerebellar peduncles (Fig. 4–7E). Microscopic examination revealed lipid-laden macrophages and scattered reactive axonal swellings (Fig. 4-7F) in and around the foci of necrosis. The reactive axons were better demonstrated in sections stained with the Bodian silver technique. This procedure showed the enlargements to be at the ends of disrupted axons (Fig. 4–7G).

COMMENT

In this patient with diffuse axonal injury, the longer period of survival allowed the histological changes to become more conspicuous. In individuals dying shortly after the injury, perivascular petechial hemorrhages may be the only histological abnormalities. After a few days to weeks, increasing numbers of lipid-laden macrophages and reactive axons can be detected, as in the present case. Eventually, the damaged white matter becomes reduced in volume. This is conspicuously reflected by thinning of the corpus callosum and enlargement of the ventricular system. The atrophy of the brain stem may be accentuated by enlargement of the aqueduct and fourth ventricle.

REFERENCE

Adams JH, Gennarelli TA, Graham DI: Brain damage in non-missile head injury: Observations in man and subhuman primates. In Smith WT, Cavanagh JB (eds): Recent Advances in Neuropathology, Number 2. Edinburgh, Churchill Livingstone, 1982, chap 7, pp 165-190.

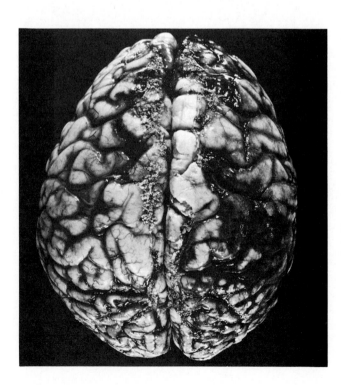

Figure 4–7A. Dorsal surface of brain showing a small amount of subarachnoid hemorrhage.

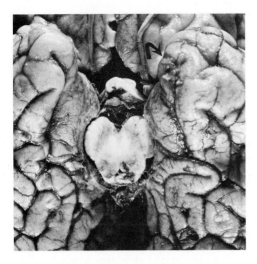

Figure 4–7B. Ventral surface of brain with caudal brain stem and cerebellum removed. Note the contusion of the left temporal lobe (curved arrrow) and foci of hemorrhagic necrosis in the mesencephalic tectum and tegmentum.

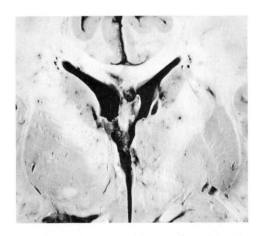

Figure 4–7D. A more caudal coronal section showing foci of hemorrhagic necrosis in the corpus callosum, right fornix, and leaves of septum pellucidum.

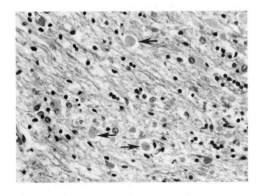

Figure 4–7F. Microscopic section showing multiple reactive axonal swellings that appear as eosinophilic spheroids (arrows).

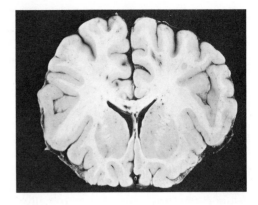

Figure 4–7C. Coronal section showing small foci of hemorrhagic necrosis in the corpus callosum, and minimal cortical contusions.

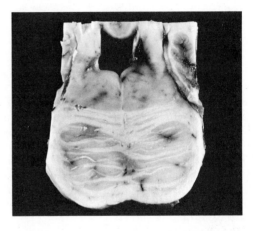

Figure 4–7E. Transverse section of pons showing foci of hemorrhagic necrosis in superior cerebellar peduncles.

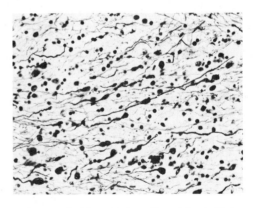

Figure 4–7G. Microscopic section, stained with the Bodian silver technique, showing the reactive axonal swellings at the ends of disrupted axons.

4.8   Vertebral Artery Dissection

Traumatic

CLINICAL

This 75-year-old male pedestrian was struck by a motor vehicle. He had multiple contusions on his face and neck and fractures of both legs. Initially, he was awake and responsive to commands. Computerized tomography showed no intracranial hemorrhage. Subsequently, his cardiorespiratory status deteriorated and he died 3 days after the accident.

PATHOLOGY

Examination of the brain showed no subarachnoid hemorrhage or cerebral contusions. The right vertebral artery, proximal to the origin of the posterior inferior cerebellar artery was distended and discolored. Sections through the proximal right vertebral artery disclosed intramural dissection (Fig. 4–8A) and partial thrombosis. No grossly discernible lesions were evident in the cerebral hemispheres, cerebellum, or brain stem. Histological examination revealed an area of recent infarction in the right dorsolateral quadrant of the medulla (Fig. 4–8B).

COMMENT

A variety of arterial lesions have been attributed to craniocervical trauma. Intramural arterial dissection, with accompanying thrombosis and cerebral infarction, is an uncommon, but well-recognized complication of blunt or penetrating trauma. The carotid arteries are involved more commonly than the vertebral arteries. Vertebro-basilar infarcts due to vertebral artery dissection have been reported following chiropractic manipulation of the neck. However, it should be noted that arterial dissections in both the carotid

and vertebro-basilar systems can also occur without any recognized trauma. Occasionally, partial laceration of an extracranial or intracranial artery will lead to dilatation of the damaged segment, giving rise to a traumatic aneurysm. Laceration of the intracavernous portion of the internal carotid artery may give rise to a carotid–cavernous fistula. This leads to marked engorgement of the ophthalmic veins and eventually blindness from anoxic damage to the eye. Development of clinical manifestations from the fistula may be delayed for several weeks following the trauma. In recent years, laceration of either the intradural or extradural portion of the vertebral arteries has become recognized as an important cause of otherwise unexplained traumatic subarachnoid hemorrhage. Traumatic laceration seems to differ from traumatic dissection of the vertebral artery only in the degree of arterial damage.

REFERENCES

Berger MS, Wilson CB: Intracranial dissecting aneurysms of the posterior circulation. Report of six cases and review of the literature. J Neurosurg 1984; 61:882-894.

Biller J, Hingtgen WL, Adams HP Jr, et al: Cervicocephalic arterial dissections: A ten-year experience. Arch Neurol 1986; 43:1234-1238.

Deck JHN, Jagadha V: Fatal subarachnoid hemorrhage due to traumatic rupture of the vertebral artery. Arch Pathol Lab Med 1986; 110:489-493.

Katirji MB, Reinmuth OM, Latchaw RE: Stroke due to vertebral artery injury. Arch Neurol 1985; 42:242-248.

Kreuger BR, Okazaki H: Vertebral–basilar distribution infarction following chiropractic cervical manipulation. Mayo Clin Proc 1980; 55:322-332.

Sherman MR, Smialek JE, Zane WE: Pathogenesis of vertebral artery occlusion following cervical spine manipulation. Arch Pathol Lab Med 1987; 111:851-853.

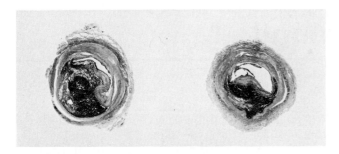

Figure 4–8A. Macrosections of the right vertebral artery showing intramural dissection and partial thrombosis.

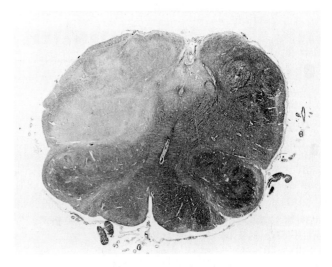

Figure 4–8B. Macrosection of brain stem showing a recent infarct in the right dorsolateral quadrant of the medulla.

4.9 Gunshot Wound

CLINICAL

This 21-year-old man was found slumped on a couch with a contact gunshot entrance wound above his eyebrow. A .22-caliber pistol was at his side.

PATHOLOGY

A parasagittal section of the brain shows the wound tract extending from the inferior surface of the frontal lobe to the vicinity of the parieto-occipital notch where the missile was recovered (Fig. 4–9A).

COMMENT

This is a typical example of a low-velocity gunshot wound of the head. When gunshot wounds of the head are examined, close attention must be paid to the skin and skull injuries as well as the missile tract within the brain. The skin lesions will often provide significant information regarding the proximity of the weapon. If the weapon is distant from the skin surface, the entrance wound may even be smaller than the diameter of the bullet. The skin immediately around the entrance wound will often show a so-called abrasion ring. If the weapon is at close range, the skin surrounding the entrance wound will usually show deposits of soot and grains of unburned powder. With loose contact, the entrance wound in the skin may be irregular or stellate. If the weapon is in tight contact with the head, the skin surface may show marks from the end of the gun barrel and gases will be forced into the subcutaneous tissue. As in this case, there may be little or no soot and powder on the surface of the skin.

Defects in the skull vary in appearance depending on whether they are entrance or exit sites. At the site of entrance, the defect in the outer table of the skull is smaller than the defect in the inner table and there is internal beveling. If the missile perforates the head, the exit wound in the skull will show the opposite features, that is, the defect in the inner table will be smaller than the defect in the outer table and there will be external beveling.

The tissue destruction resulting from the passage of a bullet through the brain is determined to a greater extent by the velocity of the missile rather than its mass, since the energy transfer is proportional to the velocity squared. In the case of low velocity, civilian weapons, the tract through the brain is often of relatively uniform diameter. The center of the tract contains a variable quantity of blood and fragmented tissue. The brain tissue immediately surrounding the wound tract is contused and discolored. Fragments of bone and foreign material may act as secondary missiles producing additional wound tracts. The sudden increase in intracranial pressure during the passage of the bullet may cause herniation and contusions remote from the wound tract. Sites of predilection for the contusions include the unci and cerebellar tonsils. The sudden pressure against the floor of the frontal fossa may lead to fractures of the orbital plates even when the wound tract is far removed from these structures.

In this case, the bullet had produced a penetrating wound of the head inasmuch as it entered, but did not pass through the head. If the bullet had passed completely through the head, the injury would have been described as a perforating wound of the head. In some cases of penetrating wounds, the bullet is deflected and continues its passage in another direction. This is referred to as "internal ricochet." Figure 4–9B is an oblique section of a brain that illustrates this phenomenon. The bullet entered low on the right and passed upward and to the left through the frontal lobes. After striking the dura on the left, the bullet ricocheted and its path continued caudally along the dorso-lateral surface of the left cerebral hemisphere.

REFERENCES

Freytag E: Autopsy findings in head injuries from firearms. Statistical evaluation of 254 cases. Arch Pathol 1963; 76:215-225.

Rose EF: Medicolegal autopsy of gunshot wound victims. In Race GR (ed): Laboratory Medicine. Hagerstown, Md, Harper & Row, 1973, vol 3, chap 13A-2, pp 21-36.

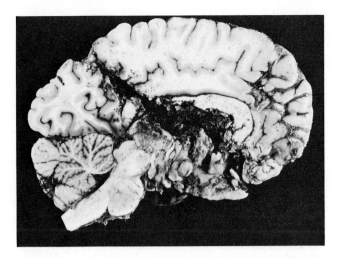

Figure 4–9A. Parasagittal section of brain showing a gunshot wound tract extending from the inferior surface of the left frontal lobe to the vicinity of the parieto-occipital notch.

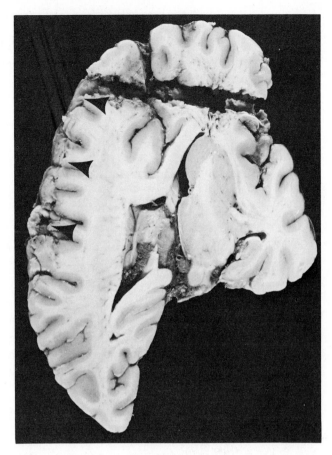

Figure 4–9B. Oblique section of brain showing a gunshot wound tract traversing the frontal lobes, followed by internal ricochet along the surface of the left frontal lobe (arrowheads).

4.10 Traumatic Myelomalacia

Acute

CLINICAL

This 16-year-old boy dove into shallow water. He immediately complained of neck pain and was quadriplegic. On examination, he was found to have a C5–C6 sensory level to touch and pinprick. A fracture–dislocation was demonstrated radiologically. The patient had a cardiac arrest and died a few days later.

PATHOLOGY

The ventral surface of the spinal cord showed a short segment of discoloration and focal compression at the level of the fracture (Fig. 4–10A). A longitudinal section of the spinal cord (Fig. 4–10B) showed that this area of traumatic myelomalacia (upper lesion) was much more extensive than was evident from the exterior. In addition, there was a second, smaller area of myelomalacia in the thoracic spinal cord (lower lesion).

COMMENT

Traumatic myelomalacia frequently results from severe fracture – dislocation injuries of the spine. In the cervical spine, these are most commonly encountered at the C5–C6 level following hyperflexion injuries. Fracture–dislocations of the lower thoracic and lumbar spine are more commonly the result of crushing injuries. The degree of spinal cord injury varies from minimal contusion to complete transection. As in the present case, cord injuries may occur at several levels. Although the external evidence of injury may be quite focal, the hemorrhagic necrosis in the interior of the spinal cord may extend for a considerable distance above and below the point of compression. Figures 4–10C through 4–10E illustrate a lumbar cord injury resulting from a fall. Although the exterior of the spinal cord showed only irregular swelling and faint discoloration of the dorsal surface, transverse sections showed extensive myelomalacia involving especially the spinal gray matter.

In the civilian population, penetrating lesions of the spinal cord from stabbings or gunshot wounds are less common than crushing injuries associated with fracture–dislocations. Figure 4–10F shows a shotgun pellet embedded in the spinal cord.

REFERENCES

Bailey FW: Trauma of the spinal cord. In Minckler J (ed): Pathology of the Nervous System. New York, McGraw-Hill, 1971, vol 2, chap 134, pp 1765-1774.

Hughes JT: Disorders of the spine and spinal cord. In Adams JH, Corsellis JAN, Duchen LW (eds): Greenfield's Neuropathology, 4th ed. New York, Wiley, 1984, chap 17, pp 779-806.

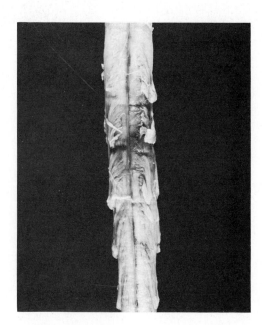

Figure 4–10A. Ventral surface of the spinal cord showing a focal area of compression and discoloration at the level of the fracture–dislocation.

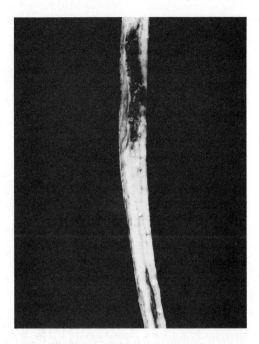

Figure 4–10B. Sagittal section of the spinal cord showing hemorrhage and traumatic myelomalacia (upper lesion) at the level noted externally. In addition, there is a second, smaller area of myelomalacia in the thoracic cord (lower lesion).

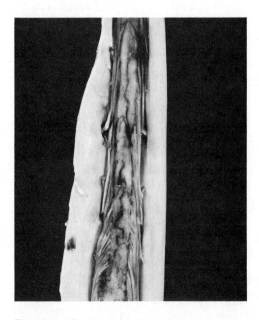

Figure 4–10D. Dorsal surface of lumbosacral spinal cord showing swelling and mild discoloration.

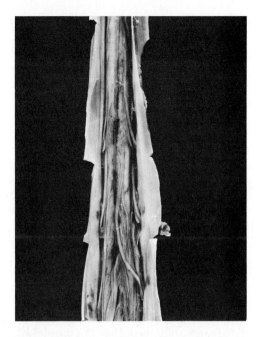

Figure 4–10C. Ventral surface of lumbosacral spinal cord showing only minimal swelling and discoloration.

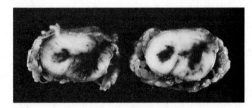

Figure 4–10E. Transverse sections of spinal cord illustrated in Figures 4–10C and 4–10D. Note the extensive traumatic myelomalacia that was barely perceptible from the exterior of the spinal cord.

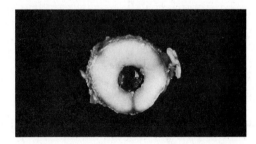

Figure 4–10F. Transverse section of spinal cord with a shotgun pellet. This was found adjacent to a shotgun wound that had transected the spinal cord.

4.11 Spinal Cord Trauma

Remote

CLINICAL

This 24-year-old woman suffered a burst fracture of the C5 vertebral body in a motorcycle accident and was left essentially quadriplegic. She died of pneumonia approximately 1 year later.

PATHOLOGY

The lower cervical spinal cord contained a markedly flattened segment (Fig. 4–11A). A sagittal section through this area showed almost complete transection of the cord with an intervening cyst (Fig. 4–11B). Histological examination disclosed small neuromas within the wall of the cyst. The cyst was bounded by gliotic neural parenchyma and fibrous tissue (Fig. 4–11C).

COMMENT

During the relatively prolonged period of survival, the necrotic spinal cord parenchyma was removed by phagocytosis, leaving behind a cystic cavity. This was accompanied by a moderate amount of fibrous scarring of the meninges. The less severely damaged portions of the spinal cord immediately above and below the site of injury showed the expected loss of neurons and gliosis. The neuromas are similar to traumatic neuromas that develop in peripheral nerves. They are thought to arise from aberrant regeneration of the centrally directed processes of dorsal root ganglia or disrupted ventral roots. The nerve fibers are ensheathed by myelin that has the staining characteristics of peripheral nerve myelin. Other patients with prolonged survival following severe spinal cord trauma may develop posttraumatic syringomyelia.

In the past, obstetrical trauma occasionally resulted in spinal cord injuries. These were usually the result of excess traction during forceps deliveries and generally involved term infants. Figures 4–11D and 4–11E illustrate a case of nearly complete cervical cord disruption in an infant. The infant had been postmature and was delivered following a midforceps rotation. The infant survived for 2 months, during which time he was quadriplegic and maintained on a respirator.

REFERENCES

Hughes JT: Disorders of the spine and spinal cord. In Adams JH, Corsellis JAN, Duchen LW (eds): Greenfield's Neuropathology, 4th ed. New York, Wiley, 1984, chap 17, pp 779-806.

Schwartz P: Birth injuries. In Minckler J (ed): Pathology of the Nervous System. New York, McGraw-Hill, 1971, vol 2, chap 135, pp 1774-1806.

Sung JH, Mastri AR, Chen KTK: Aberrant peripheral nerves and neuromas in normal and injured spinal cords. J Neuropathol Exp Neurol 1981; 40:551-565.

Wolman L: Post-traumatic regeneration of nerve fibres in the human spinal cord and its relation to intramedullary neuroma. J Pathol Bact 1967; 94:123-129.

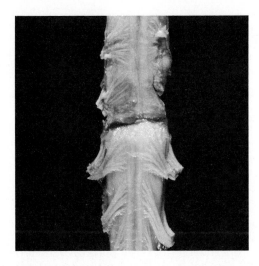

Figure 4–11A. Ventral surface of spinal cord showing an area of remote traumatic injury. This was adjacent to the site of a vertebral body fracture that had been sustained 1 year previously.

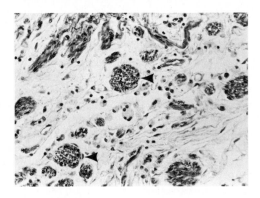

Figure 4–11C. Microscopic section showing small neuromas (arrowheads) within the wall of the cyst shown in Figure 4–11B.

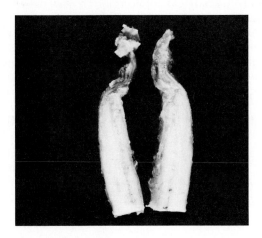

Figure 4–11E. Sagittal section of the spinal cord shown in Figure 4–11D.

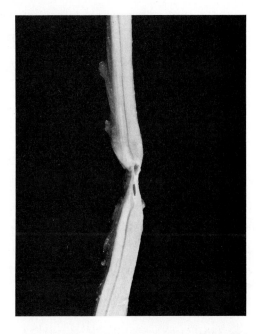

Figure 4–11B. Sagittal section of spinal cord showing the area of partially cystic, remote myelomalacia.

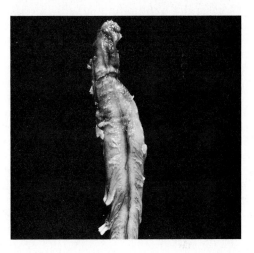

Figure 4–11D. Ventral surface of spinal cord from an infant who suffered nearly complete disruption of the cervical spinal cord at the time of delivery.

4.12 Sequelae Of Surgical Procedures

Optic Nerve Atrophy
Psychosurgery
Thalamotomies

CLINICAL

This 43-year-old man died following coronary artery bypass surgery. As a youth, his right eye had been enucleated.

PATHOLOGY

Examination of the brain showed the right optic nerve (Figs. 4–12A and 4–12B) to be markedly atrophic and less than one half the size of the left optic nerve. A macrosection of the chiasm, stained for myelin (Fig. 4–12C), showed demyelination of the atrophic nerve except for a small area immediately distal to the chiasm. This region corresponded to the genu of Wilbrand. By contrast, the optic tracts were of equal size and heavily stained. Grossly, no abnormalities were evident in the lateral geniculate bodies (Fig. 4–12D); however, microscopically they showed atrophy and loss of the neurons in selected layers. Figure 4–12E illustrates the neuronal loss and atrophy of the few remaining large neurons in layer 1 of the left lateral geniculate body.

COMMENT

Axons arising from retinal ganglion cells in the temporal half of the retina pass through the optic nerve and ipsilateral optic tract to the lateral geniculate body. By contrast, the axons arising from retinal ganglion cells in the nasal half of the retina decussate in the chiasm before continuing caudally in the contralateral optic tract. In addition, some of the fibers from the inferior nasal portion of the retina turn rostrally for a short distance in the contralateral optic nerve before projecting caudally in the optic tract to the lateral geniculate body. These fibers comprise the so-called genu of Wilbrand. Thus, enucleation of the eye eventually leads to axonal degeneration and demyelination of the ipsilateral optic nerve, sparing only fibers in the genu of Wilbrand from the contralateral eye.

The neurons in the lateral geniculate bodies are arranged in six distinct laminae. Normally, the neurons in the outer two laminae are considerably larger than the neurons in the deeper laminae. Neurons in layers 2, 3, and 5 receive input from the ipsilateral eye while the neurons in layers 1, 4, and 6 receive input from the contralateral eye. Following the loss of afferent fibers, the lateral geniculate neurons undergo transsynaptic degeneration. Initially, this is manifested by a reduction in size; later there is also a reduction in the number of neurons. These alterations are most readily seen among the neurons in the outer two magnocellular layers. Axons from the lateral geniculate neurons project through the optic radiations to the visual cortex. No changes are evident by routine histological techniques in the visual cortex following enucleation of the eye.

Other surgical procedures that result in grossly distinctive lesions include psychosurgical operations and thalamotomies. Various surgical techniques had been devised to isolate portions of the frontal lobes, especially the medial orbital cortex, by disrupting cortical projections. Although the use of psychosurgery has been largely superseded by drug therapy,

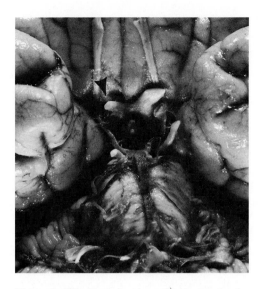

Figure 4–12A. Ventral surface of brain showing the atrophic right optic nerve (arrowhead).

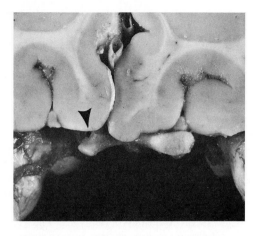

Figure 4–12B. Coronal section, viewed from the front, showing the atrophic right optic nerve (arrowhead).

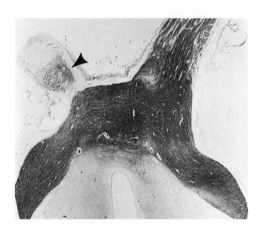

Figure 4–12C. Macrosection of optic nerves and chiasm showing demyelination of the atrophic right optic nerve except for fibers within the genu of Wilbrand (arrowhead).

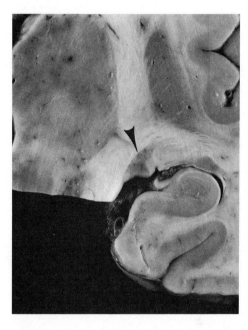

Figure 4–12D. Coronal section showing the grossly normal appearance of the right lateral geniculate body.

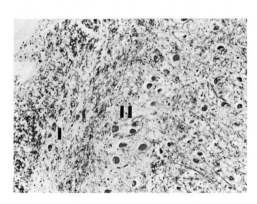

Figure 4–12E. Microsection of left lateral geniculate body showing loss of neurons from the first layer (I) in contrast to the normal neuronal population of the second layer (II).

the residua of these procedures are occasionally encountered in autopsy specimens. Figure 4–12F is from a patient with a long-standing history of psychiatric illness. A transorbital psychosurgical procedure had been performed in the remote past. There were surgical defects on the inferior surface of each frontal lobe. Horizontal sections of the cerebral hemispheres disclosed irregular cavities in the frontal white matter adjacent to the caudate nuclei.

Various types of thalamotomies have been performed to treat movement disorders and to provide relief from intractable pain. Figure 4–12G illustrates the lesions produced by recent bilateral electrolytic thalamotomies. Each of the lesions consists of a discrete focus of coagulative necrosis. Figure 4–12H shows a spherical lesion in the left thalamus produced by cryogenic thalamotomy. This procedure had been performed for the treatment of a movement disorder in a woman with multiple sclerosis.

REFERENCES

Bond MR: Psychosurgery. In Critchley M, O'Leary JL, Jennett B (eds): Scientific Foundations of Neurology. Philadelphia, Davis, 1972, Section VI, chap 9, pp 227-232.

Brodal A: Neurological Anatomy in Relation to Clinical Medicine, 3rd ed. New York, Oxford University Press, 1981, chap 8, pp 578-601.

Lindenberg R, Walsh FB, Sacks JG: Neuropathology of Vision: An Atlas. Philadelphia, Lea & Febiger, 1973.

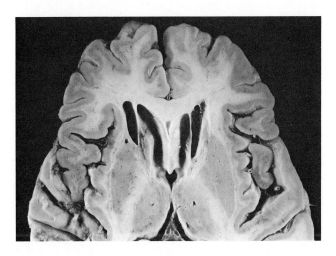

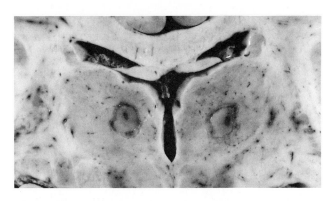

Figure 4–12G. Coronal section showing lesions produced by recent bilateral electrolytic thalamotomies.

Figure 4–12F. Horizontal section of the brain showing the cystic lesions remaining from a transorbital psychosurgical procedure performed many years previously.

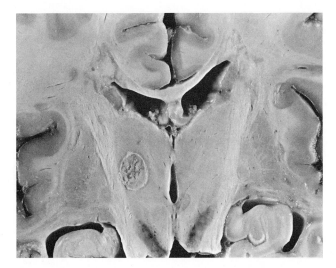

Figure 4–12H. Coronal section showing lesion produced by cryogenic thalamotomy in a woman with multiple sclerosis. Note the demyelinated plaques about the lateral angles of the lateral ventricles.

5

Intoxications and Deficiency States

5.1   Asphyxia

CLINICAL

This 30-year-old woman died acutely from asphyxia.

PATHOLOGY

Externally the brain showed edema, manifested by swelling of gyri and narrowing of sulci. Coronal sections of the cerebral hemispheres disclosed swelling of the subcortical and central white matter (Fig. 5–1). The cortex had a dusky discoloration secondary to congestion.

COMMENT

Cerebral hypoxia, the inadequate supply of oxygen to the metabolically active brain, has been described in a variety of somewhat overlapping categories.

- Ischemic or oligemic hypoxia result from interrupted or reduced supply of blood to all or part of the brain.
- Anoxic or hypoxic hypoxia result from the absence or reduction of oxygen in the lungs.

- Anemic hypoxia results from reduced blood hemoglobin content or, more commonly, from impaired transport of oxygen, for example, carbon monoxide poisoning.
- Histotoxic hypoxia results from reduced use of oxygen because of toxic interruption of critical enzyme systems, for example, cyanide poisoning.

Almost all forms of cerebral hypoxia are accompanied by impaired cerebral perfusion because of the associated myocardial damage. The brains from asphyxiated individuals reflect effects of both the inadequate oxygenation and cardiac injury. When death occurs acutely, as in the present case, edema and congestion are the principal findings. Only in cases with more prolonged survival will necrosis of the cerebral cortex, hippocampi, basal ganglia, loss of Purkinje cells and demyelination be encountered.

REFERENCE

Brierley JB, Graham DI: Hypoxia and vascular disorders of the central nervous system. In Adams JH, Corsellis JAN, Duchen LW (eds): Greenfield's Neuropathology, 4th ed. New York, Wiley, 1984, chap 4, pp 125-207.

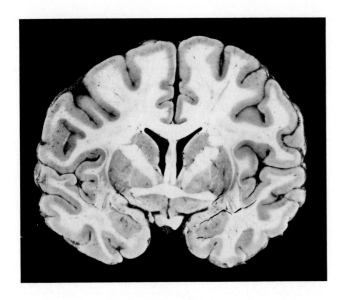

Figure 5-1. Coronal section of brain from a patient who died of acute asphyxia. Note the congestion of the cortex and swelling of the white matter.

5.2   Anoxic Encephalopathy

Delayed Death

CLINICAL

This woman suffered a cardiorespiratory arrest. She remained in a coma until she died 1 year later.

PATHOLOGY

The brain was reduced in weight and externally showed narrowing of gyri and widening of sulci, especially over the parietal and occipital lobes. Horizontal sections of the cerebral hemispheres showed thinning of the cerebral cortex, especially in the parietal and occipital lobes (Fig. 5–2A). The thinning was more marked in the depths of sulci than on the banks and crowns of affected gyri. The basal ganglia, especially the caudate and putamen, were shrunken and focally cavitated (Fig. 5–2B). The cerebral white matter was diffusely reduced in volume and abnormally firm due to secondary gliosis. The hippocampi were reduced in size, altered in color and abnormally firm. The cerebellum showed narrowed, sclerotic folia, atrophic firm white matter, and small central nuclei (Fig. 5–2C).

COMMENT

This specimen vividly demonstrates the effects of severe cerebral hypoxia followed by a prolonged period of survival. The cortical necrosis is typically more severe in the parietal and occipital lobes and may be accentuated in the depths of the sulci. Often the necrosis is more severe in the third, fifth, and sixth layers of the cortex and may result in the formation of a slit-like cavity between the more superficial and deeper layers of the cortex. This is referred to as laminar or pseudolaminar necrosis. The basal ganglia often show maximal damage in the outer portions of the caudate and putamen. This may be accompanied by atrophy or necrosis of the pallidum. Some authors have attempted to correlate pallidal damage with anoxia and cortical, putamenal, and caudate damage with impaired perfusion. The white matter is both partially demyelinated and gliotic. The reduction in volume of the white matter contributes to the ventricular enlargement. The changes in the hippocampi show regional variation in the degree of damage, illustrating one aspect of so-called selective vulnerability. The H1 sector and the end plate are the more severely affected regions, as shown in a macrosection from another case (Fig. 5–2D).

In the cerebellum, loss of Purkinje cells and other neurons, along with proliferation of glia, result in shrunken, sclerotic folia. The deep nuclei often become discolored as they become shrunken.

REFERENCES

Cole G, Cowie VA: Long survival after cardiac arrest: Case report and neuropathological findings. Clin Neuropathol 1987; 6:104-109.

Ginsberg MD, Hedley-Whyte T, Richardson EP Jr: Hypoxic–ischemic leukoencephalopathy in man. Arch Neurol 1976; 33:5-14.

Petito CK, Feldmann E, Pulsinelli WA, Plum F: Delayed hippocampal damage in humans following cardiorespiratory arrest. Neurology 1987; 37:1281-1286.

Raichle ME: The pathophysiology of brain ischemia. Ann Neurol 1983; 13:2-10.

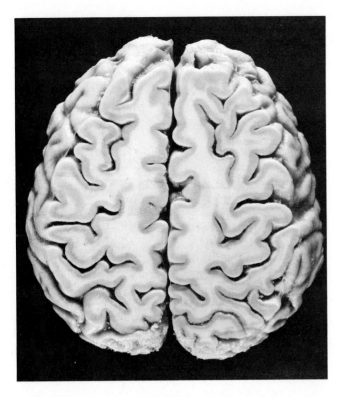

Figure 5–2A. Horizontal section of brain from a patient who survived for 1 year following a cardiac arrest. Note the thinning of the cortex, most pronounced in parietal and occipital lobes.

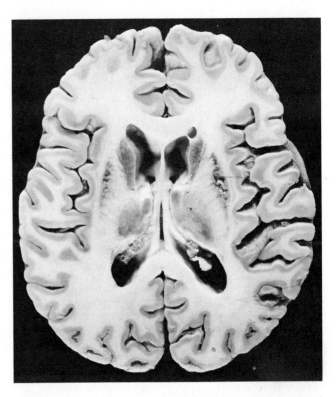

Figure 5–2B. Horizontal section showing shrunken and discolored basal ganglia and thalamus. The putamena are focally cavitated.

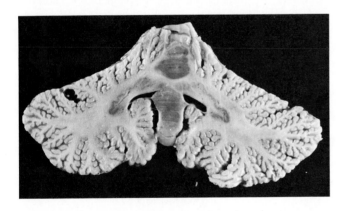

Figure 5–2C. Section of cerebellum showing severe folial sclerosis.

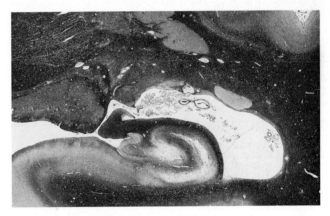

Figure 5–2D. Macrosection showing hypoxic damage most severe in the H1 sector and end plate.

5.3 Carbon Monoxide Intoxication

Acute

CLINICAL

This 49-year-old man was found dead in his automobile with the engine running. There was a leak between the exhaust manifold and the exhaust pipe. At the time of autopsy, the carbon monoxide level was 85 percent saturation.

PATHOLOGY

When fresh, the brain had a "cherry-red" color, reflecting the presence of carboxyhemoglobin in the blood. The red color tends to be leached out during fixation and the formalin often becomes strikingly discolored. Externally, the fixed brain showed cerebral edema with swollen gyri and narrowed sulci. The leptomeningeal vessels were prominently congested and there was a small amount of subarachnoid blood on the dorsal and lateral surfaces of the cerebral hemispheres (Fig. 5–3A). In addition to swelling, coronal sections (Fig. 5–3B) revealed a reddish color in the infolded portions of the cortex, the white matter, the basal ganglia, and, especially, the choroid plexi.

COMMENT

The most striking gross neuropathological feature in patients dying from acute carbon monoxide poisoning is the red color, reflecting the presence of the carboxyhemoglobin. Congestion of meningeal and intraparenchymal blood vessels with or without hemorrhages are common findings. Destructive lesions in the basal ganglia are not seen unless the patient has survived for several days. Acute deaths are often attributed to cardiac involvement. This is supported by electrocardiagraphic evidence of arrhythmias. Even with relatively short survival, myocardial necrosis, especially in the papillary muscles, is a common pathological finding.

REFERENCE

Ginsberg MD: Carbon monoxide. In Spencer PS, Schaumburg HH (eds): Experimental and Clinical Neurotoxicology. Baltimore, Williams & Wilkins, 1980, chap 26, pp 374-394.

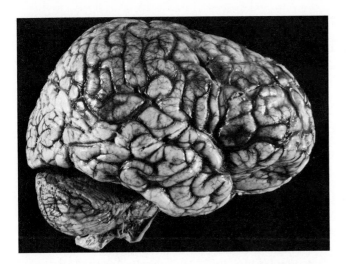

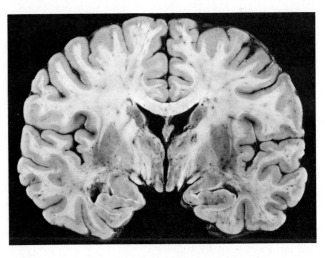

Figure 5–3A. Lateral view of brain from a man who died of acute carbon monoxide intoxication. Note the swelling and congestion of leptomeningeal blood vessels. The specimen had a cherry-red color due to the presence of carboxyhemoglobin.

Figure 5–3B. Coronal section of the brain shows swelling, congestion and reddish discoloration. The basal ganglia are intact.

5.4 Carbon Monoxide Intoxication

Delayed Death

CLINICAL

This man had been working on an automobile in a closed garage.

He was unconscious when found and remained comatose until his death 5 days later. The carbon monoxide level was 38 percent saturation shortly after initiation of resuscitation.

PATHOLOGY

Coronal sections of the cerebral hemispheres revealed bilateral pallidal necrosis (Fig. 5–4A). In this case, the small necrotic areas were faintly discolored and discontinuous.

COMMENT

Although pallidal necrosis is commonly associated with carbon monoxide intoxication, this alteration is seen only when the patient survives for more than 1 or 2 days. Pallidal necrosis can also be seen following delayed death from other causes of hypoxia, for example, anesthetic accidents, drug overdoses, and cardiac arrests. There has been much controversy regarding the pathogenesis of these lesions. Some authors have postulated selective vulnerability on the basis of physiochemical characteristics of the neurons in the pallidum. Other authors have attributed the pallidal damage to impaired perfusion through the pallidal branches of the choroidal arteries. Extension of the necrosis, although less marked, beyond the confines of the pallidum seems to support the latter hypothesis.

Another important pathological feature of delayed deaths from carbon monoxide poisoning is demyelination and necrosis of the cerebral white matter (Figs. 5–4B and 5–4C). Several patterns of white matter damage have been delineated:

- Small perivascular foci of demyelination and necrosis scattered throughout the central white matter, corpus callosum and internal capsules
- Diffuse destruction of the central white matter and corpus callosum. These lesions may extend throughout most of the hemispheres but are more severe near the ventricles and tend to spare the subcortical arcuate fibers
- Plaque-like areas of demyelination and necrosis. These lesions tend to be more severe in the caudal portions of the central white matter but spare the arcuate fibers, corpus callosum, and internal capsules. The latter lesions are the type most often associated with the biphasic clinical course described as Grinker's myelinopathy

White matter lesions have been attributed in part to the direct histotoxic effects of carbon monoxide on the oligodendroglial cells, although they can also result from other causes of cerebral hypoxia and impaired cerebral perfusion. In an experimental study, Ginsberg et al found close correlation between the size of the white matter lesions and the degree of metabolic acidosis and systolic hypotension.

REFERENCES

Brucher JM: Neuropathological problems posed by carbon monoxide poisoning and anoxia. Prog Brain Res 1967; 24:75-100.

Choi IS: Delayed neurologic sequelae in carbon monoxide intoxication. Arch Neurol 1983; 40:433-435.

Ginsberg MD, Myers RE, McDonagh BF: Experimental carbon monoxide encephalopathy in the primate. Arch Neurol 1974; 30:209-216.

Lapresele J, Fardeau M: The central nervous system and carbon monoxide poisoning. II. Anatomical study of brain lesions following intoxication with carbon monoxide (22 cases). Prog Brain Res 1967; 24:31-74.

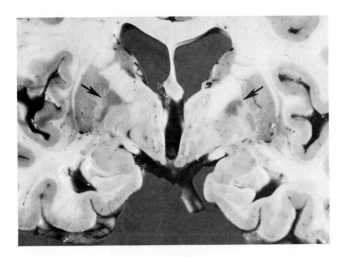

Figure 5–4A. Coronal section of the brain from a man who died 5 days after carbon monoxide intoxication. Note the discolored foci of necrosis in the pallida (arrows).

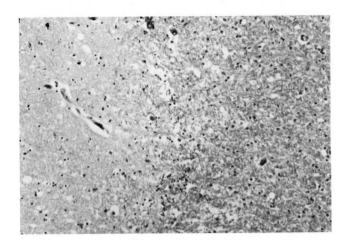

Figure 5–4C. Microscopic section showing the margin of one of the necrotic areas in the white matter.

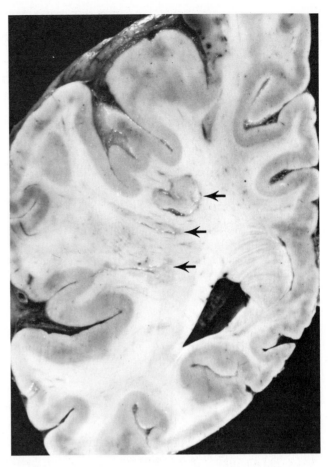

Figure 5–4B. Coronal section of a cerebral hemisphere from a patient who died 6 days after carbon monoxide intoxication. Note the foci of demyelination and necrosis in the white matter (arrows).

5.5   Wernicke's Encephalopathy

Associated with Alcoholism

CLINICAL

This 50-year-old man had a long-standing history of alcohol abuse and a 10-year history of seizures. During the previous 4 years, the seizures had become more frequent and occurred daily during the week prior to admission. He was weak and had been nonambulatory for several days.

On admission, he had a blood pressure of 70/40 mm Hg and was mildly tachypneic. He had a body temperature of 34C and a pulse of 100. Examination of the eyes revealed no abnormalities. The heart and abdomen were normal except for the elevated pulse rate. A chest x-ray revealed consolidation of the left lower lobe. While in the emergency room, the patient suffered a cardiorespiratory arrest.

PATHOLOGY

Coronal sections of the cerebral hemispheres revealed diffusely discolorated, mildly softened mammillary bodies (Fig. 5–5A). Another example from a similar case is shown in Fig. 5–5B. In macroscopic sections, the mammillary bodies appeared extensively demyelinated (Fig. 5–5C). Microscopic examination disclosed unusually prominent dilated capillaries, with swollen endothelial cells, increased numbers of macrophages including some containing hemosiderin, demyelination, decreased numbers of neurons, and mild gliosis (Fig. 5–5D).

COMMENT

Classically, Wernicke's encephalopathy is characterized by an abrupt onset of abnormalities of ocular motility, ataxia, and confusion. Horizontal nystagmus and impairment of lateral gaze are the more common ocular abnormalities. However, in recent years it has become apparent that a significant proportion of patients with Wernicke's encephalopathy do not manifest the full spectrum of symptoms. Despite atypical clinical findings, this patient displayed typical gross and microscopic features of Wernicke's encephalopathy.

Patients with Wernicke's encephalopathy may have grossly detectable lesions in the mammillary bodies, walls of the third ventricle, about the aqueduct, and beneath the floor of the fourth ventricle. The mammillary bodies are the most consistently involved site. In the acute cases, now relatively unusual, lesions in all of these sites may contain petechial hemorrhages. More often, the sites of predilection are merely softened and discolored from nonhemorrhagic necrosis.

The major histopathological changes seem to involve the blood vessels and are manifested by unusually prominent capillaries with swollen endothelial cells. The hemosiderin within some of the perivascular macrophages reflects previous, small hemorrhages. Loss of neurons is often less pronounced than demyelination.

REFERENCES

Harper CG, Giles M, Finlay-Jones R: Clinical signs in the Wernicke-Korsakoff complex: A retrospective analysis of 131 cases diagnosed at necropsy. J Neurol Neurosurg Psychiatry 1986; 49:341-345.

Reuler JB, Girard DE, Cooney TG: Current Concepts: Wernicke's encephalopathy. N Engl J Med 1985; 312: 1035-1039.

Torvik A: Topographic distribution and severity of brain lesions in Wernicke's encephalopathy. Clin Neuropathol 1987; 6:25-29.

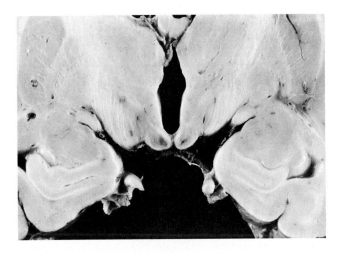

Figure 5–5A. Coronal section showing discolored and focally softened mammillary bodies in a patient with Wernicke's encephalopathy.

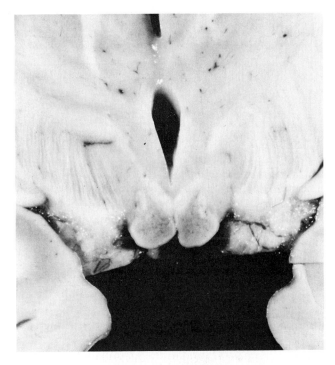

Figure 5–5B. Diffusely discolored and softened mammillary bodies from another case of Wernicke's encephalopathy.

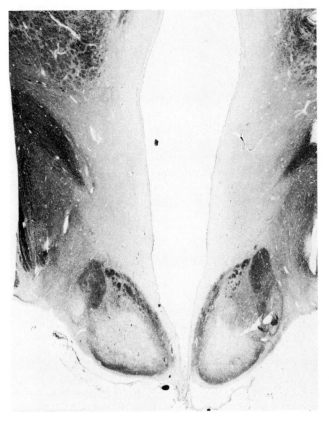

Figure 5–5C. Macrosection showing demyelination and partial necrosis of mammillary bodies.

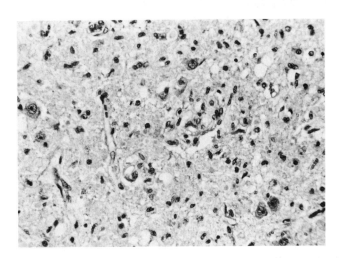

Figure 5–5D. Microscopic section of mammillary body from patient with Wernicke's encephalopathy showing prominent capillaries, macrophages, and gliosis but relatively well preserved neurons.

5.6   Wernicke's Encephalopathy

Complicating Parenteral Nutrition

CLINICAL

This 29-year-old woman had nasopharyngeal carcinoma for which she had received radiation and chemotherapy. During her terminal illness she became acutely confused and eventually comatose. She had been maintained on intravenous fluids.

PATHOLOGY

Sections of the brain revealed hemorrhagic lesions in the mammillary bodies (Fig. 5–6A), walls of the third ventricle (Fig. 5–6B), beneath the floor of the fourth ventricle (Fig. 5–6C), and in the medullary tegmentum (Fig. 5–6D).

COMMENT

This case illustrates the development of acute Wernicke's encephalopathy in a patient while on total parenteral nutrition. Patients with acute Wernicke's encephalopathy are often stuporous or comatose, obscuring the other more characteristic features of the disease. Wernicke's encephalopathy has also been reported in infants on total parenteral nutrition and as a complication of hemodialysis.

Wernicke's encephalopathy is due to thiamine deficiency. Thiamine is an essential cofactor for several enzymes involved in carbohydrate metabolism, including the pyruvate dehydrogenase complex, alpha-ketoglutarate dehydrogenase, and transketolase. Although Wernicke's encephalopathy is encountered most commonly in alcoholics, it may result from other causes of thiamine deficiency, including persistent vomiting, dialysis, or inadequate parenteral nutrition.

REFERENCES

Haid RW, Gutmann L, Crosby TW: Wernicke–Korsakoff encephalopathy after gastric plication. JAMA 1982; 247:2566-2567.

Jagadha V, Deck JHN, Halliday WC, Smyth HS: Wernicke's encephalopathy in patients on peritoneal dialysis or hemodialysis. Ann Neurol 1987; 21:78-84.

Nadel AM, Burger PC: Wernicke encephalopathy following prolonged intravenous therapy. JAMA 1976; 235:2403-2405.

Oczkowski WJ, Kertesz A: Wernicke's encephalopathy after gastroplasty for morbid obesity. Neurology 1985; 35:99-101.

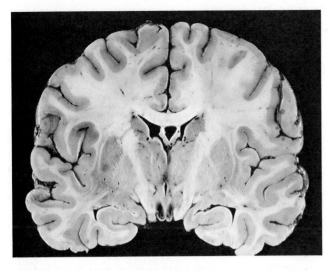

Figure 5–6A. Acute Wernicke's encephalopathy with petechial hemorrhages in mammillary bodies.

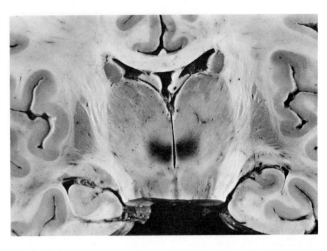

Figure 5–6B. Acute Wernicke's encephalopathy with hemorrhagic discoloration of walls of the third ventricle.

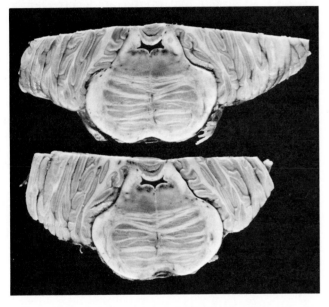

Figure 5–6C. Acute Wernicke's encephalopathy with small petechiae in pontine tegmentum beneath the fourth ventricle.

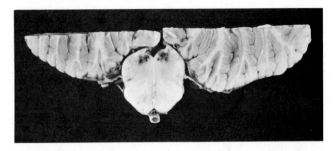

Figure 5–6D. Acute Wernicke's encephalopathy with petechial hemorrhages in medullary tegmentum.

5.7 Cerebellar Vermal Atrophy

Associated with Alcoholism

CLINICAL

This 51-year-old known alcohol abuser was found dead. General autopsy disclosed micronodular cirrhosis and alcoholic hepatitis. His postmortem blood alcohol level was 0.34 g/dL.

PATHOLOGY

Examination of the cerebellum disclosed atrophy of the anteriomedial portion of the superior surface and especially the vermis. The vermal atrophy is best seen in sagittal section where the preferential involvement of the rostral portion of the vermis is evident (Fig. 5–7A). The atrophy of the adjacent portions of the cerebellar hemisphere is seen in Fig. 5–7B. Similar vermal atrophy from another case is shown in Figure 5–7C.

COMMENT

Atrophy of the rostral vermis and adjacent portions of the superior surface of the cerebellum occurs commonly in patients with chronic alcoholism. This may be an isolated lesion or associated with other alcohol-related lesions such as Wernicke's encephalopathy. In the more severely affected areas, there is atrophy of the molecular layer, loss of Purkinje cells, and a variable loss of internal granular layer cells. The neuronal loss is accompanied by gliosis with proliferation of the Bergmann glia. The clinical manifestations attributed to this lesion include truncal instability, leg ataxia, and a wide-based gait. The atrophy can be demonstrated antemortem by computerized tomography.

In the past, cerebellar vermal atrophy has been attributed to the toxic effects of alcohol or to associated nutritional deficiencies with alcohol serving as a predisposing factor. More recently, experimental studies have suggested that overly rapid correction of hyponatremia may be responsible for this lesion as well as central pontine myelinolysis.

REFERENCES

Kleinschmidt-DeMasters BK, Norenberg MD: Cerebellar degeneration in the rat following rapid correction of hyponatremia. Ann Neurol 1981; 10:561-565.

Koller WC, Glatt SL, Perlik S, et al: Cerebellar atrophy demonstrated by computed tomography. Neurology 1981; 31:405-412.

Valsamis MP, Mancall E: Toxic cerebellar degeneration. Hum Pathol 1973; 4:513-520.

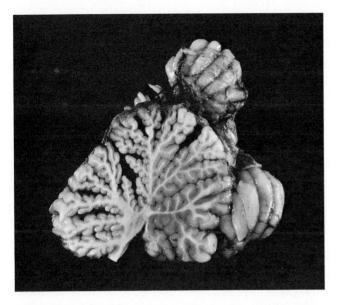

Figure 5–7A. Superior vermal atrophy in an alcoholic patient.

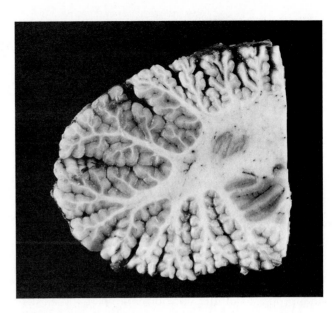

Figure 5–7B. The vermal atrophy is accompanied by atrophy of the adjacent portions of the cerebellar hemisphere.

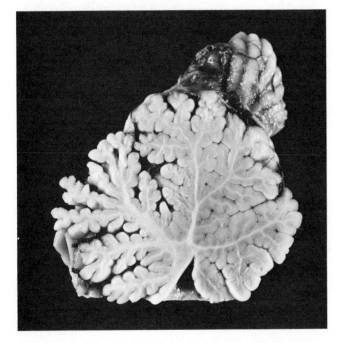

Figure 5–7C. Another example of superior vermal atrophy in an alcoholic patient.

5.8   Central Pontine Myelinolysis

Associated with Alcoholism

CLINICAL

This 59-year-old man with chronic alcoholism had been admitted to a detoxification unit where he began having generalized seizures. He was intubated and transferred to a medical intensive care unit because of respiratory distress. At the time of transfer, he was described as postictal with dysconjugate gaze and hyporeflexia. His serum sodium was 105 mEq/L. The hyponatremia was attributed to the syndrome of inappropriate antidiuretic hormone secretion (SIADH) and he was treated with normal saline, fluid restriction, and eventually oxytetracycline. He died from bronchopneumonia 3 weeks after admission.

PATHOLOGY

Transverse sections of the brain stem demonstrated the central portion of the basis pontis to be slightly softened and granular in texture (Fig. 5–8A). There was no discoloration, swelling, or cavitation. Macrosections disclosed central demyelination with relative preservation of the pontine tegmentum and periphery of the basis pontis (Fig. 5–8B). There were numerous lipid-laden macrophages in the demyelinated area; however, neurons were well preserved (Fig. 5–8C).

COMMENT

The clinical and pathological features of central pontine myelinolysis were originally described by Adams, Victor, and Mancall. Three of their four cases were alcoholics, and all were severely malnourished. Patients with central pontine myelinolysis display a wide range of clinical manifestations, depending in part on the size and location of the lesion. Some of the patients are asymptomatic while others display pseudocoma, pseudobulbar palsy, or quadriparesis. Often signs and symptoms that might be referable to the pontine demyelination are obscured by coma from associated disease. Formerly, many of the cases were undiagnosed until autopsy. More recently, the diagnosis has been established antemortem by computerized tomography and magnetic resonance imaging.

The demyelinated areas tend to involve the central portion of the basis pontis. Some have a roughly diamond or "T" shape, as shown in a microsection from another case (Fig. 5–8D). They range from small focal lesions to very large lesions that involve almost the entire cross section of the basis pontis. Characteristically, the tegmentum is relatively preserved and there is at least a thin rim of intact myelin at the periphery of the pons. These features, along with the preservation of the pontine neurons, help to distinguish central pontine myelinolysis from multiple sclerosis and pontine infarcts.

REFERENCES

Adams RD, Victor M, Mancall EL: Central pontine myelinolysis: A hitherto undescribed disease occuring in alcoholic and malnourished patients. Arch Neurol Psychiatry 1959; 81:154-172.

DeWitt LD, Buonanno FS, Kistler JP, et al: Central pontine myelinolysis: Demonstration by nuclear magnetic resonance. Neurology 1984; 34:570-576.

Gerber O, Geller M, Stiller J, Yang W: Central pontine myelinolysis: Resolution shown by computed tomography. Arch Neurol 1983; 40:116-118.

Thompson DS, Hutton JT, Stears JC, et al: Computerized tomography in the diagnosis of central and extrapontine myelinolysis. Arch Neurol 1981; 38:243-246.

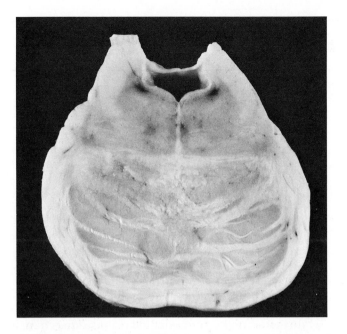

Figure 5–8A. Transverse section of pons showing central area of softening and discoloration due to central pontine myelinolysis.

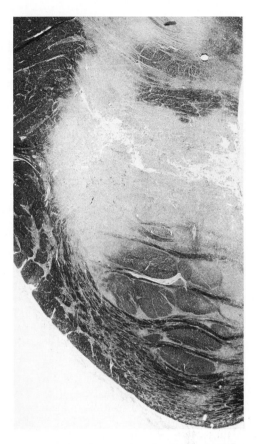

Figure 5–8B. Macrosection showing central pontine myelinolysis with preservation of the periphery of the basis pontis.

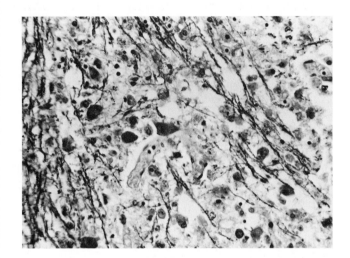

Figure 5–8C. Microscopic section showing demyelination, infiltration with macrophages, and relative preservation of neurons.

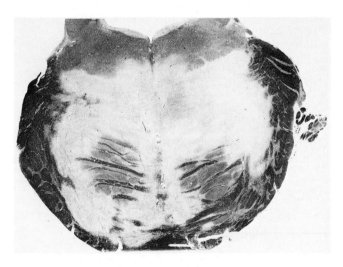

Figure 5–8D. Macrosection showing extensive demyelination in another case of central pontine myelinolysis.

5.9   Central Pontine Myelinolysis

Nonalcoholic Patient

CLINICAL

This 54-year-old woman was admitted to a hospital with gastritis, dehydration, and electrolyte imbalance presumably related to the use of thiazide diuretics for hypertension. Initially she was obtunded, responding only to painful stimuli. Laboratory studies revealed a serum sodium of 104 mEq/L. She was treated with normal saline and dopamine for hypotension. She became oliguric and remained comatose until her death 11 days after admission.

PATHOLOGY

Sagittal section of the brain stem disclosed a poorly defined, softened area in the basis pontis that extended rostrally to the ponto-mesencephalic junction and caudally to the ponto-medullary junction (Fig. 5–9A). A narrow band of tissue with a normal consistency remained at the periphery of the pons. Macrosections of the pons disclosed extensive demyelination (Fig. 5–9B). Microscopic examination disclosed numerous lipid-laden macrophages, small numbers of perivascular mononuclear cells, and relatively well preserved neurons.

COMMENT

Although many cases of central pontine myelinolysis have occurred in malnourished and alcoholic patients, these factors are no longer regarded as the immediate cause of the disease. Currently, central pontine myelinolysis is attributed to the overly rapid correction of chronic hyponatremia or the presence of severe hyperosmolality.

It has been postulated that the demyelination is due to edema that results from osmotic vascular injury. The selective involvement of the ventral pons has been attributed to the detrimental effect of edema within the grid-like anatomic structure formed by transverse and longitudinal myelinated fibers with interposed gray matter. In some cases, there are also extrapontine lesions in the internal and external capsules, striatum, thalami, lateral geniculate bodies, and white matter of the cerebellar folia. These areas have a similar admixture of gray and white matter.

REFERENCES

Goldman JE, Horoupian DS: Demyelination of the lateral geniculate nucleus in central pontine myelinolysis. Ann Neurol 1981; 9:185-189.

McKee AC, Winkelman MD, Banker BQ: Central pontine myelinolysis in severely burned patients: Relationship to serum hyperosmolality. Neurology 1988; 38:1211-1217.

Norenberg MD: A hypothesis of osmotic endothelial injury: A pathogenetic mechanism in central pontine myelinolysis. Arch Neurol 1983; 40:66-69.

Norenberg MD, Papendick RE: Chronicity of hyponatremia as a factor in experimental myelinolysis. Ann Neurol 1984; 15:544-547.

Sterns RH, Riggs JE, Schochet SS Jr: Osmotic demyelination syndrome following correction of hyponatremia. N Engl J Med 1986; 314:1535-1542.

Wright DG, Laureno R, Victor M: Pontine and extrapontine myelinolysis. Brain 1979; 102:361-385.

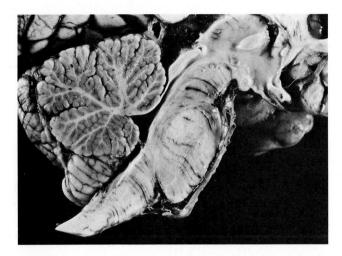

Figure 5–9A. Sagittal section showing softening and discoloration of the central portion of the pons in a nonalcoholic patient with central pontine myelinolysis.

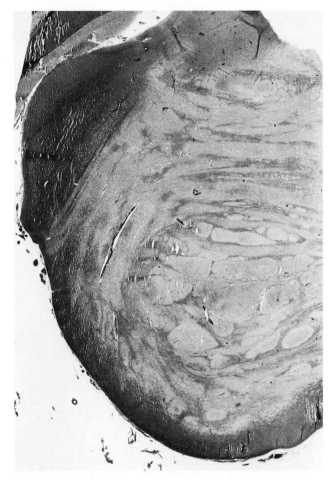

Figure 5–9B. Macrosection showing extensive demyelination of the central portion of the pons. Note the relative preservation of the periphery of the basis pontis.

5.10 Methanol Intoxication

CLINICAL

This 62-year-old man ingested 8 oz of a heating agent that contained 85 percent methanol. When found 1 hour later, he was drowsy and disoriented. Vision was reduced to counting fingers. He was treated with intravenous fluids, ethanol, and bicarbonate but died 7 days after the ingestion.

PATHOLOGY

Coronal sections of the cerebral hemispheres revealed bilateral areas of hemorrhagic necrosis involving the putamena, external capsules, and claustra (Fig. 5–10A). The optic nerves, tracts, and cerebral white matter were grossly intact.

COMMENT

There is wide variation in individual susceptibility to methanol. Although blindness may follow the ingestion of as little as 4 mL, the usual lethal dose is in the range of 100 to 250 mL. The methanol itself causes depression of the central nervous system. However, the more serious sequelae are caused by the formaldehyde and formates that are produced as the methanol is oxidized by hepatic alcohol dehydrogenase. The formates inhibit cellular respiration contributing to the systemic acidosis and blindness.

Although older reports attributed the blindness to degeneration of the retinal ganglion cells and photoreceptors, more recent studies have emphasized retrolaminar demyelination and necrosis. These are attributed to impaired axonal transport in the distal optic nerve.

Pathological changes in the brain include edema and, when death is delayed, necrosis of the putamena, external capsules, and claustra. The initial involvement is in the lateral portion of the putamen. The putamenal lesions typically become hemorrhagic while the necrotic external capsules and claustra remain ischemic. Patients with prolonged survival may show cystic degeneration of the lateral ganglionic structures and areas of necrosis in the white matter of the cerebrum and cerebellum. Both the ganglionic and white matter lesions have been demonstrated antemortem by computerized tomography.

Ethylene glycol, a major component of certain antifreezes and coolants, is another alcohol that is responsible for occasional deaths. Initially, this dihydroxy alcohol causes mild central nervous system depression. However, it is oxidized to various aldehydes and eventually oxalic acid. These catabolites are considerably more toxic than the parent compound. Ethylene glycol intoxication is accompanied by a wide variety of neurological complications, including meningismus, seizures, ocular abnormalities, and cranial nerve palsies. Death is usually the result of renal failure or cardiopulmonary toxicity.

The most distinctive pathological changes result from the combination of oxalic acid with ionic calcium to form insoluble calcium oxalate crystals. These can be seen in various body fluids and tissues including the urine, kidneys, and brain. In the nervous system, the crystals are typically encountered in the walls of blood vessels and surrounding perivascular spaces where they may be accompanied by an inflammatory cell response (Fig. 5–10B).

REFERENCES

Berger JR, Ayyar DR: Neurological complications of ethylene glycol intoxication: Report of a case. Arch Neurol 1981; 38:724-726.

McLean DR, Jacobs H, Mielke BW: Methanol poisoning: A clinical and pathological study. Ann Neurol 1980; 8:161-167.

Sharpe JA, Hostovsky M, Bilbao JM, Rewcastle NB: Methanol optic neuropathy: A histopathological study. Neurology 1982; 32:1093-1100.

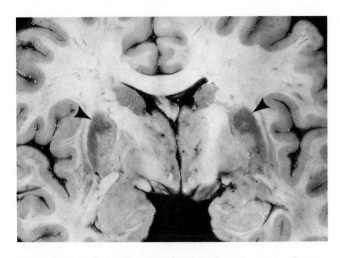

Figure 5–10A. Coronal section showing bilateral putamenal necrosis (arrowheads) due to methanol intoxication.

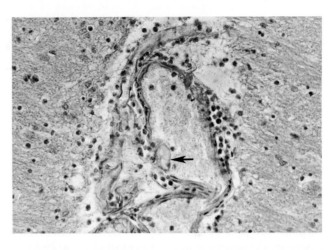

Figure 5–10B. Microscopic section showing calcium oxalate crystal (arrow) and perivascular inflammatory cell infiltrate secondary to ethylene glycol intoxication.

5.11   Epilepsy

Hippocampal Sclerosis
Cerebellar Atrophy

CLINICAL

This 31-year-old woman had had a seizure disorder since the age of 3 when she had meningitis. Over the years, she had been treated with anticonvulsants including phenytoin. She was found dead in bed.

PATHOLOGY

Externally, the cerebrum was unremarkable. On coronal sections, the only abnormality was striking atrophy of the right hippocampal formation (Fig. 5–11A). Microscopically, the involved hippocampus showed widespread neuronal loss and gliosis in all three sectors. The cerebellum was moderately atrophic with maximal sclerosis of folia on the ventral surface of the cerebellar hemispheres (Fig. 5–11B). Microscopically, there was severe loss of Purkinje cells, even in folia where the atrophy was inconspicuous grossly (Fig. 5–11C).

COMMENT

Over the years, many studies on epileptic patients have reported varying degrees of neuronal loss and gliosis. These changes are often most striking on the medial aspect of the temporal lobes including the hippocampal formation and the cerebellum. Hippocampal sclerosis has been seen in 50 to 60 percent of patients with cryptogenic epilepsy and is usually unilateral. It has been argued whether this lesion is the result of birth injury (so-called mesial sclerosis) and is a cause of seizures or whether it is the direct result of seizures, or the result of hypoxia secondary to seizures.

The cerebellar sclerosis is even more difficult to interpret. Anoxia associated with seizures is often considered to be the cause of the cerebellar damage. Nevertheless, several studies have shown cerebellar sclerosis following therapy with phenytoin in individuals who have few or no seizures. Futhermore, it has been stated that cerebellar sclerosis is more prevalent among epileptics who have received phenytoin. Finally, the very widespread, diffuse loss of Purkinje cells has been purported to favor a toxic injury rather than hypoxic damage.

Sudden unexpected deaths among epileptics are being documented with greater frequency. Some are being attributed to neurogenic pulmonary edema or cardiac arrhythmia.

REFERENCES

Dasheiff RM, Dickinson LJ: Sudden unexpected death of epileptic patients due to cardiac arrhythmia after seizure. Arch Neurol 1986; 43:194-196.

Gessaga EC, Urich H: The cerebellum of epileptics. Clin Neuropathol 1985; 4:238-245.

Lindvall O, Nilsson B: Cerebellar atrophy following phenytoin intoxication. Ann Neurol 1984; 16:258-260.

Meldrum BS, Corsellis JAN: Epilepsy. In Adams JH, Corsellis JAN, Duchen LW (eds): Greenfield's Neuropathology, 4th ed. New York, Wiley, 1984, chap 19, pp 921-950.

Rapport RL, Shaw C-M: Phenytoin-related cerebellar degeneration without seizures. Ann Neurol 1977; 2:437-439.

Terrence CF, Rao GR, Perper JA: Neurogenic pulmonary edema in unexpected, unexplained death of epileptic patients. Ann Neurol 1981; 9:458-464.

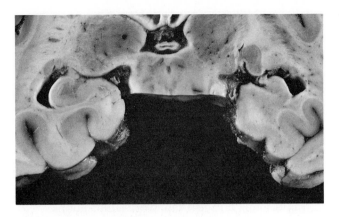

Figure 5–11A. Coronal section showing sclerosis of the right hippocampus.

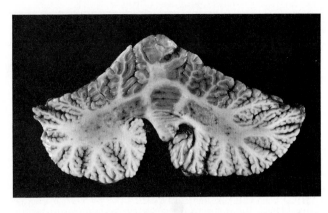

Figure 5–11B. Section of the cerebellum showing folial sclerosis that was most severe on the inferior surface.

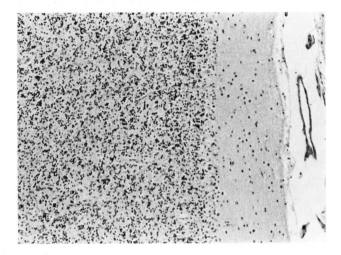

Figure 5–11C. Microscopic section showing complete loss of Purkinje cells and a reduction in the number of neurons in the internal granular cell layer.

5.12 Subacute Combined Degeneration

Vitamin B₁₂ Deficiency

CLINICAL

This 74-year-old man had a history of deteriorating gait, dementia, and urinary incontinence. He was thought to have normal pressure hydrocephalus and underwent a ventriculoperitoneal shunting procedure. This temporarily improved his gait and incontinence but his dementia remained unchanged. When re-evaluated, he was noted to have diminished position sense, hyperactive deep tendon reflexes at the knees, and absent reflexes at the ankles. Laboratory studies disclosed a mild anemia with macrocytic indices and hypersegmented polymorphonuclear leukocytes in a peripheral blood smear. A vitamin B_{12} assay revealed a level of 50 pg/mL with a low normal being 200 pg/mL. The patient died of cardiac disease shortly after completion of his evaluation.

PATHOLOGY

Grossly, the brain and spinal cord were unremarkable except for the shunt tract. Histologically, there were foci of demyelination in the posterior and lateral columns of the spinal cord (Fig. 5–12A). At higher magnification, the demyelinated areas appeared finely vacuolated and contained scattered macrophages with only minimal astrocytosis (Figs. 5–12B and 5–12C).

COMMENT

Vitamin B_{12} is an essential cofactor for two enzymatic reactions, the conversion of l-methylmalonyl-CoA to succinyl-CoA and for the methylation of homocysteine to methionine. Deficiency of this vitamin has deleterious effects on the hematopoietic system, nervous system, and epithelial surfaces. The precise mechanisms by which this deficiency adversely affects the nervous system are incompletely elucidated.

Prior to absorption through the ileum, vitamin B_{12} combines with intrinsic factor, a glycoprotein, produced by the gastric parietal cells. Dietary deficiency of vitamin B_{12} is extremely rare and seen only in individuals who are strict vegans. Individuals with pernicious anemia have inadequate production of intrinsic factor secondary to an autoimmune gastritis and thus, have inadequate absorption of vitamin B_{12}. Vitamin B_{12} deficiency can also result from intestinal diseases that impede the absorption of the vitamin from the ileum. These disorders include malabsorption syndromes, inflammatory bowel diseases, and lymphomas. Other cases have resulted from competitive utilization of the vitamin by bacterial overgrowth in blind loops and fish tapeworm infestations.

Some authors regard peripheral neuropathy as the most common form of neurological disease associated with this deficiency. Both segmental demyelination and axonal degeneration have been described in peripheral nerve specimens. The classical myelopathy, so-called subacute combined degeneration of the spinal cord, typically involves the thoracic segments of the spinal cord most severely, with lesser degrees of involvement in the cervical and lumbar segments. The initial pathological changes consist of vacuolation of myelin sheaths in small foci. These coalesce to become larger lesions. The vacuolation imparts the characteristic spongy appearance to the lesions in the dorsal and lateral columns. The vacuolation of the myelin sheaths is followed by demyelination and infiltration by lipid-laden macrophages. Some of the axons within the demyelinated lesions are destroyed, leading to Wallerian degeneration. Initially, there is only minimal astrocytosis; however, gliosis may become prominent in long-standing cases.

Occasionally, similar appearing demyelinative and destructive lesions are seen in the cerebral white matter where they are designated as Lichtheim plaques. The optic nerves may show selective involvement of the papillomacular bundles. The neurological manifestations are not consistently accompanied by hematological abnormalities. Nevertheless, determination of the mean corpuscular volume is regarded as a useful screening test.

REFERENCES

Duchen LW, Jacobs JM: Nutritional deficiencies and metabolic disorders. In Adams JH, Corsellis JAN, Duchen LW (eds): Greenfield's Neuropathology, 4th ed. New York, Wiley, 1984, chap 13, pp 585-592.

Lindenbaum J, Healton EB, Savage DG, et al: Neuropsychiatric disorders caused by cobalamin deficiency in the absence of anemia or macrocytosis. N Engl J Med 1988; 318:1720-1728.

Pallis CA, Lewis PD: The Neurology of Gastrointestinal Disease. London, Saunders, 1974, chap 5, pp 30-97.

Pant SS, Asbury AK, Richardson EP Jr: The myelopathy of pernicious anemia. A neuropathological reappraisal. Acta Neurol Scand 1968; 44 (Suppl 35):1-36.

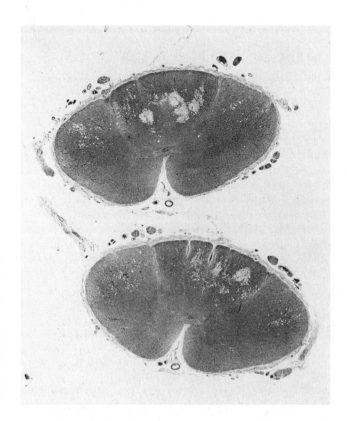

Figure 5–12A. Macrosections of spinal cord from a patient with B_{12} deficiency. Note the demyelination and vacuolar degeneration in the posterior and lateral columns.

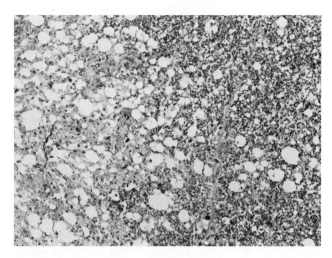

Figure 5–12B. Microscopic section showing the demyelination and vacuolar degeneration in the posterior column.

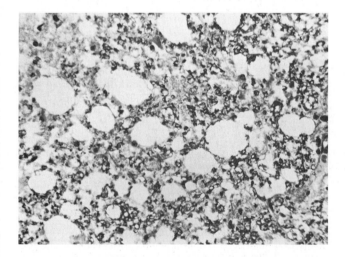

Figure 5–12C. Microscopic section at higher magnification showing the mild macrophagic response and minimal astrocytosis.

5.13   Methotrexate Radiation

CLINICAL

This 21-year-old woman had been diagnosed as having acute leukemia when she was 10 years old. She was initially treated with prednisone and vincristine and maintained on 6-mercapto-purine. At age 19, she presented with headaches and meningismus and was found to have leukemic involvement of the central nervous system. She was treated with craniospinal irradiation and intrathecal methotrexate. She became obtunded and developed diverse focal neurological deficits. Cranial CT showed multiple localized areas of decreased attenuation in the white matter of both hemispheres. She eventually died from systemic infections.

PATHOLOGY

Coronal sections of the cerebral hemispheres disclosed multiple areas of demyelination and necrosis within the white matter (Fig. 5–13A). Histologically, these areas showed gliosis, numerous reactive axons, and foci of mineralization (Fig. 5–13B). There was only minimal inflammation.

COMMENT

Intrathecal and/or intravenous methotrexate are often combined with craniospinal irradiation in the treatment of and prophylaxis against CNS involvement by acute leukemia. This regimen has contributed to cures in patients with a disease that previously was uniformly lethal. Nevertheless, the therapy may be accompanied by neurological complications. The best known of the resulting lesions has been designated as disseminated necrotizing leukoencephalopathy by Rubinstein et al and as subacute leukoencephalopathy by Price and Jamieson. The lesions consist of multiple discrete or confluent areas of coagulative necrosis and demyelination scattered throughout the white matter, especially in the cerebral hemispheres. Histologically, the lesions show coagulative necrosis, demyelination, gliosis, and, occasionally, mineralization of reactive axons and cellular debris. Lipid-laden macrophages may be abundant but inflammatory cells are generally sparse. Vascular changes are inconsistently encountered. The pathogenesis of the disorder is uncertain but may be the result of excessive quantities of methotrexate gaining access to the white matter through vessels that have been damaged by the irradiation.

The Vinca alkaloids, including vincristine and vinblastine, are also neurotoxic. Development of a peripheral neuropathy with axonal degeneration, is often the limiting factor with the use of systemic vincristine. On a few occasions, vincristine has been inadvertently administered intrathecally. This has been followed by ascending paralysis, sensory deficits, and death from respiratory failure. Histological studies have disclosed swollen, chromatolytic motor neurons with aggregates of neurofilaments. At least one case also showed eosinophilic crystals that were thought to be derived from reaggregated microtubule proteins (Fig. 5–13C).

REFERENCES

Price RA, Jamieson PA: The central nervous system in childhood leukemia. II. Subacute leukoencephalopathy. Cancer 1975; 35:306-318.

Rubinstein LJ, Herman MM, Long TF, Wilbur JR: Disseminated necrotizing leukoencephalopathy: A complication of treated central nervous system leukemia and lymphoma. Cancer 1975; 35:291-305.

Slyter H, Liwnicz B, Herrick MK, Mason R: Fatal myeloencephalopathy caused by intrathecal vincristine. Neurology 1980; 30:867-871.

Young DE, Posner JB: Nervous system toxicity of chemotherapeutic agents. In Vinken PK, Bruyn GW (eds): Handbook of Clinical Neurology. Amsterdam, Elsevier, 1980, vol 39, chap 4, pp 91-129.

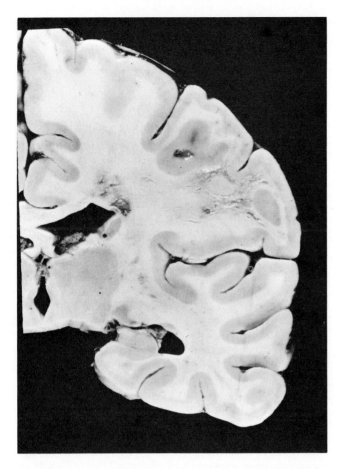

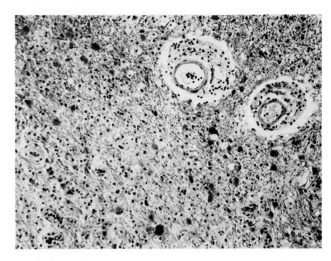

Figure 5–13B. Microscopic section showing the resulting necrosis and gliosis.

Figure 5–13A. Coronal section of the cerebral hemisphere showing necrosis of the periventricular and convolutional white matter in a woman who received cranial radiation and intrathecal methotrexate therapy for leukemia.

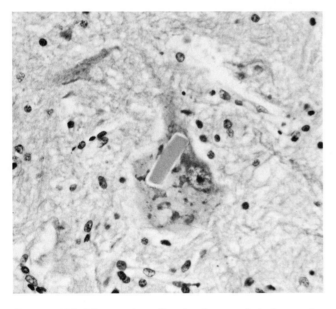

Figure 5–13C. Microscopic section showing an anterior horn motor neuron containing an eosinophilic crystal and aggregates of neurofilaments following intrathecal administration of vincristine.

5.14 Radiation Necrosis

CLINICAL

This 32-year-old woman had a chronically draining right ear. She also had a right Horner's syndrome, palsies of the right ninth and twelfth cranial nerves, and papilledema. Angiography showed thrombosis of the right lateral sinus. Computerized tomograms demonstrated erosion of the lateral portion of C1 and floor of the right middle fossa. A subtemporal craniotomy and extradural exploration of the middle fossa revealed metastatic moderately well differentiated squamous cell carcinoma. She was given 6000 rads of radiation over a 6-week period.

One year later she developed ataxia, dysarthria, and dysphagia. The right side of her tongue was atrophic and had fasciculations. Computerized tomograms showed further destruction of the skull base. During her hospitalization, the patient developed aspiration pneumonia and died.

PATHOLOGY

The inferior surface of the medulla was slightly softened (Fig. 5–14A). Transverse sections revealed a partially cystic area of necrosis at the level of the inferior olivary nuclei (Fig. 5–14B). Macrosections showed extensive involvement of the central white matter and the right olivary nucleus (Fig. 5–14C). Histologically, the lesion showed coagulative necrosis with numerous reactive axons, gliosis, and prominent vascular changes. The vessels showed varying degrees of endothelial proliferation, fibrinoid necrosis and perivascular fibrosis (Fig. 5–14D). Some of the vessels were also surrounded by amorphous proteinaceous material.

COMMENT

Radiation causes cellular injury through direct effects on macromolecules such as DNA and through indirect effects mediated by free radicals, especially those derived from water. Tissues with a high cell turnover rate are especially vulnerable. Within the central nervous system, glia and endothelial cells are regarded as the most susceptible components.

Both early and late effects have been described. The early delayed reactions occur within a few weeks to a few months after irradiation and are usually transient and nonlethal. Limited pathological studies have shown predominantly demyelinated areas within the white matter. The late delayed reactions occur several months to several years after irradiation. The lesions are dose related, progressive, and may be lethal. The resulting signs and symptoms may mimic an intraparenchymal neoplasm. The lesions are found predominantly in the white matter. Histologically, they are characterized by necrosis that is accompanied by prominent vascular alterations. These include endothelial proliferation, fibrinoid necrosis and perivascular fibrosis. The vessels appear to be abnormally permeable and may be surrounded by prominent amorphous proteinaceous exudates. Foci of mineralization may be encountered. Toward the periphery of the lesions, vessels may have enlarged lumina and appear telangiectatic. The lesions may be focally hemorrhagic.

REFERENCES

Groothuis DR, Vick NA: Radionecrosis of the central nervous system. The perspective of the clinical neurologist and neuropathologist. In Gilbert HA, Kagan AR (eds): Radiation Damage to the Nervous System. A Delayed Therapeutic Hazard. New York, Raven Press 1980, pp 93-106.

Rottenberg DA, Chernick NL, Deck MDF, et al: Cerebral necrosis following radiotherapy of extracranial neoplasms. Ann Neurol 1979; 1:339-357.

Sheline GE: Irradiation injury of the human brain. A review of clinical experience. In Gilbert HA, Kagan AR (eds): Radiation Damage to the Nervous System. A Delayed Therapeutic Hazard. New York, Raven Press, 1980, pp 39-58.

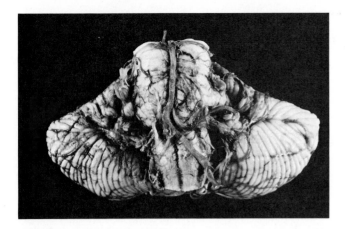

Figure 5–14A. Ventral surface of brain stem from a patient who had received cranial radiation for carcinoma of the ear. The medulla was slightly softened.

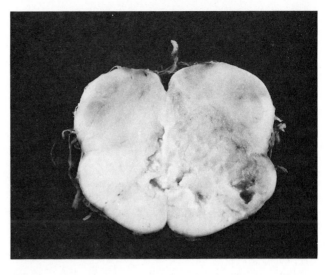

Figure 5–14B. Transverse section of medulla showing extensive area of radiation necrosis.

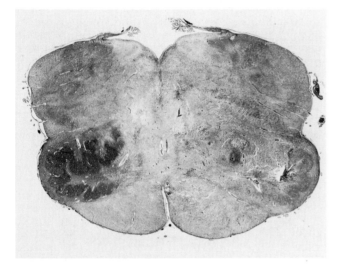

Figure 5–14C. Macrosection of medulla showing demyelination and necrosis secondary to the radiation.

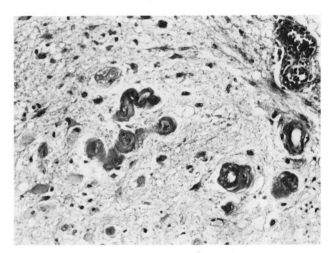

Figure 5–14D. Microscopic section showing the gliosis and thickened blood vessels in the area of radiation necrosis.

6

Demyelinating and Metabolic Diseases

6.1   Multiple Sclerosis

CLINICAL

This 33-year-old woman had a 4-year history of multiple neurological deficits. Her illness began at 29 years of age with a 2½ week episode of diplopia that resolved spontaneously. Later that year, she had difficulty focusing her eyes and examination demonstrated both horizontal and vertical nystagmus. One year later, she complained of an unsteady gait and was found to have a right extensor toe sign. Urinary incontinence developed at 31 years of age. The following year, head and hand tremors were noted. She was bedridden at the time of her death. The family history was remarkable in that her mother, sister, and brother also had multiple sclerosis.

PATHOLOGY

The brain weighed 1300 grams and appeared normal externally. Horizontal sections of the cerebral hemispheres revealed numerous demyelinated plaques within the convolutional and central white matter (Figs. 6–1A and 6–1B). The plaques varied in appearance from faintly discolored and poorly defined to dark gray and distinctly demarcated. The plaques were especially numerous around the angles of the ventricular system (Fig. 6–1C). Some of the plaques extended from the white matter into the cortex and basal ganglia. Plaques were also present in the brain stem. A large plaque was found in the pontine tegmentum beneath the floor of the fourth ventricle (Fig. 6–1D).

Histologically, most of the plaques appeared as distinctly demarcated, sparsely cellular areas that were almost completely devoid of myelin and oligodendrocytes (Fig. 6–1E). Some of the plaques contained lipid-laden macrophages and mononuclear inflammatory cells. The mononuclear cells consisted predominantly of lymphocytes and rare plasma cells and tended to be most numerous around blood vessels and at the margins of the plaques. Other plaques contained reactive astrocytes (Fig. 6–1F). Some

of the astrocytes contained relatively large, bizarre nuclei. Axons were generally intact.

COMMENT

Multiple sclerosis is the most common primary demyelinating disease involving the central nervous system. The disease is more prevalent among women than men, and generally becomes clinically apparent between the ages of 20 and 40 years. The signs and symptoms are highly variable, reflecting the development of lesions that are separated in time and location. The most frequent clinical manifestations are referable to involvement of the spinal cord, visual system, brain stem, and cerebellum. Paresthesias, spasticity, Babinski signs, and weakness eventually develop in more than 90 percent of the patients. In some cases, the spinal cord involvement can be demonstrated by electrical sensations that are elicited upon flexing the neck, the so-called Lhermitte's sign. Visual disturbances including scotomata, blurred vision, and impaired eye movements are common features. In particular, the development of an internuclear ophthalmoplegia in a young individual is highly suggestive of multiple sclerosis. Impairment of ocular motility reflects the presence of plaques in the brain stem. Nearly 20 percent of patients with multiple sclerosis will have impaired vision as the result of optic neuritis. Although the majority of the individuals recover almost normal vision, recurrences may occur in the same eye or other eye. Cerebellar dysfunction, manifested by ataxia, intention tremor, dysmetria, and incoordination, constitutes another important group of abnormalities. The course of the disease is generally characterized by exacerbations and remissions, although some patients may show steadily progressive deterioration.

The cerebrospinal fluid generally shows a normal cell count, although there may be a mild increase in the number of cells during acute exacerbations. The protein is normal or only slightly elevated but often contains an increased proportion of IgG. Electrophoresis of the cerebrospinal fluid will usually dem-

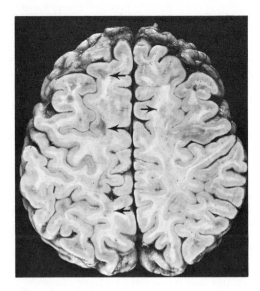

Figure 6–1A. Horizontal section of brain from patient with multiple sclerosis showing numerous plaques (arrows) in the convolutional and central white matter.

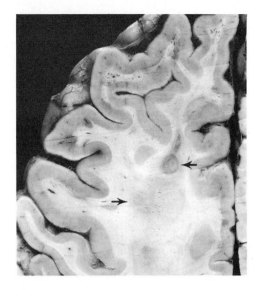

Figure 6–1B. Horizontal section showing both faintly demarcated (arrow on left) and sharply demarcated (arrow on right) plaques.

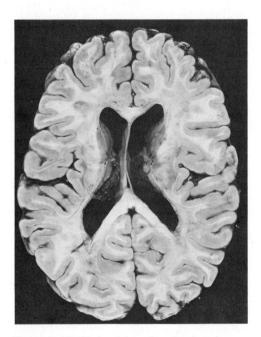

Figure 6–1C. Horizontal section showing plaques about the angles of the lateral ventricles.

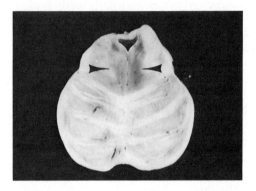

Figure 6–1D. Transverse section of brain stem showing a plaque (arrows) in pontine tegmentum.

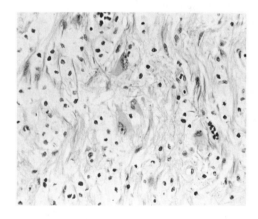

Figure 6–1F. Microscopic section showing reactive astrocytes in the interior of another plaque.

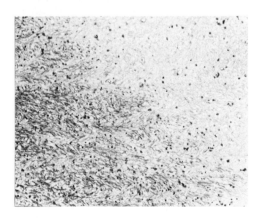

Figure 6–1E. Microscopic section showing margin of demyelinated plaque.

onstrate the presence of oligoclonal bands. Computerized tomography with contrast enhancement has demonstrated the demyelinated plaques in some patients, but more often shows only mild cerebral atrophy. Magnetic resonance imaging has been shown to be much more effective in demonstrating the demyelinated areas (Fig. 6–1G).

The prevalence of multiple sclerosis shows striking geographical variations. In general, the disease is much more common in the colder northern areas than in the warmer southern areas. The variations in prevalence have been attributed to environmental factors, especially exposure to infectious diseases during childhood. This interpretation has been supported by certain epidemiological studies. Individuals who have migrated from northern, high-risk areas to southern, low-risk areas before the age of 15 have a lower incidence of multiple sclerosis than individuals who have migrated as older adults. Between 15 and 20 percent of cases of multiple sclerosis show familial aggregation. This has been variously interpreted as supportive evidence for genetic predisposition or common exposure. There is a higher prevalence of multiple sclerosis among individuals with certain histocompatibility antigens such as HLA-3 and B7. Despite extensive investigation, the etiology and pathogenesis of multiple sclerosis remain unsettled. A viral infection or an immunologically mediated process are the most likely causes.

REFERENCES

Cook SD, Dowling PC: Multiple sclerosis and virus: An overview. Neurology 1980; 30:80-91.

Ebers GC: Multiple sclerosis and other demyelinating diseases. In Asbury AK, McKhann GM, McDonald WI (eds): Diseases of the Nervous System: Clinical Neurobiology. Philadelphia, Saunders, 1986, vol II, chap 102, pp 1268-1281.

Jacobs L, Kinkel WR, Polachini I, Kinkel P: Correlation of nuclear magnetic resonance imaging, computerized tomography, and clinical profiles in multiple sclerosis. Neurology 1986; 36:27-34.

Kurtzke JF: Epidemiologic contributions to multiple sclerosis: An overview. Neurology 1980; 30:61-79.

McFarlin DE, McFarland HF: Multiple sclerosis. N Engl J Med 1982; 307:1183-1188, and 1982; 307:1246-1251.

Paty DW, Oger JJF, Kastrukoff LF, et al: MRI in diagnosis of MS: A prospective study with comparison of clinical evaluation, evoked potentials, oligoclonal banding, and CT. Neurology 1988; 38:180-185.

Raine CS: Demyelinating diseases. In Davis RL, Robertson DM (eds): Textbook of Neuropathology. Baltimore, Williams & Wilkins, 1985, chap 11, pp 468-547.

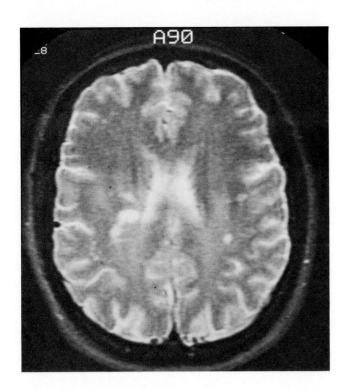

Figure 6–1G. Magnetic resonance imaging scan showing multiple lesions in the white matter of a patient with multiple sclerosis.

6.2 Multiple Sclerosis

Late Onset

CLINICAL

This 80-year-old woman was in good health until age 55 when she developed blurred vision in the left eye that did not resolve. Five years later, she fell and sustained a fractured leg. She attributed the fall to an unsteady gait and continued to complain of unsteadiness for the following 3 years. She was evaluated at age 64 for double vision. Examination demonstrated diplopia on left lateral and upward gaze. There was a decrease in fine motor movements of the left hand and foot. She had an extensor toe sign on the left and mild hyperreflexia in the left upper and lower extremities. Her signs and symptoms were attributed to a brain stem vascular accident. The diplopia subsequently resolved. Later that year, she developed difficulty walking and was thought to have a cervical myelopathy secondary to cervical spondylosis. She developed increasing weakness in her left leg and associated clumsiness of gait. She was ultimately confined to a nursing home where she died.

PATHOLOGY

The brain weighed 1167 grams and showed atrophy of the frontal lobes. Coronal sections of the cerebral hemispheres showed convolutional atrophy with widening of the intervening sulci. There were scattered demyelinated plaques in the white matter. The largest plaques were in periventricular locations about the angles of the lateral horns, temporal horns and occipital horns of the lateral ventricles (Figs. 6–2A and 6–2B). In addition, there were smaller plaques in the centrum semiovale, convolutional white matter, and corpus callosum. Histologically, the periventricular plaques showed extensive demyelination (Fig. 6–2C). No grossly discernible lesions were evident within the brain stem or cerebellum, although small plaques were seen histologically. The cervical and thoracic portions of the spinal cord were flattened. The spinal white matter was discolored and histologically showed extensive demyelination (Fig. 6–2D). Small foci of demyelination were demonstrable in the optic nerves and chiasm (Fig. 6–2E).

COMMENT

Although multiple sclerosis is generally regarded as a disease of young adults, occasional cases with typical exacerbations and remissions may be encountered in older individuals. In other older patients, the disease may be manifested by a steadily progressive myelopathy, sometimes complicating the diagnosis. In addition, there is a small but well documented group of patients in whom the disease is clinically asymptomatic and diagnosed only at the time of autopsy. Cerebral atrophy as demonstrated in the present case may be seen in association with multiple sclerosis and should not be misinterpreted as another disease process.

Certain demyelinating diseases that have been described as separate entities may be variants of multiple sclerosis. Neuromyelitis optica or Devic's syndrome may be a relatively acute form of multiple sclerosis with preferential involvement of the optic pathways and spinal cord. Balo's syndrome, a very rare disorder characterized morphologically by alternating concentric bands of demyelination and intact myelin, also may be a variant of multiple sclerosis. The concentric lesions have been interpreted as intermediate stages in the development of plaques. Other rare cases of multiple sclerosis may be accompanied by demyelination of peripheral nerves resembling an inflammatory neuropathy.

REFERENCES

Filley CM, Sternberg PE, Norenberg MD: Neuromyelitis optica in the elderly. Arch Neurol 1984; 41:670-672.

Gilbert JJ, Sadler M: Unsuspected multiple sclerosis. Arch Neurol 1983; 40:533-536.

Moore GRW, Neumann PE, Suzuki K, et al: Balo's concentric sclerosis: New observations on lesion development. Ann Neurol 1985; 17:604-611.

Rubin M, Karpati G, Carpenter S: Combined central and peripheral myelinopathy. Neurology 1987; 37:1287-1290.

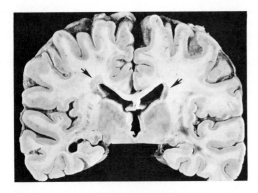

Figure 6–2A. Coronal section of brain from elderly woman with multiple sclerosis. Note the plaques (arrows) about the angles of the lateral ventricles.

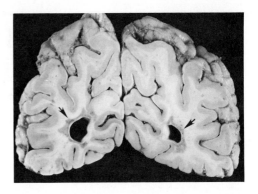

Figure 6–2B. Coronal section showing large plaques (arrows) about the occipital horns of the lateral ventricles.

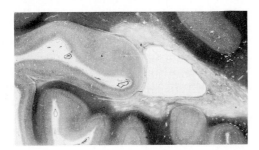

Figure 6–2C. Macrosection showing a demyelinated plaque about the occipital horn of the lateral ventricle.

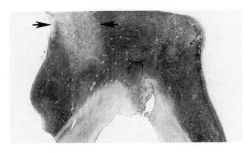

Figure 6–2E. Macrosection of optic chiasm showing demyelinated plaque (arrows).

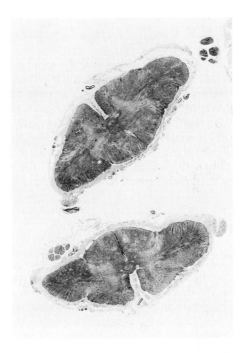

Figure 6–2D. Macrosections showing extensive demyelination of the spinal cord.

6.3 Acute Disseminated Encephalomyelitis

Postinfectious Encephalomyelitis
Acute Hemorrhagic Encephalomyelitis

CLINICAL

This 8-year-old boy suddenly developed fever, lapsed into coma, and died within 1 week of having measles.

PATHOLOGY

The brain was mildly swollen and the leptomeningeal blood vessels were congested. Other than mild swelling, no abnormalities were evident grossly. Histological examination showed numerous vessels, predominantly venules, to be surrounded by infiltrates of mononuclear cells consisting of lymphocytes, occasional plasma cells, and macrophages (Fig. 6–3A). When stained for myelin, these areas of perivascular inflammation also showed demyelination (Fig. 6–3B).

COMMENT

Acute disseminated encephalomyelitis or postinfectious encephalomyelitis is a rare but potentially serious complication of exanthematous infections of childhood, especially measles (rubeola). Formerly, nearly 1 per 1000 cases of measles were complicated by this disorder. In addition, the resulting encephalomyelitis was often more severe following rubeola than other viral exanthemata. Acute disseminated encephalomyelitis has also been described following *Mycoplasma* pneumonia, vaccination, and immunizations. The clinical symptoms begin abruptly and include fever, headache, meningismus, and a decreased level of consciousness. When the disease follows chickenpox (varicella), cerebellar ataxia may be a prominent feature. Computerized tomography may show enhancing lesions in the cortex and low-density areas in the white matter and basal ganglia.

Grossly, brains from patients with acute disseminated encephalomyelitis usually show only swelling and congestion. Occasionally, there may be slight discoloration of the white matter. Since the disease is generally monophasic, the histological features are similar and at the same stage of evolution in all of the lesions. Inflammatory cell infiltrates are found predominantly around small veins and venules within the white matter. The inflammatory cells include lymphocytes, plasma cells, and macrophages. The lymphocytes and plasma cells are generally most numerous in close proximity to the vessel whereas the macrophages are more peripherally situated in the area of demyelination. Occasionally there are also subpial inflammatory cell infiltrates. Axons tend to be preserved. Cases with a somewhat longer period of survival may show reactive astrocytes and occasional larger cells with multiple small nuclei in the perivascular demyelinated zones. The multinucleated cells have been variously interpreted as mesodermal or astrocytic.

Acute hemorrhagic encephalomyelitis is probably a fulminant variant of acute disseminated encephalomyelitis. It has the additional gross pathological feature of petechial hemorrhages in the white matter. Histologically, the walls of small vessels may appear necrotic and there are erythrocytes, deposits of fibrin, and polymorphonuclear leukocytes within perivascular inflammatory cell infiltrates (Fig. 6–3C). Both acute disseminated encephalomyelitis and acute hemorrhagic encephalomyelitis are probably mediated by immunologic mechanisms. In only very rare instances have viruses been isolated from the brains of these individuals.

REFERENCES

Bauman M, Bergman I: Postvaricella encephalitis. Arch Neurol 1984; 41:556-558.

Fenichel GM: Neurological complications of immunization. Ann Neurol 1982; 12:119-128.

Fisher RS, Clark AW, Wolinsky JS, et al: Postinfectious leukoencephalitis complicating *Mycoplasma pneumoniae* infection. Arch Neurol 1983; 40:109-113.

Hart MN, Earle KM: Haemorrhagic and perivenous encephalitis: A clinical–pathological review of 38 cases. J Neurol Neurosurg Psychiatry 1975; 38:585-591.

Lukes SA, Norman D: Computed tomography in acute disseminated encephalomyelitis. Ann Neurol 1983; 13:567-572.

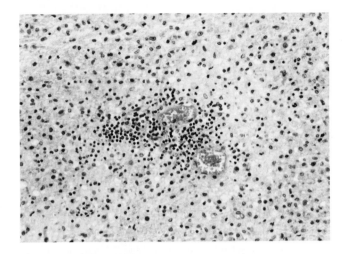

Figure 6–3A. Microscopic section showing perivenular infiltrate of mononuclear inflammatory cells and macrophages.

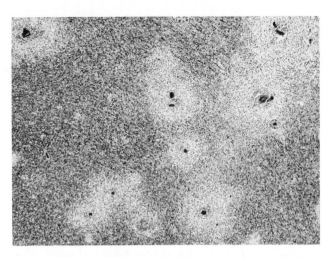

Figure 6–3B. Microscopic section showing demyelination in the areas of perivenular inflammation.

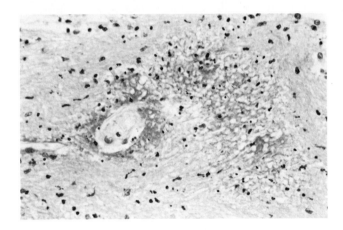

Figure 6–3C. Microscopic section showing intramural and perivascular deposits of fibrin with occasional polymorphonuclear leukocytes in a brain from a patient with acute hemorrhagic encephalomyelitis.

6.4 Krabbe's Disease

Globoid Cell Leukodystrophy

CLINICAL

This female infant had been delivered by cesarean section because of premature rupture of membranes. Her initial development was normal but by the age of 3 months, spontaneous movements had nearly stopped. She became excessively irritable, cried constantly, and occasionally displayed opisthotonic posturing. She fed poorly and at 7 months, required a feeding tube gastrostomy. By age 9 months, she had become hypotonic and had episodes of irregular respirations. At 10 months of age, it was noted that her pupils responded poorly to light. She had no organomegaly. Lumbar punctures revealed elevated cerebrospinal fluid protein content (170 to 210 mg/dL) and enzyme studies on fibroblasts cultured from a skin biopsy specimen revealed the galactocerebroside β-galactosidase activity to be less than 5 percent of normal. The child died at age 11 months.

PATHOLOGY

The brain was moderately atrophic and, prior to fixation, had an abnormally firm consistency. Coronal sections revealed a diffuse reduction in the volume of the cerebral white matter. This was especially marked in the corpus callosum and internal capsules (Fig. 6–4A). These white matter structures also contained small cystic spaces (Fig. 6–4B). The ventricular system was mildly enlarged. Sections of the brain stem disclosed a diffuse reduction in the volume of white matter and additional small cystic spaces within the pyramidal tracts (Fig. 6–4C). The cerebellar white matter was diffusely discolored, reduced in volume, and focally cystic (Fig. 6–4D).

Histological examination revealed a reduction in the number of oligodendroglial cells and the quantity of stainable myelin. However, the most striking feature was the presence of numerous large macrophages,

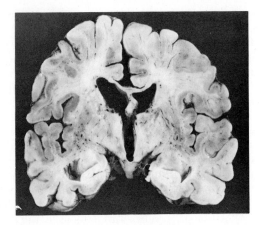

Figure 6–4A. Coronal section of a brain from a child with Krabbe's disease showing diffuse reduction in white matter.

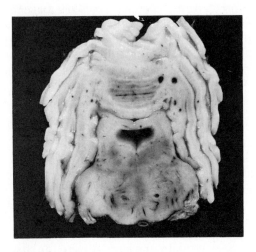

Figure 6–4C. Transverse section of pons showing reduction in volume of white matter.

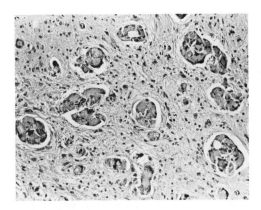

Figure 6–4E. Microscopic section showing numerous globoid cells aggregated about blood vessels in the demyelinated white matter.

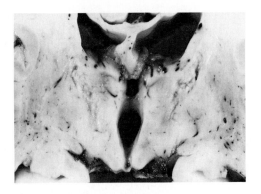

Figure 6–4B. Coronal section showing cavitation in white matter of the internal capsules.

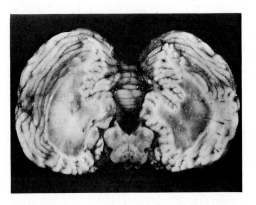

Figure 6–4D. Transverse section of brain stem and cerebellum. Note the diffuse discoloration and focal cystic alteration of the cerebellar white matter. Note also the cystic degeneration within the medullary pyramidal tracts.

the so-called globoid cells, that tended to aggregate around blood vessels (Fig. 6–4E). The globoid cells were further characterized by intense staining of their cytoplasm with the periodic acid–Schiff technique. Electron microscopy disclosed striated, multiangular profiles within the cytoplasm of the globoid cells. Some of these profiles were membrane bound whereas others were free in the cytoplasm (Fig. 6–4F).

COMMENT

The leukodystrophies are rare, genetically determined metabolic disorders that involve predominantly the white matter of the central nervous system. Some of the leukodystrophies also involve the peripheral nervous system and visceral organs to a varying extent. Krabbe's disease is an autosomal recessive disease due to deficiency of galactocerebroside β-galactosidase. Since galactocerebroside is a normal constituent of myelin, the clinical manifestations reflect involvement of the brain and peripheral nerves.

Krabbe's disease generally becomes manifest clinically between the ages of 3 and 6 months with excessive irritability and progressive hypertonia. Some of the individuals also have episodes of fever in the absence of infection. Later in the course of the disease, spasticity gives way to hypotonia. Optic atrophy is another common manifestation, reflecting white matter involvement. The cerebrospinal fluid consistently shows an elevated protein content. Computerized tomography has shown decreased attenuation in the central white matter and unexplained densities in the deep gray matter. Magnetic resonance imaging has demonstrated large plaque-like areas in the centrum semiovale.

Grossly, the brains are small and abnormally firm. The cortex and basal ganglia are relatively normal appearing. The white matter is reduced in volume, discolored, and may be focally cavitated. The alterations in the white matter tend to be more severe caudally and are especially pronounced in the corpus callosum, internal capsules, and pyramidal tracts. The characteristic globoid cells result from accumulation of undegraded galactocerebroside in macrophages. Ultrastructurally, this material appears as striated, multiangular or twisted tubular profiles (Fig. 6–4F). Although the globoid cells result from intracellular accumulation of galactocerebroside, the overall brain content of this material is not increased. The paucity of myelin, reduction in the number of oligodendrocytes, and foci of cystic degeneration have been attributed to the presence of small but significant amounts of psychosine. This is a highly toxic material that would normally have been catabolized by galactocerebroside β-galactosidase, the enzyme that is deficient in Krabbe's disease.

In addition, peripheral nerve involvement is common and leads to depression or even absence of deep tendon reflexes. Since the neuropathy is due to demyelination, nerve conduction velocities are slowed. Histologically, the nerves are abnormally cellular and contain lipid-laden cells but no true globoid cells.

REFERENCES

Baram TZ, Goldman AM, Percy AK: Krabbe disease: Specific MRI and CT findings. Neurology 1986; 36:111-115.

Becker LE, Yates A: Inherited metabolic diseases. In Davis RL, Robertson DM (eds): Textbook of Neuropathology. Baltimore, Williams & Wilkins, 1985, chap 8, pp 284-371.

Suzuki K, Suzuki Y: Galactosylceramide lipidosis: Globoid cell leukodystrophy (Krabbe's disease). In Stanbury JB, Wyngaarden JB, Fredrickson DS, et al (eds): The Metabolic Basis of Inherited Diseases, 5th ed. New York, McGraw-Hill, 1983, chap 43, pp 857-880.

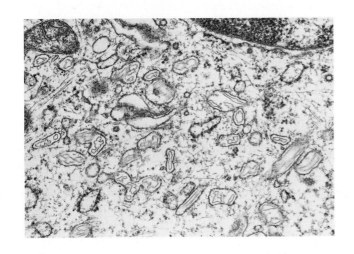

Figure 6–4F. Electron micrograph of a globoid cell showing the membrane-bound, multiangular profiles of galactocerebroside.

6.5 Metachromatic Leukodystrophy

Sulfatide Lipidosis

CLINICAL

This boy had been the product of a normal pregnancy and delivery. His early development had been considered to be normal. At 19 months of age, he began to have difficulty walking. Within 1 month, he was unable to sit without assistance. Over the next year, he lost the ability to feed himself and became mute. His vision gradually deteriorated and he was blind by the age of 4. He died when he was 5 years old.

PATHOLOGY

The brain was mildly atrophic with moderate enlargement of the ventricular system. The cerebral white matter had a gray discoloration and was reduced in volume. Macrosections, stained for myelin, disclosed extensive demyelination of the central white matter with relative preservation of the subcortical arcuate fibers (Fig. 6–5A). Within the demyelinated areas, the number of oligodendrocytes were reduced and there were intracellular and extracellular deposits of sulfatide (Fig. 6–5B). The sulfatide appeared as eosinophilic granular material and was further characterized by staining dark red with the periodic acid–Schiff reaction (Fig. 6–5C). In frozen sections, the sulfatide stained brown with acidified cresyl violet, the so-called Hirsch–Peiffer reaction. Although much of the sulfatide was in the cytoplasm of macrophages, especially around blood vessels, other deposits were within glial cells and in the form of small extracellular globules. Peripheral nerves showed segmental demyelination with abnormal deposits of sulfatide in Schwann cells and perivascular macrophages.

COMMENT

Metachromatic leukodystrophy, or sulfatide lipidosis, is a group of autosomal recessive disorders characterized by the abnormal accumulation of sulfatide, especially in the white matter of the brain and in peripheral nerves. Other tissues are also involved to varying degrees and excess sulfatide may be excreted in the urine. The various forms of metachromatic leukodystrophy differ in usual age of onset, course, and enzymatic abnormalities.

The late infantile form generally becomes manifest clinically during the first 2 years of life. Infants with this form of the disease often have gait impairment that is due, in part, to the peripheral nerve involvement. They also have intellectual deterioration, impaired speech, and loss of vision. Laboratory studies show an elevated cerebrospinal fluid protein content and slowed nerve conduction velocities. Most of these patients die within the first decade.

The juvenile form of the disease generally becomes evident between the ages of 5 and 7 years but may be delayed until adolescence. The clinical features are similar to the late infantile form but the intellectual deterioration may be the dominant feature. Furthermore, the course of the disease is generally more slowly progressive. The adult form is dominated by mental deterioration and is accompanied by pyramidal tract and cerebellar dysfunction. In all of these forms, there is deficient activity of aryl sulfatase A. This may be due to the presence of a functionally abnormal enzyme or deficiency of an activator protein, rather than actual deficiency of the enzyme itself.

There is also a very rare form of metachromatic leukodystrophy that is characterized by multiple sulfatase deficiencies (aryl sulfatase A, B, and C). Clinically, these patients resemble the late infantile form of the disease, but they also have skeletal anomalies, visceromegaly, ichthyosis, and urinary excretion of mucopolysaccharides.

The neuropathological alterations in the late infantile, juvenile, and adult forms are similar. The cerebral white matter shows demyelination with relative preservation of the arcuate fibers. There are intracellular and extracellular deposits of granular, metachromatic sulfatide. The term "metachromatic"

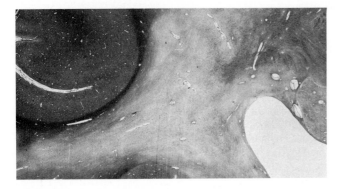

Figure 6–5A. Macrosection showing extensive demyelination in the central white matter but relative preservation of the myelin in the subcortical arcuate fibers.

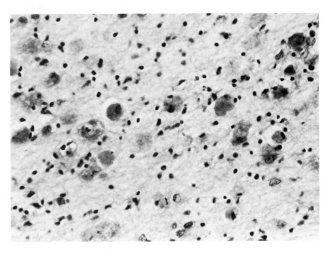

Figure 6–5B. Microscopic section showing accumulation of sulfatide, predominantly in macrophages.

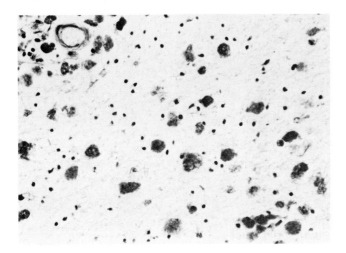

Figure 6–5C. Microscopic section showing intense staining of the sulfatide deposits by the periodic acid–Schiff technique.

refs to color alterations caused by the highly acidic sulfate group on the sulfatide. The identification of sulfatide can be confirmed by the brown color obtained when frozen sections are stained with acidified cresyl violet, the so-called Hirsch–Peiffer reaction. Ultrastructurally, the sulfatide has a variety of appearances, including concentric lamellae and stacks of lamellae with a herring-bone pattern (Fig. 6–5D). Patients with the multiple sulfatase deficiencies also have intraneuronal storage of sulfatide and gangliosides. The exact mechanism by which the excess sulfatide leads to the demyelination is unknown.

REFERENCES

Becker LE, Yates A: Inherited metabolic diseases. In Davis RL, Robertson DM (eds): Textbook of Neuropathology. Baltimore, Williams & Wilkins, 1985, chap 8, pp 284-371.

Glew RH, Basu A, Prence EH, Remaley AT: Lysosomal storage diseases. Lab Invest 1985; 53:250-269.

Kolodny EH, Moser HW: Sulfatide lipidosis: Metachromatic leukodystrophy. In Stanbury JB, Wyngaarden JB, Frederickson DS et al (eds): The Metabolic Basis of Inherited Disease, 5th ed. New York, McGraw-Hill, 1983, chap 44, pp 881-905.

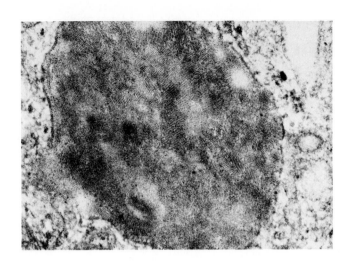

Figure 6–5D. Electron micrograph of a sulfatide deposit showing a stacked lamellae with a herring-bone pattern.

6.6   Adrenoleukodystrophy

CLINICAL

This 24-year-old man developed adrenal cortical insufficiency at age 13. His electrolyte abnormalities and hyperpigmentation responded to treatment with steroids, and he appeared to be well for the next 10 years. At age 23, he experienced the insidious onset of progressive difficulty in reading and recalling recent events. Following a generalized seizure, he was found to have a right homonymous hemianopsia. The remainder of his neurological examination was normal. A computerized tomogram revealed large areas of decreased attenuation with foci of enhancement in the left posterior frontal, parietal, and occipital lobes (Fig. 6–6A). There was no mass effect. Punctate calcifications were evident on a lateral skull x-ray.

The patient was rehospitalized after having two more seizures. His general physical examination revealed hyperpigmentation of palmar creases on both hands. Neurological examination revealed his homonymous hemianopsia to be unchanged, but he had developed a questionable right facial palsy, aphasia, alexia, apraxia, and decreased graphesthesia in the right upper extremity. A repeat computerized tomogram revealed enlargement of the lesions in the left posterior parietal and occipital lobes. A brain biopsy was performed.

PATHOLOGY

Grossly, the tissue had a gray-white color and was abnormally firm. Histological examination showed extensive demyelination and gliosis of the white matter. There were numerous lipid-laden macrophages in the demyelinated tissue. Some of the macrophages stained strongly with the periodic acid–Schiff reaction. In addition, there were infiltrates of small mononuclear cells (Figs. 6–6B and 6–6C) around blood vessels. Ultrastructural examination revealed acicular clefts and trilaminar leaflets in the cytoplasm of the macrophages (Figs. 6–6D and 6–6E). Subsequent biochemical assays of the plasma fatty acids showed abnormally high proportions of very long-chain fatty acids.

COMMENT

Adrenoleukodystrophy and adrenomyeloneuropathy are a group of X-linked recessive disorders of lipid metabolism that are fully expressed only in males. The classic, childhood form of adrenoleukodystrophy usually presents between the ages of 5 and 15 years with behavioral changes, loss of vision and hearing, and gait abnormalities. Seizures may occur as a late manifestation. In addition to the neurological dysfunction, the patients often have evidence of adrenal cortical insufficiency. This form of the disease is rapidly progressive and leads to death in 3 to 5 years. In a few patients, like the present case, the cerebral manifestations do not become apparent until adulthood.

Brains from these individuals typically show extensive demyelination and gliosis that is most pronounced in the parieto-occipital regions. This is demonstrated in an autopsy specimen from another case (Fig. 6–6F). The demyelinated tissue is infiltrated by numerous lipid-laden macrophages. Some of the macrophages have striated appearing cytoplasm that stains weakly with the periodic acid–Schiff reaction. These cells contain the distinctive trilaminar leaflets. Other macrophages stain intensely with the periodic acid–Schiff reaction. Blood vessels are typically surrounded by mononuclear cell infiltrates composed of lymphocytes and plasma cells. The demyelinated tissue shows a variable degree of gliosis and may

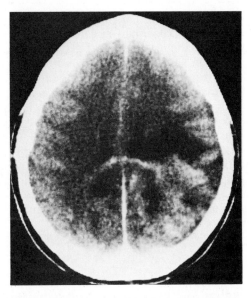

Figure 6–6A. Computerized tomogram showing decreased attenuation and irregular foci of enhancement in the left parietal lobe.

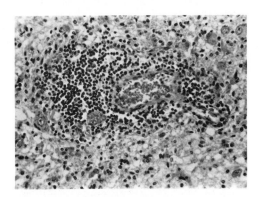

Figure 6–6C. Microscopic section, at higher magnification, showing the perivascular mononuclear inflammatory cell infiltrate.

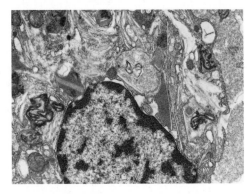

Figure 6–6E. Higher-magnification electron micrograph showing the trilaminar leaflets and osmiophilic granular material.

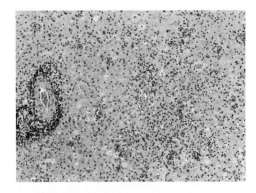

Figure 6–6B. Microscopic section showing lipid-laden macrophages, gliosis, and perivascular mononuclear cell infiltrates in the demyelinated white matter.

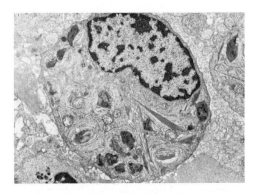

Figure 6–6D. Electron micrograph showing osmiophilic granular material, membranous whorls and trilaminar leaflets in the cytoplasm of a macrophage.

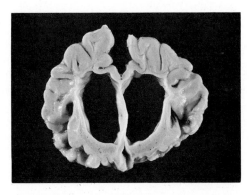

Figure 6–6F. Coronal section of the brain of another patient with adrenoleukodystrophy. Note the extensive loss of white matter and ventricular dilatation.

contain foci of mineralization. Axons are generally spared, although cavitation may be encountered in more advanced cases. The adrenal cortex may be hypertrophied or atrophic and infiltrated by mononuclear cells. However, the characteristic pathological alteration is the presence of cortical cells with striated cytoplasm (Fig. 6–6G). Similar appearing cells have also been noted in the testes.

By contrast, adrenomyeloneuropathy usually presents in early adult life with clinical manifestations that are predominantly those of a myelopathy, such as spastic paraparesis. These are usually accompanied or preceded by evidence of adrenal insufficiency. This form of the disease pursues a more indolent course than the classic childhood adrenoleukodystrophy. Female heterozygotes are usually asymptomatic but some show clinical features that are similar to males with adrenomyeloneuropathy.

Pathological changes in patients with adrenomyeloneuropathy are most pronounced in the long tracts of the spinal cord. Histological changes consist of demyelination with perivascular accumulations of macrophages and small mononuclear cells. The cerebral changes are relatively mild. Peripheral nerves show variable degrees of demyelination. The adrenals and testes show changes that are similar to those seen in childhood adrenoleukodystrophy.

Very rare cases of neonatal adrenoleukodystrophy have been described. This form of the disease is inherited as an autosomal recessive trait. The pathological findings include abnormal gyri and gray matter heterotopias in addition to the characteristic features of leukodystrophy.

All forms of adrenoleukodystrophy are characterized by abnormal lipid metabolism. This is reflected by the accumulation of very long chain fatty acids in blood plasma and in tissues. The abnormal fatty acids are contained in gangliosides and cholesterol esters. The accumulation of very long chain fatty acids has been attributed to abnormal beta-oxidation in peroxisomes. The exact mechanisms by which the cellular damage is produced in the brain and adrenals remains incompletely elucidated.

REFERENCES

Moser HW, Moser AE, Singh I, O'Neill BP: Adrenoleukodystrophy: Survey of 303 cases: Biochemistry, diagnosis, and therapy. Ann Neurol 1984; 16:628-641.

Powers JM: Adreno-leukodystrophy (Adreno-testiculo-leuko-myelo-neuropathic-complex). Clin Neuropathol 1985; 4:181-199.

Powers JM, Moser HW, Moser AB, et al: Pathologic findings in adrenoleukodystrophy heterozygotes. Arch Pathol Lab Med 1987; 111:151-153.

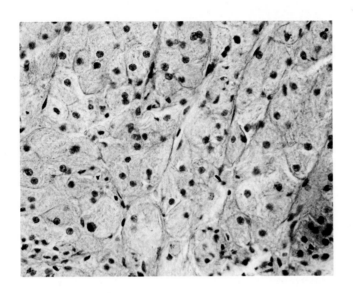

Figure 6–6G. Microscopic section of the adrenal cortex showing the striated appearance of the cells within the zona fasciculata.

6.7   Zellweger's Syndrome

CLINICAL

This 2-month-old girl was hospitalized for evaluation of abnormal bruising. She was the product of an uncomplicated pregnancy. At birth, she was noted to have multiple congenital anomalies including an abnormal head shape, dislocated hips, and clubbed feet. As a neonate, she developed seizures and fed poorly.

Physical examination revealed a small child with low set ears, a high forehead, and a flattened occiput. She was markedly hypotonic, had poor head control, and exhibited no spontaneous movements. She would not follow objects, her pupillary responses were sluggish, and she had a poor gag reflex. Her liver was enlarged. Laboratory studies revealed a hemoglobin of 8.0 g/dL and hematocrit of 26 percent. White blood cell and platelet counts were normal. The partial thromboplastin time was prolonged. A liver biopsy revealed increased iron stores in hepatocytes and Kupffer cells. The child died a few weeks later at the age of 3 months.

PATHOLOGY

The most striking visceral abnormalities were in the kidneys and liver. There were multiple small subcortical cysts in both kidneys. The liver also contained a small number of widely scattered cysts and showed moderately severe hepatic fibrosis.

Examination of the brain revealed blunting of the frontal poles and gyral abnormalities. There were excessively complex convolutions in the frontal lobes, on the superior aspect of the parietal lobes, and on the inferior surface of the temporal lobes. Other gyri in the same areas were abnormally broad (Fig. 6–7A). Coronal sections confirmed the gyral abnormalities (Fig. 6–7B) and disclosed bilateral germinal matrix cysts (Fig. 6–7C). The basal ganglia and thalami were grossly normal. Histological examination revealed a paucity of myelin and scattered lipid-laden macrophages, especially in the periventricular regions. The inferior olivary nuclei were malformed and had simplified convolutions (Fig. 6–7D).

COMMENT

Zellweger's syndrome is a rare autosomal recessive disorder. The clinical manifestations are evident from the time of birth and include weakness, hypotonia, and hyporeflexia. The infants often have seizures. These neurological manifestations are accompanied by a distinctive craniofacial configuration. This is caused by a high forehead, hypoplastic supraorbital ridges, hypertelorism, low set ears, and a flattened occiput. Other common skeletal anomalies include dislocated hips, camptodactyly, and clubbed feet. The individuals often have hepatomegaly and evidence of hepatic dysfunction in the form of elevated serum enzymes. Many of the infants develop cutaneous and gastrointestinal bleeding.

Due to the gyral abnormalities, Zellweger's disease had been regarded as an inherited disorder of neuronal migration. In more recent years, the disease has been reinterpreted as a metabolic disorder involving peroxisomes. This newer concept was initiated when it was demonstrated, by ultrastructural studies, that peroxisomes were absent from the kidney and liver of patients with this disorder.

Subsequently, it was shown that certain metabolic functions attributed to peroxisomes, including synthesis of plasmalogen and bile acids and oxidation of very long chain fatty acids, are abnormal in these patients. The deficiency of this organelle is also seen in the neonatal form of adrenoleukodystrophy. By contrast, patients with the classical juvenile form of adrenoleukodystrophy and with adrenomyeloneuropathy have the organelles, but the organelles do not function properly. Other diseases that have now been attributed to abnormal metabolism of peroxisomes include Refsum's disease and cerebrotendinous xanthomatosis.

REFERENCES

Aubourg P, Robain O, Rocchioccioli F, et al: The cerebro-hepato-renal (Zellweger) syndrome: Lamellar lipid profiles in adrenocortical, hepatic mesenchymal, astrocyte cells and increased levels of very long chain fatty acids and phytanic acid in the plasma. J Neurol Sci 1985; 69:9-25.

Moser HW: The peroxisome: Nervous system role of a previously underrated organelle. Neurology 1988; 38: 1617-1627.

Powers JM, Moser HW, Moser AB, et al: Fetal cerebro-hepatorenal (Zellweger) syndrome: Dysmorphic, radiologic, biochemical, and pathologic findings in four affected fetuses. Hum Pathol 1985; 16:610-620.

Volpe JJ, Adams RD: Cerebro-hepato-renal syndrome of Zellweger: An inherited disorder of neuronal migration. Acta Neuropathol 1972; 20:175-198.

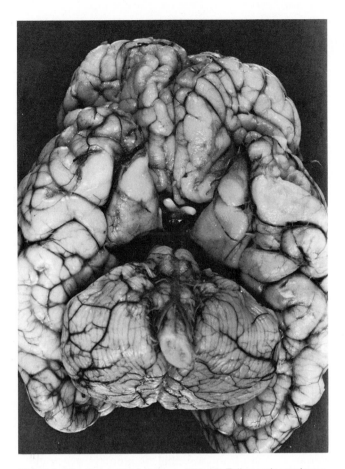

Figure 6–7A. Base of brain from a child with Zellweger's syndrome.

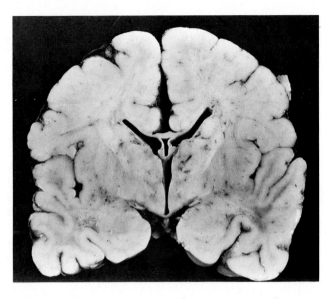

Figure 6–7B. Coronal section showing gyral abnormalities.

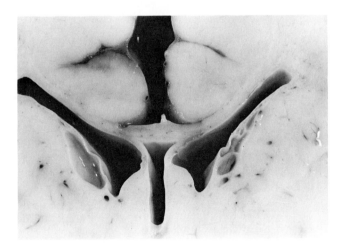

Figure 6–7C. Coronal section showing germinal matrix cysts.

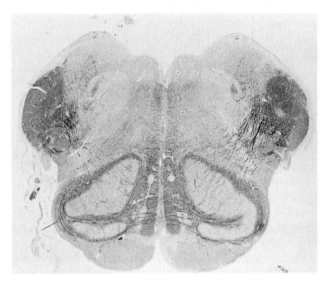

Figure 6–7D. Macrosection of the medulla showing malformed inferior olivary nuclei with simplified convolutions.

6.8 Alexander's Disease

CLINICAL

This female infant had been born prematurely. At birth she weighed 1162 grams and had a head circumference of 26 cm. She would not smile or cry but would turn toward a loud noise. She was hospitalized at age 4 months because of an enlarging head that by then measured 42 cm. A pneumoencephalogram showed enlarged ventricles, and a ventriculoatrial shunt was inserted. Shunt failure was suspected when she was readmitted at age 6 months with a head circumference of 45 cm. She developed seizures that persisted until her death at age 8 months.

PATHOLOGY

The brain was moderately enlarged and weighed 780 grams. The gyri and sulci were of normal proportions and distribution. Coronal sections revealed the cortex and basal ganglia to be intact. The white matter was soft but rubbery and retracted from the cut surface (Fig. 6–8A). The ventricles were only slightly enlarged. Histological examination revealed many small, round to elongated, eosinophilic bodies. These so-called Rosenthal fibers formed a continuous band beneath pial surfaces (Fig. 6–8B), surrounded blood vessels (Fig. 6–8C), and aggregated beneath the ependyma. They were present in smaller numbers throughout the gliotic and sparsely myelinated white matter. Variable numbers of Rosenthal fibers were also present in the gray matter, especially the thalamus and brain stem nuclei. Ultrastructurally, the Rosenthal fibers appeared as variable-sized masses of osmiophilic granular material within the cytoplasm of astrocytes (Fig. 6–8D).

COMMENT

Alexander's disease is a rare neurodegenerative disorder. Although it is generally discussed among the leukodystrophies, it is best regarded as a metabolic disorder of astrocytes. The disease can be divided into several more or less distinct clinical forms but all have similar histopathological features.

The originally described and most common type is the infantile form. These individuals have an early onset of symptoms and a rapidly progressive course. The clinical manifestations include severe psychomotor retardation, seizures, spasticity, and often megalencephaly. At least some of these cases appear to be familial. Individuals with the juvenile form of the disease have a somewhat later onset of symptoms and a more indolent course. The clinical manifestations are dominated by long-tract and bulbar signs, with less pronounced psychomotor retardation. Some adults with the histopathological features of Alexander's disease have symptoms resembling multiple sclerosis while others remain asymptomatic. Still other adults with diverse neurological and nonneurological diseases have focal or multifocal deposits of Rosenthal fibers. It remains to be determined which if any of these adult cases should be regarded as a form of Alexander's disease.

The most characteristic pathological feature of Alexander's disease is extensive deposition of Rosenthal fibers predominantly in subpial, perivascular, and subependymal locations. The white matter shows a variable degree of demyelination and cavitation and contains scattered Rosenthal fibers. Rosenthal fibers are also found in gray matter, especially the basal ganglia, thalami, and brain stem nuclei.

The pathogenesis of the Rosenthal fibers is unclear. Ultrastructurally, they appear as masses of osmiophilic granular material associated with glial filaments and are contained in the cytoplasm of astrocytes. However, Rosenthal fibers probably do not arise directly from the glial filaments since they are not stained by immunoperoxidase reactions for antibodies to glial fibrillary acidic protein.

It should be noted that small focal deposits of Rosenthal fibers are encountered in a wide variety of neoplastic and nonneoplastic disease processes involving astrocytes. Rosenthal fibers were originally described in the walls of syringomyelic cavities. They are commonly seen in cerebellar and diencephalic astrocytomas, in cysts associated with hemangioblastomas, in the glial tissue adjacent to craniopharyngiomas, in the glial core of the pineal, and in ependymal granulations. They are seen less often around remote contusions and vascular lesions.

REFERENCES

Borrett D, Becker LE: Alexander's disease: A disease of astrocytes. Brain 1985; 108:367-385.

Janzer RC, Friede RL: Do Rosenthal fibers contain glial fibrillary acid protein? Acta Neuropathol 1981; 55:75-76.

Riggs JE, Schochet SS Jr, Nelson J: Asymptomatic adult Alexander disease: Entity or nosological misconception? Neurology 1988; 38:152-154.

Russo LS Jr, Aron A, Anderson PJ: Alexander's disease: A report and reappraisal. Neurology 1976; 26:607-614.

Towfighi J, Young R, Sassani J, et al: Alexander's disease: Further light- and electron-microscopic observations. Acta Neuropathol 1983; 61:36-42.

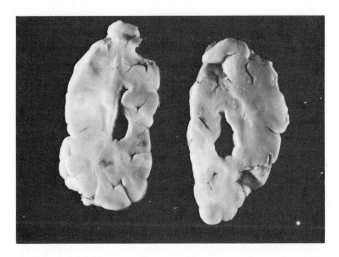

Figure 6–8A. Coronal sections of cerebral hemispheres from a child with Alexander's disease.

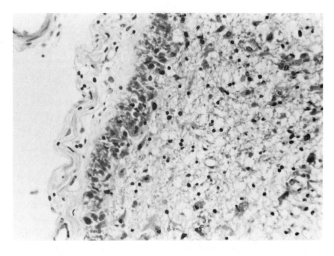

Figure 6–8B. Microscopic section showing accumulation of Rosenthal fibers beneath the pia.

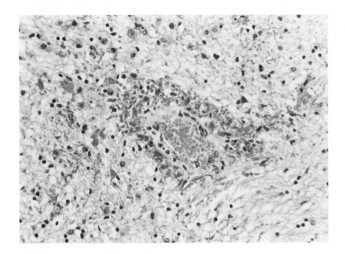

Figure 6–8C. Microscopic section showing perivascular accumulation of Rosenthal fibers.

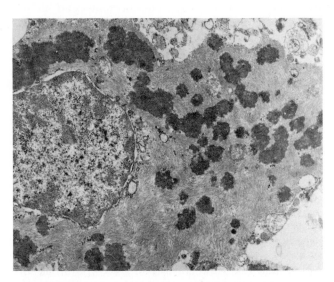

Figure 6–8D. Electron micrograph showing osmiophilic granular material, corresponding to Rosenthal fibers, within the cytoplasm of an astrocyte.

6.9 Other Leukodystrophies

Canavan's Disease
Pelizaeus–Merzbacher's Disease
Seitelberger's Disease

Canavan's disease or infantile spongy degeneration of the white matter is a rare autosomal recessive disorder that occurs predominantly among infants of Ashkenazi Jewish descent. Symptoms usually appear during the first 6 months of life and include psychomotor retardation, hypotonia, and blindness. Later, the infants develop seizures and spasticity. The infants typically develop macrocephaly; however, computerized tomography demonstrates normal sized ventricles and symmetrical low-density white matter lesions.

Brains from infants with Canavan's disease are large and have diffusely discolored, softened white matter. There is moderate demyelination and gliosis of the central white matter. The most striking histological feature is vacuolization of the subcortical white matter and deeper layers of the cortex (Fig. 6–9A). This is in contrast to most other leukodystrophies where the arcuate fibers tend to be spared. The vacuolization in the white matter is due to accumulation of fluid between myelin lamellae, so-called intramyelinic edema. The vacuolization in the cortex is due to swelling of astrocytic cytoplasm. When examined by electron microscopy, these cells are found to contain very large mitochondria with abnormal cristae (Fig. 6–9B). It has been suggested that the intramyelinic edema and the astrocytic swelling result from abnormal movement of electrolytes and impaired regulation of intracellular water content. Nevertheless, biochemical studies have failed to demonstrate consistent abnormalities in mitochondrial adenosine triphosphatase, despite their structural aberrations. Cortical neurons tend to be unaffected.

Pelizaeus–Merzbacher's disease is another rare leukodystrophy that occurs in several forms. The classic, juvenile form is an X-linked recessive disorder that becomes manifest during the first decade. The clinical manifestations include psychomotor retardation, choreoathetosis, and nystagmus. The brains from these individuals are characterized by a marked deficiency of myelin except for patches that tend to occur around blood vessels. This imparts a distinctive appearance to the white matter and has been described as "tigeroid." The pathogenesis of this disorder has not been established.

Seitelberger's disease is generally considered to be an infantile form of Pelizaeus–Merzbacher's disease. The brains and spinal cords from these infants contain virtually no myelin, but show normal myelination of the peripheral nervous system. The specimen illustrated in Figure 6–9C has been stained for myelin. It shows normal myelin staining in the spinal roots; however, practically no myelin staining in the cord itself. This disease has been interpreted as a disorder of oligodendrocytes that leads to failure of central nervous system myelination.

REFERENCES

Adachi M, Schneck L, Cara J, Volk BW: Spongy degeneration of the central nervous system (van Bogaert and Bertrand type; Canavan's disease): A review. Hum Pathol 1973; 4:331-347.

Adornato BT, O'Brien JS, Lampert PW, et al: Cerebral spongy degeneration of infancy: A biochemical and ultrastructual study of affected twins. Neurology 1972; 22:202-210.

Koeppen AH, Ronca NA, Greenfield EA, Hans MB: Defective biosynthesis of proteolipid protein in Pelizaeus–Merzbacher disease. Ann Neurol 1987; 21:159-170.

Seitelberger F: Pelizaeus–Merzbacher disease. In Vinken PJ, Bruyn GW (eds): Handbook of Clinical Neurology. Amsterdam, Elsevier, 1970, vol 10, chap 10, pp 150-202.

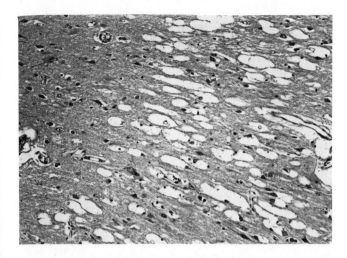

Figure 6–9A. Microscopic section from the brain of an infant with Canavan's disease, showing vacuoles in the deeper layers of the cortex and outer portion of the white matter.

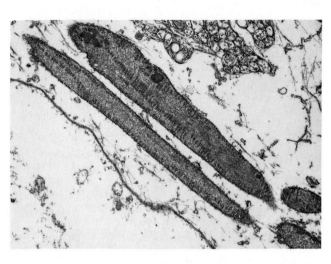

Figure 6–9B. Electron micrograph showing large mitochondria with aberrant cristae within a swollen astrocyte.

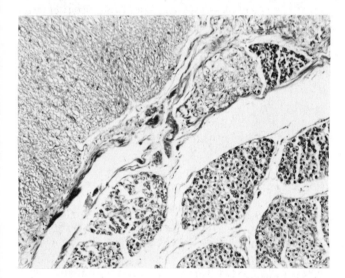

Figure 6–9C. Microscopic section of spinal cord and nerve root from an infant with Seitelberger's disease. Note the lack of myelin staining in the spinal cord (upper left) in contrast to the normal myelin staining of the nerve root (lower right).

Dementias and Degenerations

7.1 Alzheimer's Disease

CLINICAL

This 79-year-old woman, who was a nursing home resident, was hospitalized with confusion, fever, and decreased appetite. She had a 10-year history of memory loss. Laboratory studies revealed pyuria and hypernatremia. Despite antibiotics and rehydration, she died 1 week later.

PATHOLOGY

The brain weighed 1100 grams and, externally, showed convolutional atrophy that was most marked in the frontal lobes (Fig. 7–1A). In coronal sections, the gyri appeared moderately atrophic but the cortical gray matter was not conspicuously thinned. Widening of the sulci was especially obvious in the insulae (Figs. 7–1B and 7–1C). The volume of the subcortical and central white matter was markedly reduced and the ventricular system was enlarged (Figs. 7–1B and 7-1C). The lateral angles of the lateral horns were broadly rounded and the temporal horns were prominently enlarged. The ventricular enlargement was less evident in the third ventricle. The hippocampi were atrophic but the basal ganglia and thalami were of normal size. The cerebellum and brain stem were not significantly affected.

Histologically, there were numerous neurofibrillary tangles and senile plaques in the isocortex, hippocampi, and, to a lesser extent, the basal ganglia. Occasional neurofibrillary tangles (Fig. 7–1D, curved arrow) and senile plaques (Fig. 7–1E) could be seen in sections stained with hematoxylin–eosin. However, they appeared far more numerous and were much more readily demonstrated in sections stained with silver techniques, such as the Bodian stain (Fig. 7–1F). Sections of the hippocampi also showed occasional neurons with granulovacuolar degeneration (Fig. 7–1D, arrowheads) and occasional Hirano bodies (Fig. 7–1G). Sections through the basal nucleus of Meynert showed a reduction in the neuronal population and occasional globose neurofibrillary tangles in the remaining neurons (Fig. 7–1H). Additional globose neurofibrillary tangles were present in the brain stem.

COMMENT

Alzheimer's disease, including senile dementia of the Alzheimer type, is the most common form of dementia and probably affects more than 5 percent of the population over the age of 65. Although the majority of cases of Alzheimer's disease appear to be sporadic, there are well documented familial cases. Often these individuals manifest the disease at a younger age and some show especially severe pathological changes. The possibility of significant genetic contribution is supported by the frequent occurrence of dementia and histopathological alterations of Alzheimer's disease in older individuals with Down's syndrome.

The clinical diagnosis of Alzheimer's disease is generally made after excluding less common causes of dementia such as Parkinson's disease, Huntington's disease, Pick's disease, Creutzfeldt–Jakob disease, and certain metabolic derangements. Another important but less common type of dementia among the older population is so-called multi-infarct dementia. However, many individuals with advanced arteriosclerosis and multiple infarcts also have pathological changes of Alzheimer's disease.

Most patients with Alzheimer's disease have some degree of cerebral atrophy and ventricular enlargement. However, the extent of these changes is highly variable and in some patients, the gross alterations are not striking. Quantitative studies of the cerebral cortex from patients with Alzheimer's disease have shown a marked decrease in the number of cortical neurons although the extent of the reduction is often not readily apparent in routine sections. By contrast, similar studies on brains from elderly, nondemented individuals have shown a reduction in the size of the cortical neurons but a less marked reduction in their number. The loss of neurons is accompanied by an increase in the number of fibrous astrocytes.

The most conspicuous histopathological changes in the isocortex and the hippocampi are the presence of senile plaques and neurofibrillary tangles. Small numbers of these structures may be encountered in elderly nondemented individuals, especially in the hippocampi. However, in patients with Alzheimer's disease, senile plaques and neurofibrillary tangles are far more numerous and widespread in the isocortex. Some patients with Alzheimer's disease, especially older patients, may have numerous senile plaques but few if any neurofibrillary tangles. The senile plaques are typically composed of a core of extracellular amyloid surrounded by degenerating neurites. Microglial cells and astrocytes may be present at the periphery of the plaques. Occasionally, plaques can be seen in sections stained with hematoxylin–eosin but are seen better with the periodic acid–Schiff stain.

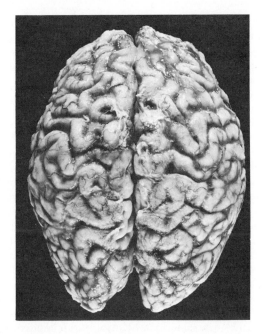

Figure 7–1A. Dorsal surface of brain from patient with Alzheimer's disease showing convolutional atrophy most marked in frontal lobes.

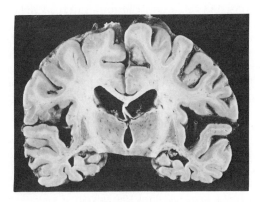

Figure 7–1C. Coronal section showing especially pronounced enlargement of the subarachnoid space over the insulae.

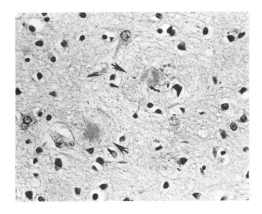

Figure 7–1E. Senile plaques (arrows) in a section of cortex stained with hematoxylin–eosin.

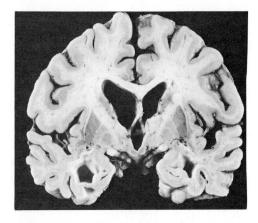

Figure 7–1B. Coronal section showing widened sulci, decreased volume of white matter, and enlargement of the ventricles.

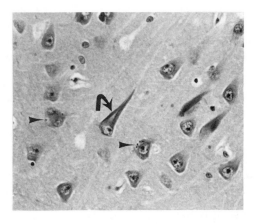

Figure 7–1D. Neurofibrillary tangles (curved arrow) and granulovacuolar degeneration (arrowheads) in a section of hippocampus stained with hematoxylin–eosin.

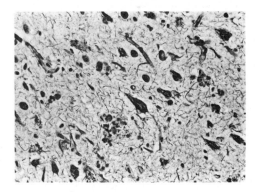

Figure 7–1F. The neurofibrillary tangles and senile plaques are more conspicuous with the Bodian silver stain.

They are best demonstrated in sections stained with various silver techniques or stains for amyloid. Additional deposits of amyloid may be present in meningeal and small cortical blood vessels. There is no correlation between these intracerebral deposits of amyloid and systemic amyloidosis. The exact pathogenesis of the plaques and the origin of the amyloid remain controversial. Neuronal fibrous proteins and hematogenous proteins, including prealbumin, have been proposed by various authors as the source of the amyloid. Recent evidence has suggested that the intracerebral amyloid deposition is under the control of a gene on chromosome 21.

Neurofibrillary tangles are found in a wide variety of disorders and are a less specific feature of Alzheimer's disease than the senile plaques. The neurofibrillary tangles tend to have a flame shape when they occur in the pyramidal neurons of the cortex and hippocampi and a globose configuration when they occur in the basal ganglia including the basal nucleus of Meynert and the brain stem. Neurofibrillary tangles are never seen among the Purkinje cells of the cerebellum and are only very rarely seen in the anterior horn motor neurons of the spinal cord. As with senile plaques, they are occasionally seen in sections stained with hematoxylin–eosin but are most readily seen in sections stained with silver or amyloid stains. Ultrastructurally, they are composed of paired helical filaments that appear as periodically constricted structures formerly described as twisted tubules (Fig. 7–1I). These structures have been observed only in human brains. The chemical composition and pathogenesis of the neurofibrillary tangles remain unsettled. Recent immunohistochemical studies have emphasized the presence of neurofilament proteins and microtubule-associated proteins in neurofibrillary tangles regardless of the disease process with which they are associated.

There are also other less specific histopathological changes. The so-called granulovacuolar degeneration of Simchowicz occurs almost exclusively among neurons in the pyramidal layer of the hippocampus. This process results in the formation of small dark granules surrounded by clear halos within the neuronal cytoplasm. It has been suggested that these structures result from autophagy since the affected neurons contain less lipofuscin than adjacent neurons. Granulovacuolar degeneration is more pronounced but not restricted to individuals with Alzheimer's disease.

Patients with Alzheimer's disease may have numerous Hirano bodies in their hippocampi. The Hirano bodies are small eosinophilic spherical to fusiform structures. They are found predominantly in neuronal perikarya and processes. The Hirano bodies are composed of filaments that are arranged in complex latticework arrays so as to produce a paracrystalline appearance when viewed by electron microscopy. Immunochemical studies have demonstrated the presence of actin in these bodies. The pathogenesis and significance of Hirano bodies remain unknown. These structures also may be found in elderly nondemented individuals and in patients with other neurodegenerative diseases.

Possibly the most significant alteration in Alzheimer's disease is the loss of neurons from the basal nucleus of Meynert. This nucleus is an indistinctly demarcated mass of large neurons located beneath the striatum at the level of the anterior commissure. The nucleus contains cholinergic neurons that project to all parts of the isocortex and hippocampus. The loss of these neurons results in decreased cortical choline acetyl transferase and acetylcholine. By contrast, the decreased levels of other neurotransmitters such as somatostatin and substance P have been attributed to the loss of intracortical neurons. The loss of these various neurotransmitters is not restricted to Alzheimer's disease. For example, a similar loss of cholinergic neurons from the basal nucleus of Meynert has been observed in demented patients with Parkinson's disease and loss of cortical somatostatin is seen in patients with Pick's disease. Recently, increased levels of a protein designated as A68 has been demonstrated in brain tissue and cerebrospinal fluid of patients with Alzheimer's disease. Trace amounts were also identified in patients with Pick's disease and Guamanian Parkinson dementia complex. Although the origin and significance of this protein remains to be established, assays for this material may be useful for clinical diagnosis.

REFERENCES

Joachim CL, Morris JH, Kosik KS, Selkoe DJ: Tau antisera recognize neurofibrillary tangles in a range of neurodegenerative disorders. Ann Neurol 1987; 22:514-520.

Katzman R: Alzheimer's disease. N Engl J Med 1986; 314:964-973.

Roberts GW, Lofthouse R, Allsop D, et al: CNS amyloid proteins in neurodegenerative diseases. Neurology 1988; 38:1534-1540.

Terry RD: Alzheimer's disease. In Davis RL, Robertson DM (eds): Textbook of Neuropathology. Baltimore, Williams & Wilkins, 1985, chap 16, pp 824-841.

Terry RD, DeTeresa R, Hansen LA: Neocortical cell counts in normal human adult aging. Ann Neurol 1987; 21:530-539.

Whitehouse PJ, Price DL, Clark AW, et al: Alzheimer disease: Evidence for selective loss of cholinergic neurons in the nucleus basalis. Ann Neurol 1981; 10:122-126.

Wolozin B, Davies P: Alzheimer-related neuronal protein A68: Specificity and distribution. Ann Neurol 1987; 22:521-526.

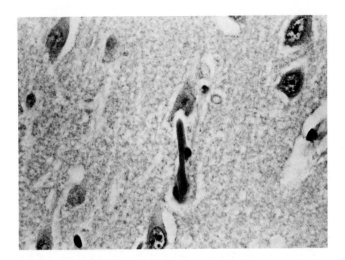

Figure 7–1G. Microscopic section of the hippocampus showing eosinophilic, rod-shaped Hirano body.

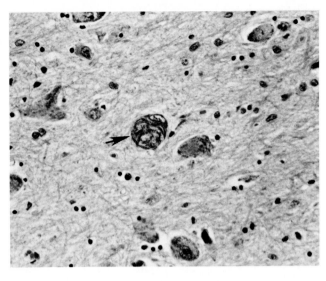

Figure 7–1H. Microscopic section of the basal nucleus of Meynert showing a globose neurofibrillary tangle (arrow).

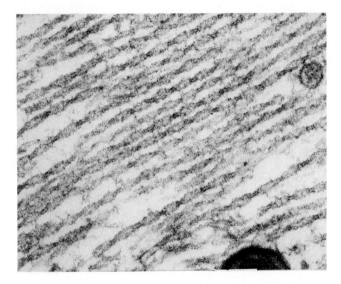

Figure 7–1I. Ultrastructurally, the neurofibrillary tangles are composed of paired helical filaments.

7.2   Pick's Disease

CLINICAL

This 69-year-old man had been institutionalized for the last 5 months of his life. His illness began at age 61 when he would wander aimlessly, get lost, and act confused. During the last months of his life, he was bedridden, mute, and could not recognize people.

PATHOLOGY

The brain was severely atrophic. The distribution and severity of the atrophy was demonstrated more clearly after removing the meninges. So-called knife-edge atrophy was apparent in the frontal, orbital, and anterior temporal convolutions (Figs. 7–2A and 7–2B). The inferior parietal lobule was moderately atrophic. The posterior portion of the superior temporal convolution, the precentral gyrus, the postcentral gyrus, the cingulate gyrus, the superior parietal lobule and the occipital lobe were conspicuously spared (Figs. 7–2A through 7–2C). The hippocampal gyrus showed only moderate atrophy. The volume of subcortical and central white matter was markedly reduced. The basal ganglia showed moderate atrophy. The ventricular system was markedly enlarged.

Histological examination revealed marked loss of cortical neurons and gliosis in all of the atrophic areas. Many of the remaining cortical neurons were enlarged and somewhat globular. These constituted the so-called Pick cells. Other neurons contained spherical intracytoplasmic inclusions, the so-called Pick bodies. The Pick bodies were more numerous in the pyramidal layer neurons of the hippocampus than in the isocortex. They were unusually small but especially numerous in the neurons of the dentate fascia. The Pick bodies appeared as amphophilic spheroids in sections stained with hematoxylin–eosin but were much more readily seen in sections stained by silver techniques such as the Bodian stain (Fig. 7–2D). Numerous Hirano bodies were also present in the hippocampus.

COMMENT

In contrast to Alzheimer's disease, Pick's disease is extremely rare. The clinical manifestations of these two diseases are very similar. However, some authors have emphasized the earlier involvement of personality, emotional behavior, and language in patients with Pick's disease. Most cases appear to be sporadic, although some familial cases have been reported.

Brains from patients with Pick's disease generally show severe symmetrical or asymmetrical lobar atrophy involving especially the frontal and temporal lobes. The gyri are often so severely atrophic that the term "knife-edge" atrophy is used to describe the process. Nevertheless, certain areas are typically spared. These include the posterior portion of the superior temporal gyrus, the precentral gyrus, the postcentral gyrus, and the cingulate gyrus. Usually, the hippocampus is only moderately atrophic. The parietal lobes show a variable degree of involvement while the occipital lobes are generally spared. The white matter is markedly reduced in volume. Recently, this has been shown to be associated with a selective loss of galactolipids including galactocerebrosides and sulfatides. In some cases the basal ganglia are severely atrophic (Fig. 7–2E), resulting in a configuration that grossly resembles Huntington's disease.

The histological findings in Pick's disease include neuronal loss, Pick cells, Pick bodies, and gliosis. The Pick cells are enlarged globular neurons that resemble chromatolytic neurons. The Pick bodies are spherical intracytoplasmic inclusions that may be found occasionally in the atrophic cerebral cortex and more often in the pyramidal neurons of the hippocampus and the entorhinal cortex. Large numbers of small Pick bodies are often found among the neurons of the dentate fascia. Although some of the inclusions may be seen in sections stained with hematoxylin–eosin, they are more clearly demonstrated with silver stains. Many authors regard the presence of Pick bodies as a prerequisite for the diagnosis of Pick's disease. By electron microscopy, Pick bodies appear as sharply demarcated but unbounded aggregates of neurofilaments, tubules, and, occasionally, paired helical filaments along with other cytoplasmic components. Immunocytochemical studies have shown that Pick bodies contain various neurofilament- and microtubule-associated proteins such as tau, similar to those found in neurofibrillary tangles. Some patients with Pick's disease have a reduced number of neurons in the nucleus basalis of Meynert. However, the cortical choline acetyltransferase tends to be less severely reduced than in Alzheimer's disease. Some patients with lobar atrophy, loss of cortical neurons, and gliosis, but without Pick bodies, have been described under the heading of dysphasic dementia.

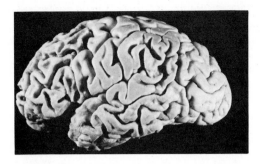

Figure 7–2A. Lateral surface of brain from patient with Pick's disease showing "knife-edge" lobar atrophy. Note the involvement of the rostral portion of the superior temporal gyrus. *(Schochet, SS Jr, Lampert, PW, & Lindenberg, R: Fine Structure of the Pick and Hirano bodies in a case of Pick's disease.* Acta Neuropathol *11:330–337, 1968.)*

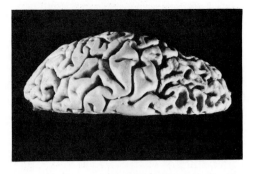

Figure 7–2B. Dorsal surface of brain showing the severe atrophy of the frontal lobe.

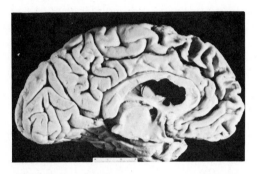

Figure 7–2C. Medial surface of the brain showing the relative preservation of the cingulate gyrus.

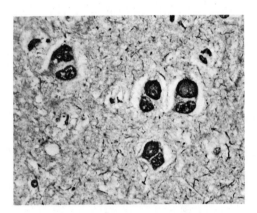

Figure 7–2D. Pick bodies appear as argentophilic intracytoplasmic spheroids when stained with the Bodian silver technique.

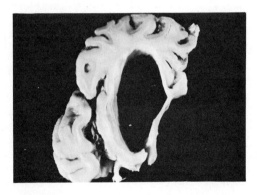

Figure 7–2E. Pick's disease with severe atrophy of basal ganglia.

REFERENCES

Cummings JL, Duchen LW: Kluver–Bucy syndrome in Pick disease: Clinical and pathological correlations. Neurology 1981; 31:1415-1422.

Mehler MF, Horoupian DS, Davies P, Kickson DW: Reduced somatostatin-like immunoreactivity in cerebral cortex in nonfamilial dysphasic dementia. Neurology 1987; 37:1448-1453.

Munoz-Garcia D, Ludwin SK: Classic and generalized variants of Pick's disease: A clinicopathological, ultrastructural, and immunochemical comparative study. Ann Neurol 1984; 16:467-480.

Rasool CG, Selkoe DJ: Sharing of specific antigens by degenerating neurons in Pick's disease and Alzheimer's disease. N Engl J Med 1985; 312:700-705.

Scicutella A, Davies P: Marked loss of cerebral galactolipids in Pick's disease. Ann Neurol 1987; 22:606-609.

Uhl GR, Hilt DC, Hedreen JC, et al: Pick's disease (lobar sclerosis): Depletion of neurons in the nucleus basalis of Meynert. Neurology 1983; 33:1470-1473.

7.3   Creutzfeldt–Jakob Disease

CLINICAL

This 70-year-old man developed ataxia followed by gait impairment and mental deterioration. One week before hospitalization, he developed jerking of his hand and forearm. On physical examination, he was found to have diffuse muscle wasting, generalized rigidity, and jerking of the hand and forearm every 1 to 2 seconds. Computerized tomograms with and without contrast revealed only generalized cerebral atrophy. Electroencephalograms showed generalized slowing and triphasic complexes of approximately 1 hertz. The patient's condition continued to deteriorate and he died 4 months after the onset of his illness.

PATHOLOGY

The brain weighed 1000 grams and showed atrophy that was most pronounced in the frontal and occipital lobes (Fig. 7–3A). Horizontal sections showed moderate convolutional atrophy and reduction in the volume of the subcortical and central white matter. The nuclear components of the basal ganglia were of normal size and intact. The ventricular system was only moderately enlarged (Fig. 7–3B). Histological examination revealed neuronal loss, gliosis, and fine vacuolation (status spongiosus) in the cerebral cortex (Fig. 7–3C) and putamen. The cerebellar cortex showed status spongiosus and gliosis (Fig. 7–3D). There were virtually no senile plaques or neurofibrillary tangles in the hippocampi or isocortex.

COMMENT

Creutzfeldt–Jakob disease is a rare cause of dementia with a worldwide prevalence of about 1 to 2 per million. It is generally a rapidly progressive dementia that is accompanied by varying degrees of cerebellar, pyramidal, extrapyramidal, visual, and lower motor neuron involvement. Myoclonus is common but may occur late in the course of the illness. Although most of the cases are sporadic, familial cases have comprised 5 to 10 percent of some series. The peak incidence is during the seventh decade; however, the onset of the disease may be as early as the teens or as late as the ninth decade. Although most patients die within 1 year of the onset, some have the disease for more than a decade. A protracted course is more apt to be encountered among familial cases or in individuals with an unusually early onset of the disease. Electroencephalography discloses characteristic periodic synchronous discharges in the majority of patients. Computerized tomography may show varying degrees of cerebral atrophy or no abnormalities.

Brain specimens from patients with Creutzfeldt–Jakob disease range from grossly normal to moderately atrophic with enlarged ventricles. In some cases, the atrophy is most pronounced in the occipital lobes. The characteristic histopathological alterations are vacuolation (status spongiosus) and gliosis of gray matter. These changes involve the cerebral cortex, basal ganglia, brain stem, and cerebellum but are variable in degree and uneven in distribution. The individual vacuoles are generally small and nearly spherical. Ultrastructural studies have shown that many of these vacuoles are within neuronal processes and perikarya. The vacuoles characteristic of Creutzfeldt–Jakob disease must be distinguished carefully from larger vacuoles that can result from cerebral hypoxia or even postmortem artifacts. The artifactual vacuoles are within astrocytes, around neurons, and around vessels. Cases of Creutzfeldt–Jakob disease with a longer course may show less vacuolation and relatively more gliosis. The status spongiosus and gliosis are accompanied by a variable loss of neurons. In some cases of Creutzfeldt–Jakob disease there are small amyloid plaques especially in the cerebellum. In contrast to senile plaques, these so-called kuru plaques are not accompanied by degenerating neurites.

Creutzfeldt–Jakob disease has been transmitted to various laboratory animals, initially primates, and, more recently, rodents. Human to human transmission has been documented following corneal transplants, implantation of depth electrodes, placement of a dura mater graft, and in recipients of growth hormone prepared from pooled autopsy pituitaries. For a number of years, 4 percent sodium hypochlorite solution was regarded as an effective disinfectant. More recently, the use of 1 N sodium hydroxide has been recommended.

Despite intensive investigation, the causative agent has not been fully characterized. Some authors have suggested that the infection is caused by prions, unique protease-resistant proteins that have been isolated from the brains of patients and animals with Creutzfeldt–Jakob disease and from animals with scrapie. Furthermore, it has been suggested that the

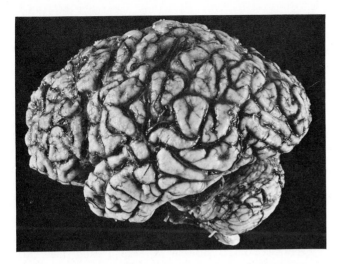

Figure 7–3A. Lateral surface of brain from patient with Creutzfeldt–Jakob disease showing atrophy of frontal and occipital lobes.

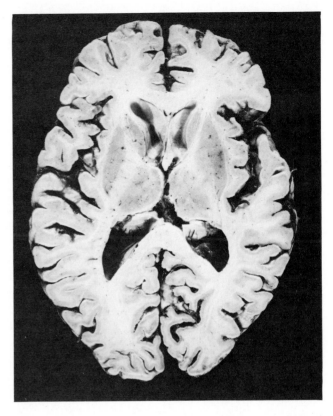

Figure 7–3B. Horizontal section showing moderate convolutional atrophy and reduction in volume of white matter.

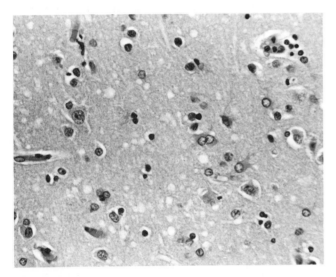

Figure 7–3C. Microscopic section of the isocortex showing small vacuoles (status spongiosus) and gliosis.

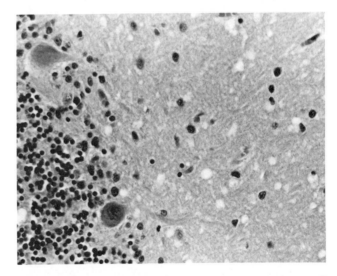

Figure 7–3D. Microscopic section of cerebellum showing small vacuoles in the molecular layer of the cerebellum.

amyloid plaques found in patients with Creutzfeldt–Jakob disease and the Gerstmann–Straussler syndrome are composed of paracrystalline aggregates of infectious prions. However, more recently, it has been suggested that these low-molecular-weight prions arise from alterations of larger proteins present in the normal host. The immunologic detection of these various abnormal proteins in brain tissue and cerebrospinal fluid may prove to be useful adjunct techniques for the diagnosis of the various spongiform encephalopathies.

REFERENCES

Brown P, Cathala F, Castaigne P, Gajdusek DC: Creutzfeldt–Jakob disease: Clinical analysis of a consecutive series of 230 neuropathologically verified cases. Ann Neurol 1986; 20:597-602.

Brown P, Cathala F, Raubertas RF, et al: The epidemiology of Creutzfeldt–Jakob disease: Conclusion of a 15-year investigation in France and review of the world literature. Neurology 1987; 37:895-904.

Brown P, Coker-Vann M, Pomeroy K, et al: Diagnosis of Creutzfeldt–Jakob disease by western blot identification of marker protein in human brain tissue. N Engl J Med 1986; 314:547-551.

Brown P, Rodgers-Johnson P, Cathala F, et al: Creutzfeldt–Jakob disease of long duration: Clinicopathological characteristics, transmissibility, and differential diagnosis. Ann Neurol 1984; 16:295-304.

Harrington MG, Merril CR, Asher DM, Gajdusek DC: Abnormal proteins in the cerebrospinal fluid of patients with Creutzfeldt–Jakob disease. N Engl J Med 1986; 315: 279-283.

7.4 Parkinson's Disease

Idiopathic Parkinsonism

CLINICAL

This 78-year-old man had a 6-year history of Parkinson's disease. This had been manifested by a tremor, stooped posture, rigidity, and a shuffling gait. He died of carcinoma of the lung.

PATHOLOGY

Externally, the brain was grossly unremarkable. Coronal sections of the cerebral hemispheres showed a mild reduction in the volume of the subcortical and central white matter. The basal ganglia were intact (Fig. 7–4A). Sections of the brain stem demonstrated abnormally light pigmentation of the substantia nigra (Fig. 7–4B) and loci caerulei. Histological examination of the pars compacta of the substantia nigra revealed a mild reduction in the number of pigmented neurons. Some of the remaining neurons harbored eosinophilic intracytoplasmic inclusions, the so-called Lewy bodies (Fig. 7–4C). In addition, there were occasional macrophages with pigmented, intracytoplasmic debris.

COMMENT

Parkinson's disease or idiopathic parkinsonism is a relatively common neurological disorder with a prevalence of 150 to 200 per 100,000. The disease is more common among men than women and affects predominantly older individuals. The onset of symptoms is usually during the sixth or seventh decades. The cardinal clinical manifestations include a resting tremor, rigidity, bradykinesia, and loss of postural reflexes. The disease begins insidiously and, initially, may be unilateral. The tremor diminishes during voluntary movements and disappears during sleep. Nearly one third of the patients show some degree of dementia in addition to the movement disorders.

In part, Parkinsonism is due to dopamine deficiency in the striatum. This results from degeneration of neurons in the substantia nigra. These neurons are known to be vulnerable to a variety of injuries. Destruction of the nigral neurons by a viral infection was the apparent cause of so-called postencephalitic parkinsonism. Exposure to toxins such as carbon monoxide and manganese has long been known to cause occasional cases of parkinsonism. In recent years, MPTP (1-methyl-4-phenyl-1,2,3,6-tetrahydropyridine), a contaminant of certain "designer drugs," has been demonstrated to selectively damage dopaminergic nigral neurons, producing an acute parkinsonian disorder. Although the pathogenesis of the neuronal degeneration in idiopathic parkinsonism remains unknown, increased emphasis is being given to a causative or contributory role of environmental toxins.

The major pathological changes in idiopathic parkinsonism are degeneration of pigmented neurons and the presence of Lewy bodies. The neuronal loss from the pars compacta of the substantia nigra is often sufficiently severe to produce gross depigmentation of this structure. Histologically, the neuronal degeneration may be accompanied by macrophages with pigmented debris in their cytoplasm. Virtually all patients with idiopathic parkinsonism have Lewy bodies in the substantia nigra. Often, additional Lewy bodies can be found in other pigmented nuclei, including the locus caeruleus and the dorsal nucleus. Occasionally, they may be encountered in the nucleus basalis, hypothalamus, and other brain stem nuclei. The Lewy bodies are spherical to elongated, laminated intracytoplasmic inclusions. Occasionally, multiple Lewy bodies are harbored by a single neuron. The inclusions are eosinophilic and stain blue or green with the trichrome stains (Fig. 7–4D). They remain unstained with the periodic acid–Schiff technique. Ultrastructurally, the core of the Lewy body contains granular material and circular profiles while the periphery contains radially oriented fibrils. Recent immunochemical studies have suggested that the Lewy bodies are derived from neurofilaments. Demented patients with idiopathic parkinsonism show a significant loss of neurons from the nucleus basalis.

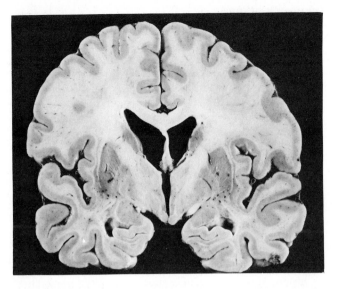

Figure 7–4A. Coronal section showing intact basal ganglia and mild ventricular enlargement.

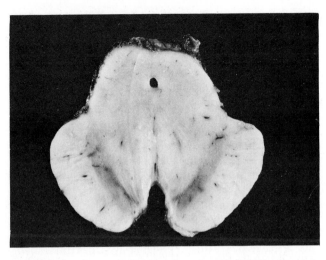

Figure 7–4B. Transverse section of mesencephalon showing moderate depigmentation of the pars compacta of the substantia nigra.

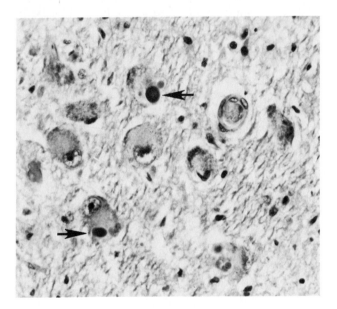

Figure 7–4C. Microscopic section showing eosinophilic intra-cytoplasmic Lewy bodies (arrows).

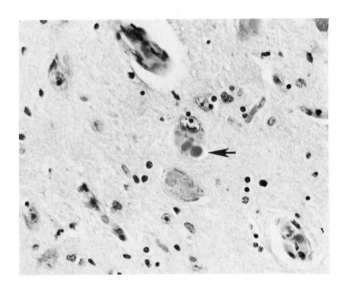

Figure 7–4D. Multiple Lewy bodies (arrow) in the cytoplasm of a single neuron. The Lewy bodies are stained green with the trichrome procedure.

Patients with postencephalitic parkinsonism generally show grossly discernible atrophy of the mesencephalon and more severe loss of neurons from the substantia nigra. The remaining neurons characteristically contain globose neurofibrillary tangles (Fig. 7–4E), instead of Lewy bodies. Additional neurofibrillary tangles may be encountered in the cerebral cortex, basal ganglia, and other brain stem nuclei. Similar changes are found in patients with Guamanian parkinsonism–dementia syndrome. Generally, the brains from patients with parkinsonism secondary to various intoxicants show degeneration of pigmented neurons but neither Lewy bodies or neurofibrillary tangles. However, structures resembling Lewy bodies have been observed in the loci caerulei of monkeys following intoxication with MPTP.

Progressive supranuclear palsy or the Steele–Richardson–Olszewski syndrome is another disorder that must be considered in the differential diagnosis of parkinsonism. The disease is characterized by rigidity, bradykinesia, postural instability, dysarthria, and vertical gaze paresis, especially of downward gaze. Many of the patients also have dystonia of the neck and trunk. In contrast to idiopathic parkinsonism, resting tremor is uncommon. The patients may develop mild dementia. The disease generally has its onset during the sixth or seventh decade and is somewhat more common among men than women.

Histopathologically, the disease is characterized by neuronal loss and gliosis involving especially the globus pallidus, substantia nigra, red nucleus, periaqueductal gray matter, and dentate nucleus. Globose neurofibrillary tangles are found in many of the remaining brain stem neurons. Ultrastructurally, the tangles are found to contain both smooth tubules and paired helical filaments. The neuronal population of the nucleus basalis is mildly reduced and some of the remaining neurons may contain neurofibrillary tangles.

REFERENCES

Ballard PA, Tetrud JW, Langston JW: Permanent human parkinsonism due to 1-methyl-4-phenyl-1,2,3,6-tetrahydropyridine (MPTP): Seven cases. Neurology 1985; 35:949-956.

Forno LS, Langston JW, DeLanney LE, et al: Locus caeruleus lesions and eosinophilic inclusions in MPTP-treated monkeys. Ann Neurol 1986; 20:449-455.

Maher ER, Lees AJ: The clinical features and natural history of the Steele–Richardson–Olszewski syndrome (progressive supranuclear palsy). Neurology 1986; 36:1005-1008.

Nakano I, Hirano A: Parkinson's disease: Neuron loss in the nucleus basalis without concomitant Alzheimer's disease. Ann Neurol 1984; 15:415-418.

Pappolla MA: Lewy bodies of Parkinson's disease: Immune electron microscopic demonstration of neurofilament antigens in constituent filaments. Arch Pathol Lab Med 1986; 110:1160-1163.

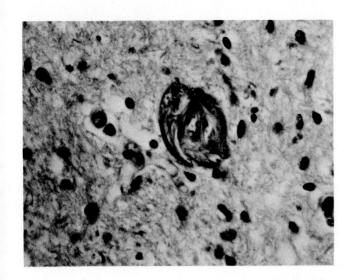

Figure 7–4E. Globose neurofibrillary tangle in brain from patient with post-encephalitic Parkinsonism.

7.5 Huntington's Disease

CLINICAL

This patient was first evaluated when he was 43 years old. At that time, he had a 1-year history of abnormal face and limb movements and mild impairment of memory. Physical examination disclosed facial grimaces and choreiform movements of his neck, tongue, and limbs. During the next 2 years, these symptoms became progressively more severe. He suffered weight loss and became withdrawn. He committed suicide by a drug overdose when he was 46 years old. The patient's mother and a maternal uncle had died of Huntington's disease. Two other maternal uncles who had become "nervous and depressed" had also committed suicide.

PATHOLOGY

The brain appeared mildly atrophic and weighed 1073 grams. Coronal sections revealed severe atrophy of the basal ganglia, especially the caudate nucleus (Fig. 7–5A). The caudate nucleus was flattened and no longer protruded into the lateral ventricle. Microscopically, both the caudate nucleus and putamen showed loss of neurons and gliosis (Fig. 7–5B).

COMMENT

Huntington's disease is a relatively common disorder with a prevalence of 4 to 7 per 100,000. It is inherited as an autosomal dominant trait with a very high degree of penetrance. Recently, the gene locus has been identified on the short arm of chromosome number 4.

The clinical manifestations usually appear during the fourth decade, although there is a rare juvenile variant of the disease. The clinical manifestations include abnormal movements that may eventually become choreiform and behavioral changes that ultimately evolve into dementia. The disease is generally slowly progressive with a protracted course averaging 12 years in length. Suicide is relatively common among individuals afflicted with Huntington's disease.

The diagnosis is generally based on the clinical features and the family history. This can be augmented by computerized tomography with demonstration of the abnormal ventricular configuration produced by the caudate atrophy (Fig. 7–5C). Various biochemical and pharmacological tests for diagnosing the disease prior to the onset of clinical manifestations are under investigation but are controversial in application.

Grossly, the most obvious pathological change is atrophy of the striatum. This may be sufficiently severe that the normal convex contour of the caudate is obliterated or replaced by a concave surface. The dorsal portion of the putamen is affected earlier than the remainder of this nucleus. The pallidum is also affected but to a lesser extent. Histologically, the striatum shows neuronal loss, generally considered to be more severe among the smaller neurons. The neuronal loss is accompanied by gliosis. Cortical neurons are lost especially from the deeper layers of the frontal and parietal lobes. The remaining neurons contain increased quantities of lipofuscin. The neuronal population of the nucleus basalis does not differ from age-matched controls.

Biochemical studies have shown a decreased level of various neurotransmitters in the basal ganglia. Gamma-aminobutyric acid (GABA) and acetylcholine are decreased in the striatum. Substance P is decreased in the pallidum and substantia nigra. In contrast to Parkinson's disease, the dopamine content is not significantly decreased.

REFERENCES

Clark AW, Parhad IM, Folstein SE, et al : The nucleus basalis in Huntington's disease. Neurology 1983; 33:1262-1267.

Martin JB: Huntington's disease: New approaches to an old problem. Neurology 1984; 34:1059-1072.

Vonsattel J-P, Myers RH, Stevens TJ, et al: Neuropathological classification of Huntington's disease. J Neuropathol Exp Neurol 1985; 44:559-577.

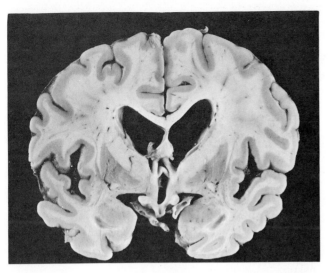

Figure 7–5A. Coronal section of brain of patient with Huntington's disease showing atrophy of the caudate nucleus.

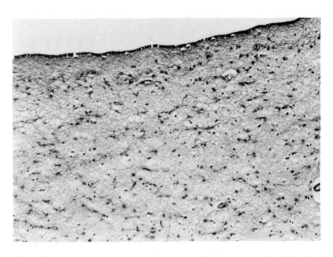

Figure 7–5B. Microscopic section of caudate nucleus showing loss of neurons and gliosis.

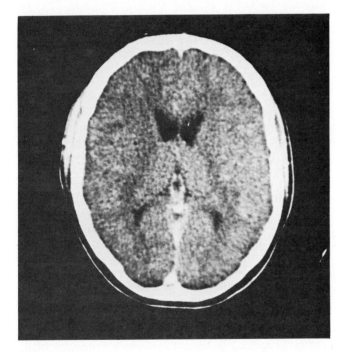

Figure 7–5C. Computerized tomogram showing flattening of caudate nucleus in patient with Huntington's disease.

7.6 Wilson's Disease

Hallervorden–Spatz Disease

CLINICAL

This 33-year-old man had been diagnosed as having Wilson's disease when he was 14 years old. He was initially evaluated for deteriorating school performance, slurred speech, and facial grimaces. Examination had revealed emotional lability, dysarthria, rigidity, an intention tremor, and a hesitant gait. He had splenomegaly but no hepatomegaly or ascites. Slit lamp examination revealed bilateral Kayser–Fleischer rings. Laboratory studies demonstrated a markedly reduced ceruloplasmin level and increased urinary copper excretion.

The patient was treated with penicillamine and a low copper diet. However, after the age of 21, he intermittently stopped his medications and refused medical care. Approximately 2 years prior to his demise, he began to abuse alcohol. He was in hepatic coma during his terminal admission and died following a massive gastrointestinal hemorrhage.

PATHOLOGY

The brain weighed 1548 grams and was externally unremarkable. Coronal sections of the cerebral hemispheres revealed large irregular cavities in both putamena (Fig. 7–6A). The caudate nuclei and pallida were grossly normal. The substantia nigra was heavily pigmented. Histologically, the cavities in the putamena were surrounded by markedly gliotic neural tissue (Fig. 7–6B). Gray matter in other areas contained scattered astrocytes, with swollen, vacuolated nuclei (Alzheimer type II astrocytes) and rare astrocytes that were unusually large and contained very large grotesque nuclei (Alzheimer type I astrocytes). The Alzheimer type I cells were especially conspicuous in the lateral geniculate bodies (Fig. 7–6C) and other thalamic nuclei. The liver showed micronodular cirrhosis.

COMMENT

Wilson's disease is an uncommon autosomal recessive disorder with a prevalence of about 1 per 200,000. The various manifestations of the disease are due to abnormal copper metabolism that probably results from decreased copper excretion in the bile. The copper initially accumulates in the liver, leading to various forms of hepatic dysfunction and cirrhosis. Liver biopsy specimens from patients with Wilson's disease have shown a wide spectrum of alterations, including steatosis, focal necrosis, chronic hepatitis, micronodular cirrhosis, and macronodular cirrhosis. Attempts to demonstrate excessive copper by histochemical techniques are less reliable than quantitative assays for total copper content in the liver tissue.

Later in the course of the disease, after hepatic binding sites have become saturated, the copper accumulates in other tissues, including kidney, cornea, and brain. As a result of deleterious effects of the copper on the kidney, the patients may have aminoaciduria and hypercalcuria as well as excessive urinary excretion of copper. The deposition of copper in Descemet's membrane of the cornea leads to the development of the Kayser–Fleischer rings. These yellow-brown to green deposits in the limbus of the cornea are generally regarded as virtually diagnostic of the disease. Although they may be absent early in the course of the disease, they are almost always present by the time that neurological involvement has developed.

The neurological manifestations typically appear during the second or third decade and include behavioral problems, dysarthria, dysphagia, mask-like facies, excessive drooling, rigidity, tremor, and an abnormal gait. Pathologically, the striatum, especially the putamen, shows the most severe alterations. The putamena may show frank cavitation as in the present case or merely shrinkage and discoloration. The pallida also may be shrunken and discolored. Lesions in the basal ganglia have been demonstrated antemortem by computerized tomography and magnetic resonance imaging. Additional features are evident histologically. Throughout the gray matter, many astrocytes have swollen, vesicular nuclei and scanty visible cytoplasm. Some also contain small intranuclear inclusions composed of glycogen. These are the so-called Alzheimer type II astrocytes and may be seen with various types of acute or chronic liver failure. By contrast, the Alzheimer type I astrocytes are very large cells with multiple nuclei or large grotesque nuclei. These are much less common but characteristic of Wilson's disease. Another relatively uncommon cell found in patients with Wilson's disease is the Opalski cell. These are large cells with brownish, granular cytoplasm and small nuclei. They have been variously

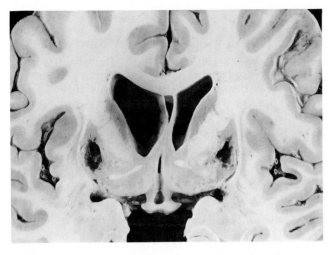

Figure 7–6A. Coronal section showing bilateral putamenal cavitation in patient with Wilson's disease.

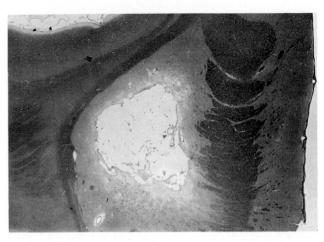

Figure 7–6B. Macroscopic section showing cavitation of putamen.

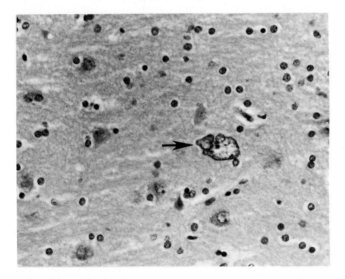

Figure 7–6C. Microscopic section showing large convoluted nucleus of an Alzheimer type I astrocyte (arrow) in the lateral geniculate nucleus.

interpreted as macrophages or derived from degenerating neurons or Alzheimer type I cells.

Most patients with Wilson's disease will have low ceruloplasmin levels. However, this is not entirely diagnostic since patients with other diseases may also have reduced ceruloplasmin levels. Furthermore, some patients with Wilson's disease have normal levels. More recently, the incorporation of radiolabeled copper into ceruloplasmin has been shown to be a more reliable indicator of Wilson's disease.

Hallervorden–Spatz disease is another rare degenerative disorder of the basal ganglia that is due, at least in part, to abnormal metal metabolism. The disease is inherited as an autosomal recessive trait. The clinical manifestations typically become apparent during late childhood or adolescence and include abnormal posture, rigidity, involuntary movements, spasticity, and decline of intellectual function. The course of the disease is protracted over a decade or more. Biochemical studies have demonstrated an increased uptake of iron in the basal ganglia, however, there is no evidence of a systemic abnormality in iron metabolism.

Brains from these individuals characteristically display a rusty brown discoloration of the globus pallidus and to a lesser extent, the substantia nigra and red nucleus. Histologically, the affected areas are characterized by the presence of dystrophic axons (Fig. 7–6D), reactive astrocytes, macrophages, and de-

posits of pigments. The pigments are both intra- and extracellular. At least some of the pigment contains iron that can be demonstrated with the Prussian blue reaction. In addition, much of the pigment is stained strongly with the periodic acid–Schiff reaction and appears to be lipofuscin. Recently, it has been suggested that the disease may involve an error in cysteine metabolism with accumulation of this amino acid and chelated iron in the globus pallidus.

REFERENCES

Danks DM: Hereditary disorders of copper metabolism in Wilson's disease and Menkes' disease. In Stanbury JB, Wyngaarden JB, Fredrickson DS, et al (eds): The Metabolic Basis of Inherited Disease, 5th ed. New York, McGraw-Hill, 1983, chap 58, pp 1251-1268.

Dooling EC, Schoene WC, Richardson EP Jr: Hallervorden–Spatz syndrome. Arch Neurol 1974; 30:70-83.

Perry TL, Norman MG, Yong VW, et al: Hallervorden–Spatz disease: Cysteine accumulation and cysteine dioxygenase deficiency in the globus pallidus. Ann Neurol 1985; 18:482-489.

Starosta-Rubinstein S, Young AB, Kluin K, et al: Clinical assessment of 31 patients with Wilson's disease: Correlations with structural changes on magnetic resonance imaging. Arch Neurol 1987; 44:365-370.

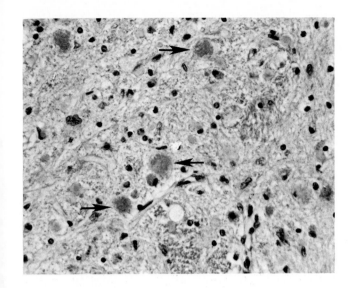

Figure 7–6D. Microscopic section showing axonal spheroids (arrows) in the pallidum of a patient with Hallervorden–Spatz disease.

7.7 Leigh's Disease

Subacute Necrotizing Encephalomyelopathy

CLINICAL

This patient was born prematurely after 35 weeks of gestation. He exhibited slow motor and verbal development. He fed poorly and was irritable but stopped crying at 13 months. A computerized tomogram at age 15 months disclosed bilateral hypodense lesions in the basal ganglia and centrum semiovale. He ceased talking at 21 months. By 2 years, he developed labored breathing and was lethargic. He had nystagmus and increased tone in all four extremities. Another computerized tomogram disclosed additional hypodense lesions in the brain stem near the red nuclei. Laboratory studies repeatedly disclosed lactic acidosis. The child subsequently developed hypotonia, respiratory depression, and died at age 25 months.

PATHOLOGY

Sections of the brain revealed roughly symmetrical areas of discoloration and softening in the centrum semiovale, caudate nuclei, putamena, walls of the third ventricle (Fig. 7–7A), substantia nigra, and mesencephalic tegmentum. Although there was demyelination and necrosis in the substantia nigra and wall of the third ventricle, the mammillary bodies were well preserved (Fig. 7–7B). Microscopically, the partially necrotic areas were characterized by relative preservation of neurons, gliosis, and proliferation of blood vessels (Fig. 7–7C).

COMMENT

Leigh's disease is a rare autosomal recessive disorder. The onset of symptoms is generally in early infancy; however, juvenile and even adult cases have been described. Most of the cases with an infantile onset die early in childhood. The clinical manifestations are protean and not diagnostic. They include psychomotor regression, feeding problems, weakness, hyper- or hypotonia, seizures, nystagmus, impaired eye movements, blindness, and respiratory difficulties. Some of the patients also have evidence of peripheral neuropathy. As in the present case, acidosis is commonly present. Bilateral, roughly symmetrical destructive lesions have been demonstrated by computerized tomography and magnetic resonance imaging in the cerebrum and brain stem.

Pathologically, the disease is characterized by discolored and partially necrotic areas in the cerebral white matter, basal ganglia, and brain stem. Usually, the lesions are bilateral and roughly symmetrical. Lesions also may be found in the cerebellum and spinal cord. Histologically, the lesions show edema, demyelination, necrosis, gliosis, and prominent proliferation of blood vessels, with relative preservation of neurons. The lesions resemble those encountered in Wernicke's encephalopathy but are distinguished by location. In particular, the mammillary bodies are generally spared while the substantia nigra, optic nerves, and spinal cord are commonly involved in Leigh's disease.

Leigh's disease is probably best regarded as a syndrome resulting from several different metabolic defects. Some, but not all patients with Leigh's disease have a substance in their urine that inhibits the phosphorylation of thiamine to thiamine triphosphate. Although the presence of this material would not account for all of the clinical and pathological features, assays for this inhibitor have been used as a screening test for Leigh's disease. More recently, cases of Leigh's disease have been attributed to defects in the pyruvate dehydrogenase complex and to cytochrome c oxidase deficiency.

REFERENCES

DeVivo DC, Haymond MW, Obert KA, et al: Defective activation of the pyruvate dehydrogenase complex in subacute necrotizing encephalomyelopathy (Leigh's disease). Ann Neurol 1979; 6:483-494.

DiMauro S, Servidei S, Zeviani M, et al: Cytochrome c oxidase deficiency in Leigh's syndrome. Ann Neurol 1987; 22:498-506.

Kissel JT, Kolkin S, Chakeres D, et al: Magnetic resonance imaging in a case of autopsy-proved adult subacute necrotizing encephalomyelopathy (Leigh's disease). Arch Neurol 1987; 44:563-566.

Montpetit VJA, Andermann F, Carpenter S, et al: Subacute necrotizing encephalomyelopathy: A review and study of two families. Brain 1971; 94:1-30.

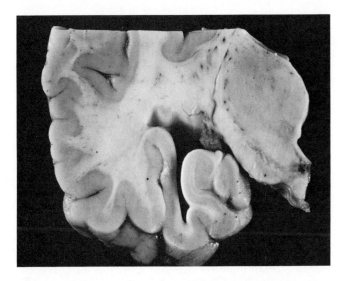

Figure 7–7A. Coronal section showing necrosis in wall of third ventricle and substantia nigra of a patient with Leigh's disease.

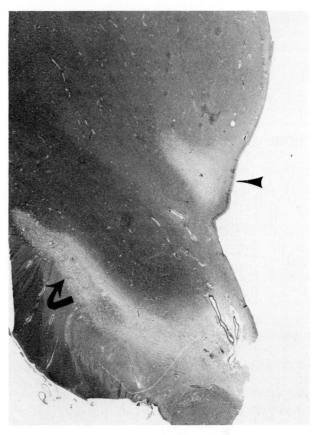

Figure 7–7B. Macrosection showing demyelination and necrosis in the wall of the third ventricle (arrowhead) and substantia nigra (curved arrow).

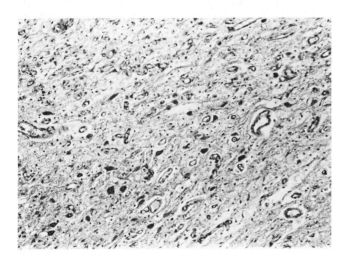

Figure 7–7C. Microscopic section showing relative preservation of neurons and proliferation of blood vessels.

7.8 Ceroid–Lipofuscinosis

Batten–Vogt Syndrome

CLINICAL

This boy was evaluated for seizures when he was 3 years old. His first seizures had occurred 6 months previously and were characterized by "staring spells" and falling limply to the floor. Subsequently, he developed generalized tonic clonic seizures that continued despite anticonvulsant medications. His birth and early development were unremarkable, although he was described as being slower than other children of his age. His neurological examination revealed an intention tremor and a wide based gait. Funduscopic examination demonstrated no abnormalities. An electroencephalogram showed frequent paroxysms of high voltage spike and 4 per second slow wave activity in all leads. Six months later, computerized tomography revealed mild ventricular enlargement and prominent cortical sulci. Assays for lysosomal enzymes and urinalyses for abnormal amino acid and mucopolysaccharide excretion were normal. Muscle and sural nerve biopsies were performed. The specimens were unremarkable by light microscopy, but electron microscopy revealed membrane bounded masses of curvilinear profiles in myofibers (Fig. 7–8A), endothelial cells and Schwann cells. On the basis of these findings, the child was diagnosed as having (neuronal) ceroid–lipofuscinosis. The child's condition continued to deteriorate and he eventually died of intercurrent infection when he was 8 years old.

PATHOLOGY

The brain was severely atrophic, abnormally firm, and faintly gray in color. All cerebral gyri were sclerotic and separated by enlarged sulci (Fig. 7–8B). Coronal sections of the cerebral hemispheres revealed diffuse atrophy of gray and white matter with ventricular enlargement (Fig. 7–8C). The cerebellum was also atrophic with sclerotic folia (Fig. 7–8D). Histologically, there was extensive neuronal loss and gliosis. Neurons remaining in the cerebral cortex and basal ganglia and the few Purkinje cells remaining in the cerebellum were mildly distended by finely granular, intracytoplasmic pigments. Some of the neurons in the thalamus and various brain stem nuclei contained unusually coarse aggregates of intracytoplasmic pigments (Fig. 7–8E). The pigments stained bright red with the periodic acid–Schiff reaction and dark blue with luxol fast blue. Sections of the retina showed loss of ganglion cells and moderate distension of those remaining.

COMMENT

The ceroid–lipofuscinoses are a group of four or more closely related neurodegenerative diseases. Most cases are inherited as an autosomal recessive trait, although some families have shown autosomal dominant inheritance. The diseases result in the accumulation of lipopigments in a wide variety of tissues, although the clinical manifestations are related predominantly to involvement of the brain and eye. The lipopigments are similar to ceroid and lipofuscin in that they are brown to yellow, autofluorescent, and stained by the periodic acid–Schiff and sudan reactions. Although ceroid and lipofuscin are in part derived from peroxidation of unsaturated fatty acids, recent studies on patients with the ceroid–lipofuscinoses have shown abnormal accumulation of dolichols. It has been suggested that the disease may be due to abnormal degradation or recycling of lysosomal membranes. Peroxidase deficiency, formerly implicated in the pathogenesis of this disease, has not been substantiated in more recent studies.

The infantile, Haltia–Santavuori, form of the disease is characterized by a very early onset of clinical symptoms, usually before the age of 2 years. The patients display rapidly progressive psychomotor retardation and early blindness with optic atrophy and retinal degeneration. The infants have myoclonus but seizures are rare. The patients may survive in a decerebrate condition for a number of years. Brains from these patients are severely atrophic. The cortex shows extensive neuronal loss and gliosis while the white matter shows loss of myelin. By electron microscopy, the pigment appears predominantly as granular osmiophilic material with only occasional lamellar profiles.

The present case is regarded as an example of the late infantile or Janksy–Bielschowsky form of ceroid–lipofuscinosis. This form of the disease is characterized by rapidly progressive psychomotor retardation and numerous, often intractable seizures. Visual impairment tends to be mild until late in the course of the illness. Brains from these patients show cerebral atrophy and especially severe cerebellar atrophy. The cerebellar atrophy has been demonstrated by com-

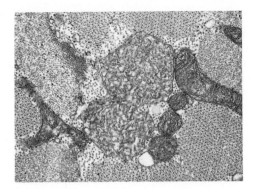

Figure 7–8A. Electron micrograph of muscle biopsy specimen showing curvilinear profiles, diagnostic of ceroid–lipofuscinosis.

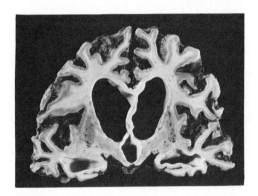

Figure 7–8C. Coronal section of brain showing severe atrophy and ventricular enlargment.

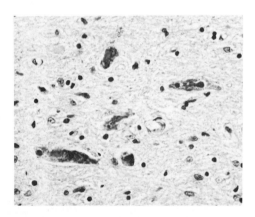

Figure 7–8E. Microscopic section showing coarse aggregates of lipopigment in the cytoplasm of thalamic neurons.

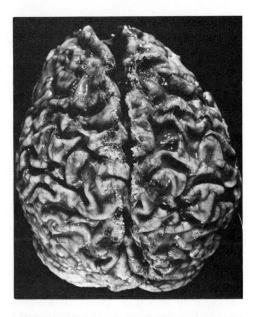

Figure 7–8B. Dorsal surface of the brain from this child with the late infantile form of ceroid lipofuscinosis. Note the severe atrophy.

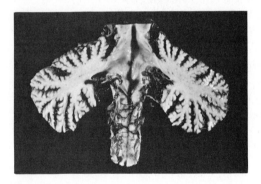

Figure 7–8D. Section showing especially severe atrophy of the cerebellum.

puterized tomography prior to the onset of intellectual deterioration or development of retinal pigmentary degeneration. The cerebral cortex shows neuronal loss, pigment accumulation in the remaining neurons, and gliosis. The cerebellum shows especially marked neuronal loss and gliosis. Large, compact aggregates of intracytoplasmic pigments may be found in the thalamus, substantia nigra, inferior olivary nuclei, and dentate nuclei. Ultrastructurally, the pigment in neurons and other tissues appears predominantly as curvilinear profiles. Smaller quantities of lamellar fingerprint profiles and granular material also may be present.

The juvenile or Spielmeyer–Sjogren form of ceroid–lipofuscinosis is characterized by onset later in childhood, severe visual impairment, and slowly progressive psychomotor retardation. Seizures occur late in the course of the disease. Brains from these individuals are less severely atrophic and show only a moderate loss of neurons. The remaining neurons may be mildly enlarged by the accumulated lipopigments (Fig. 7–8F). Ultrastructurally, the pigments in the brain and other tissues appear as both fingerprint and curvilinear profiles. Lymphocytes from these patients are often vacuolated.

Kufs' disease, the adult form of ceroid–lipofuscinosis, is very rare. The clinical manifestations are predominantly those of extrapyramidal and cerebellar involvement. Seizures are rare and visual impairment and dementia are mild. Brains from these individuals are only mildly atrophic. Pigment accumulation is mild and the affected cells are unevenly distributed in the brain. Ultrastructurally, the pigment in the brain resembles lipofuscin, although curvilinear profiles have been reported in skeletal muscle.

At the present time, the diagnosis of the ceroid–lipofuscinoses is generally confirmed by electron microscopy with demonstration of curvilinear profiles in various tissues. Skin, conjunctiva, peripheral nerve, skeletal muscle, and lymphocytes (Fig. 7–8G) are among the tissues most commonly examined.

REFERENCES

Dunn DW: CT in ceroid lipofuscinosis. Neurology 1987; 37:1025-1026.

Wolfe LS, Palo J, Santavuori P, et al: Urinary sediment dolichols in the diagnosis of neuronal ceroid–lipofuscinosis. Ann Neurol 1986; 19:270-274.

Zeman W: The neuronal ceroid–lipofuscinoses. In Zimmerman HM (ed): Progress in Neuropathology. New York, Grune and Stratton, 1976, vol III, pp 203-223.

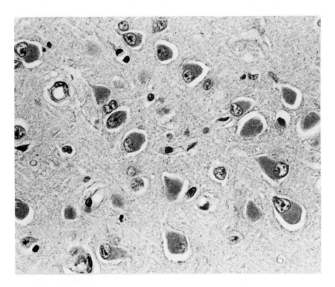

Figure 7–8F. Microscopic section of cortex from a patient with juvenile ceroid–lipofuscinosis. The cortical neurons are distended with lipopigment.

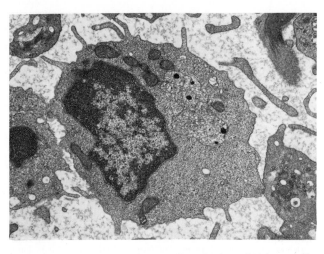

Figure 7–8G. Electron micrograph of lymphocytes showing curvilinear profiles.

7.9 Lafora's Disease

Familial Myoclonus Epilepsy

CLINICAL

This 17-year-old girl was the product of a normal gestation but a prolonged labor and delivery. As a young child, her growth and development were described as somewhat slower than others. At the age of 15, she began to have severe behavioral problems at school and was noted to have deterioration of mental function. She also began to have seizures and myoclonic jerks. These manifestations became progressively worse and were accompanied by ataxia and an unsteady gait.

When evaluated, she was noted to be alert but severely demented. She was able to speak only a few words in an infantile fashion. Neurological examination revealed poor coordination, intention tremor, and an unsteady gait. Funduscopic examination was unremarkable. Electroencephalography revealed diffuse slowing with multiple spike and wave patterns. Routine laboratory studies disclosed no abnormalities. A brain biopsy was performed.

PATHOLOGY

Examination of the brain biopsy specimen disclosed spheroidal intracytoplasmic inclusion bodies in the perikarya and processes of neurons (Fig. 7–9A). The inclusions were varying shades of blue in sections stained with hematoxylin–eosin. The larger bodies displaced the nucleus and appeared laminated with a dark core and a lighter, radially striated periphery. The inclusions stained bright red with the periodic acid–Schiff technique and appeared far more numerous since additional smaller ones could be seen. By electron microscopy they appeared as unbounded masses of branched fibrils surrounding a central core of osmiophilic granular material (Fig. 7–9B).

COMMENT

Lafora's disease or familial myoclonus epilepsy is a rare degenerative disorder that is inherited as an autosomal recessive trait. The disease generally becomes evident during the second decade and is manifested by progressive mental deterioration, seizures, myoclonus, ataxia, and dysarthria. The seizures are refractory to therapy and death generally occurs within 5 to 10 years.

Morphologically, the disease is characterized by the presence of polyglucosan deposits. In the brain, the deposits are termed Lafora bodies and are found in the perikarya and processes of neurons throughout the cerebral cortex, basal ganglia, and brain stem. The Lafora bodies within the substantia nigra are often especially large. The characteristic, large laminated Lafora bodies in neuronal perikarya are far less numerous than the smaller granular deposits in neuronal processes. The latter deposits are more readily seen when the sections are stained with the periodic acid–Schiff or silver techniques.

Patients with Lafora's disease also have polyglucosan deposits in other tissues including heart, liver, skeletal muscle, and skin. In recent years, examination of biopsy specimens from liver, and especially skin has been recommended for the diagnosis of this disease. The polyglucosan bodies are readily demonstrated with the periodic acid–Schiff stain within cells lining sweat gland ducts. Therefore, biopsy of axillary skin has been specifically recommended.

Although the accumulation of polyglucosans would suggest an abnormality of carbohydrate metabolism, the biochemical basis for Lafora's disease has not been established. Polyglucosan deposits are also seen in conditions other than Lafora's disease. They are encountered most commonly as corpora amylacea. These bodies are found within the cytoplasm of fibrous astrocytes, especially in subpial, perivascular, and subependymal locations. They tend to increase in number with aging and are not associated with any particular disease process. Polyglucosan bodies may be found in neuronal processes and astrocytes of adults with the so-called adult polyglucosan body disease. This condition is manifested by progressive upper and lower motor neuron deficits, sensory impairment, neurogenic bladder, and, occasionally, dementia. Polyglucosan deposits are found in astrocytes, skeletal muscle, and liver in patients with type IV glycogenosis. The so-called Bielschowsky bodies, found in the pallidum of certain patients with choreoathetosis, are also composed of polyglucosans.

REFERENCES

Baumann RJ, Kocoshis SA, Wilson D: Lafora disease: Liver histopathology in presymptomatic children. Ann Neurol 1983; 14:86-89.

Busard BLSM, Renier WO, Gabreels FJM, et al: Lafora's disease: Comparison of inclusion bodies in skin and brain. Arch Neurol 1986; 43:296-299.

Robitaille Y, Carpenter S, Karpati G, DiMauro S: A distinct form of adult polyglucosan body disease with massive involvement of central and peripheral neuronal processes and astrocytes. Brain 1980; 103:315-336.

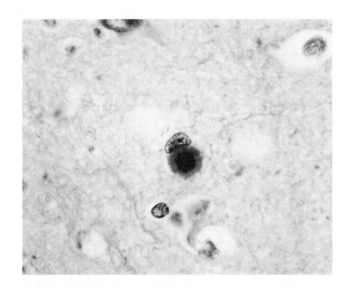

Figure 7–9A. Microscopic section showing a laminated Lafora body in the cytoplasm of a neuron.

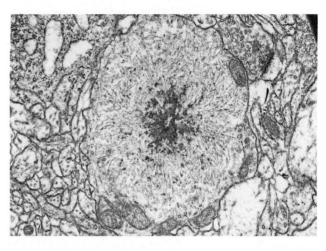

Figure 7–9B. Electron micrograph showing the granular and fibrillar ultrastructure of a Lafora body.

7.10 Amyotrophic Lateral Sclerosis

CLINICAL

This 52-year-old man was hospitalized with progressively more severe respiratory difficulties. He had a 17-month history of weakness, muscle wasting, and fasciculations and had been diagnosed as having amyotrophic lateral sclerosis.

Physical examination revealed an alert but apprehensive man with moderate weakness and generalized muscle wasting. He had fasciculations involving his tongue, neck, trunk, and extremities. His deep tendon reflexes were hyperactive, and he had bilateral Babinski signs. Sensation was intact. The patient suffered a respiratory arrest and died 6 days after being hospitalized.

PATHOLOGY

Grossly (Figs. 7–10A and 7–10B), and histologically, the brain was unremarkable. The spinal cord showed minimal atrophy in the lumbosacral region but the spinal roots were grossly normal (Fig. 7–10C). Macrosections of the spinal cord, stained for myelin, showed pallor of the lateral columns (Fig. 7–10D). The ventral spinal roots were small and stained less darkly than the dorsal roots. A reduction in the number of anterior horn motor neurons was evident when compared with control material. The anterior horns showed mild gliosis and contained a small number of argentophilic globules.

COMMENT

Amyotrophic lateral sclerosis is a progressive degenerative disease affecting predominantly motor neurons in the brain and spinal cord. Several forms of the disease have been delineated. The more common, sporadic form of the disease has a prevalence of approximately 5 per 100,000 and affects men twice as commonly as women. The clinical manifestations generally become apparent during the fifth or sixth decades and reflect varying degrees of upper and lower motor neuron involvement. Involvement of the spinal cord leads to weakness and spasticity that may be quite asymmetrical. Nevertheless, bowel, bladder, and autonomic function are generally intact. Bulbar involvement leads to dysphagia and dysarthria but the extraocular muscles are almost never affected. Although the patients may report abnormal sensations, the sensory examination is generally normal. Usually the disease is steadily progressive and generally leads to death in 3 to 5 years. About 5 percent of the cases are familial. Another variant, encountered predominantly on Guam, is more frequently accompanied by dementia.

All forms of amyotrophic lateral sclerosis show loss of motor neurons in the brain stem and spinal cord, atrophy of the ventral spinal roots, and varying degrees of degeneration and secondary demyelination of the lateral columns of the spinal cord. Many of the familial cases also show involvement of the posterior columns and spinocerebellar tracts. Motor neurons remaining in the anterior horns of the spinal cord and in bulbar nuclei may be atrophic and show

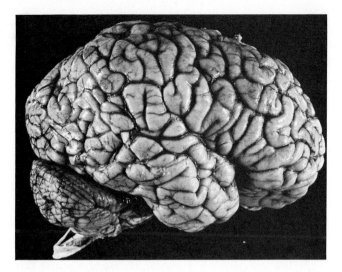

Figure 7–10A. Lateral surface of grossly normal brain from patient with amyotrophic lateral sclerosis.

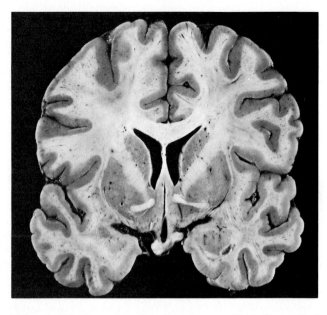

Figure 7–10B. Coronal section of grossly normal brain from patient with amyotrophic lateral sclerosis.

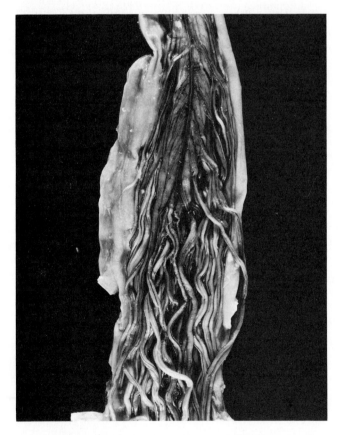

Figure 7–10C. Caudal spinal cord showing grossly normal appearance of nerve roots.

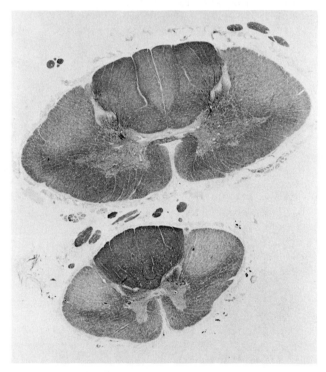

Figure 7–10D. Macrosection of spinal cord showing pale staining in the lateral columns, reflecting degeneration. The ventral roots are smaller and less darkly stained than the dorsal roots.

nonspecific alterations. These include increased lipofuscin and, occasionally, small eosinophilic granules, the so-called Bunina bodies. In addition, there may be focal accumulations of neurofilaments in proximal axons producing argentophilic spheroids (Fig. 7–10E). Less commonly, accumulations of neurofilaments may be demonstrated in the perikarya of the neurons (Fig. 7–10F). The neuronal loss is accompanied by gliosis of the anterior horns. The Guamanian cases are further characterized by having numerous neurofibrillary tangles in the cerebral cortex, hippocampi, basal ganglia, brain stem nuclei, and anterior horns of spinal cord. Skeletal muscle from patients with amyotrophic lateral sclerosis show features typical of neurogenic atrophy (Fig. 7–10G). These include large and small groups of angular atrophic myofibers and, occasionally, target fibers.

Despite intensive investigation, the etiology and pathogenesis of amyotrophic lateral sclerosis remain largely unknown. It has been suggested that impaired axoplasmic transport accounts for the accumulations of neurofilaments that are seen in the perikarya and processes of the affected motor neurons. The apparent sparing of certain motor neurons such as those innervating the extraocular muscles, bowel, and bladder are additional enigmas regarding the pathogenesis of this disease.

REFERENCES

Mitsumoto H, Hanson MR, Chad DA: Amyotrophic lateral sclerosis: Recent advances in pathogenesis and therapeutic trials. Arch Neurol 1988; 45:189-202.

Mulder DW: Motor neuron disease. In Dyck PJ, Thomas PK, Lambert EH, Bunge R (eds): Peripheral Neuropathy, 2nd ed. Philadelphia, Saunders, 1984, vol II, chap 66, pp 1525-1536.

Tandan R, Bradley WG: Amyotrophic lateral sclerosis: Part 1. Clinical features, pathology, and ethical issues in management. Ann Neurol 1985; 18:271-280.

Tandan R, Bradley WG: Amyotrophic lateral sclerosis: Part 2. Etiopathogenesis. Ann Neurol 1985; 18:419-431.

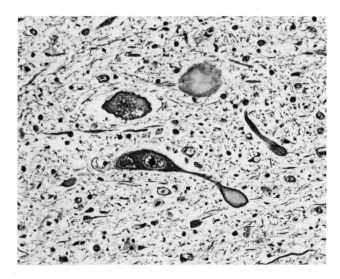

Figure 7–10E. Microscopic section showing argentophilic swellings on proximal axons of anterior horn motor neurons.

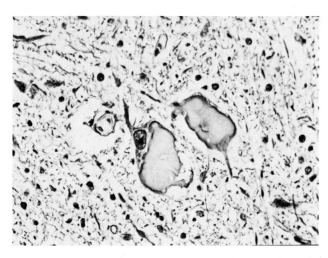

Figure 7–10F. Microscopic section showing argentophilic accumulation of neurofilaments in the perikarya of anterior horn motor neurons.

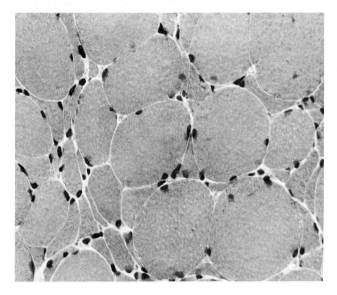

Figure 7–10G. Microscopic section of skeletal muscle showing small groups of angular atrophic myofibers.

7.11   Hereditary Neuropathies

Hereditary Sensory Neuropathy
Charcot–Marie–Tooth Disease
Dejerine–Sottas Disease

CLINICAL

This 36-year-old woman died from pneumonia. She had a long history of impaired pain and temperature perception in both the upper and lower extremities and had sustained various burns and traumatic injuries without associated pain. She had a foot ulcer and chronic osteomyelitis that required amputation of her great toe. Examination demonstrated impaired proprioception and areflexia. Her strength was normal. Electrodiagnostic studies had shown normal motor nerve conduction velocities but no sensory responses in the median, ulnar, radial, or sural nerves. Her cranial nerves were intact. Family history was unavailable.

PATHOLOGY

The brain weighed 1176 grams and was grossly normal. The spinal cord appeared slightly flattened due to mild atrophy of the posterior columns. The dorsal roots were markedly thinned and had an abnormal gray color (Figs. 7–11A and 7–11B). By contrast, the ventral roots appeared normal. Sections of the spinal cord, stained for myelin, showed degeneration of the dorsal columns (Fig. 7–11C).

COMMENT

The hereditary sensory neuropathies are rare diseases that are manifested by sensory deficits and varying degrees of autonomic dysfunction. They are generally classified according to their mode of inheritance. The so-called type I sensory neuropathy is inherited as an autosomal dominant trait. The disease usually becomes manifest in late childhood or early adult life. The sensory deficits are more severe in the lower extremities and involve predominantly pain and temperature perception. As a result, the disease often leads to recurrent foot injuries and infections. Peripheral nerve biopsy specimens usually show severe loss of small unmyelinated fibers and mild to moderate loss of myelinated fibers. The so-called type II sensory neuropathy is inherited as an autosomal recessive trait and usually becomes manifest in early childhood or infancy. Both upper and lower extremities are affected. Peripheral nerve biopsy specimens from these individuals generally show severe loss of myelinated fibers and mild loss of unmyelinated fibers. Type III sensory neuropathy or the Riley–Day syndrome is an autosomal recessive disorder that is manifested predominantly by autonomic dysfunction. Peripheral nerve specimens show loss of unmyelinated fibers.

There are also several forms of hereditary neuropathy with mixed motor and sensory deficits. Type I hereditary motor and sensory neuropathy, otherwise known as hypertrophic Charcot–Marie–Tooth disease, is inherited as an autosomal dominant trait. It is a relatively common disorder with highly variable expression. The patients typically develop weakness and atrophy of distal leg muscles. This may produce a characteristic appearance resembling "an inverted champagne bottle." Many of the patients, including less severely affected individuals, have high arched feet. Sensory deficits are generally not severe but reflexes are depressed. About one fourth of the patients develop palpably enlarged peripheral nerves. Nerve conduction velocities are abnormally slowed.

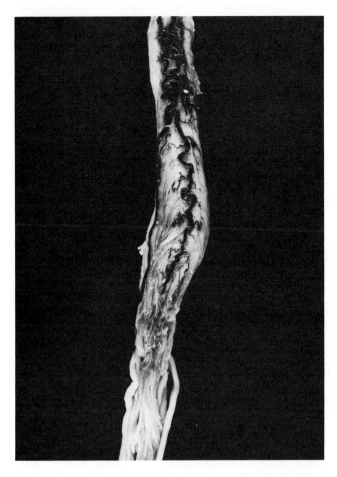

Figure 7–11A. Dorsal surface of spinal cord from patient with hereditary sensory neuropathy.

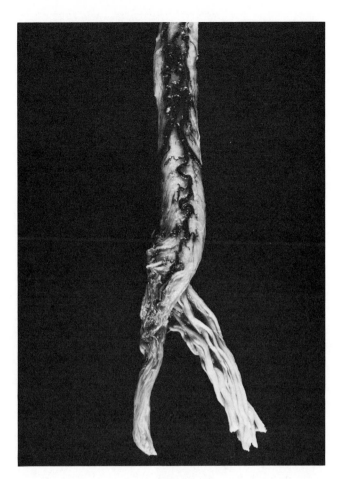

Figure 7–11B. Spinal cord from patient with hereditary sensory neuropathy. The atrophic dorsal roots have been moved to the left to contrast with the intact ventral roots on the right.

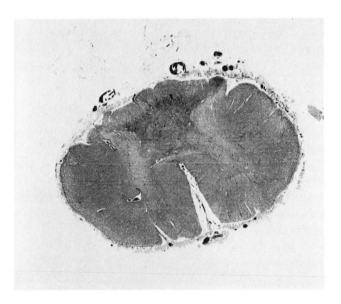

Figure 7–11C. Macrosection of the spinal cord showing atrophy of the posterior columns.

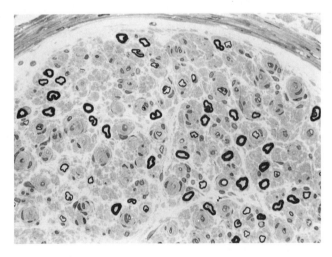

Figure 7–11D. Microscopic section of sural nerve from patient with hypertrophic Charcot–Marie–Tooth disease showing demyelination and onion bulb formations.

Peripheral nerve specimens typically show segmental demyelination and numerous onion bulb formations that are especially well seen in epoxy-embedded sections (Fig. 7–11D). Ultrastructurally, the onion bulbs are composed of concentric lamellae of Schwann cells and collagen fibers surrounding a nerve fiber (Fig. 7–11E). Type II hereditary motor and sensory neuropathy, otherwise known as neuronal Charcot–Marie–Tooth disease, is also inherited as an autosomal dominant trait but is less common and generally becomes manifest somewhat later in life. Clinically, the patients are most readily distinguished from the type I disorder by having nearly normal nerve conduction velocities. Peripheral nerve specimens from these individuals show a reduction in the number of large myelinated nerve fibers secondary to axonal atrophy (Fig. 7–11F) but only rare onion bulb formations. Type III hereditary motor and sensory neuropathy or Dejerine–Sottas disease is inherited as an autosomal recessive trait. It is a rare disorder that becomes manifest during infancy by weakness, retarded motor development, and delayed walking. The motor disability is accompanied by sensory deficits involving predominantly touch, position, and vibration. The patients often have elevated cerebrospinal fluid protein. Peripheral nerves are enlarged and show a reduction in the number of nerve fibers, demyelination, and large onion bulb formations (Fig. 7–11G).

REFERENCES

Dyck PJ: Neuronal atrophy and degeneration predominantly affecting peripheral sensory and autonomic neurons. In Dyck PJ, Thomas PK, Lambert EH, Bunge R (eds): Peripheral Neuropathy, 2nd ed. Philadelphia, Saunders 1984, vol II, chap 68, pp 1557-1599.

Dyck PJ: Inherited neuronal degeneration and atrophy affecting peripheral motor, sensory and autonomic neurons. In Dyck PJ, Thomas PK, Lambert EH, Bunge R (eds): Peripheral Neuropathy, 2nd ed. Philadelphia, Saunders, 1984, vol II, chap 69, pp 1600-1655.

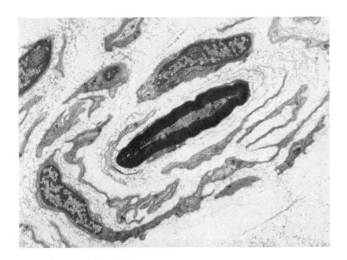

Figure 7–11E. Electron micrograph showing an onion bulb.

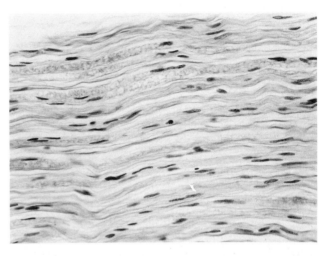

Figure 7–11F. Microscopic section from sural nerve from patient with axonal form of Charcot–Marie–Tooth disease. Note marked reduction in number of large myelinated nerve fibers but absence of onion bulbs.

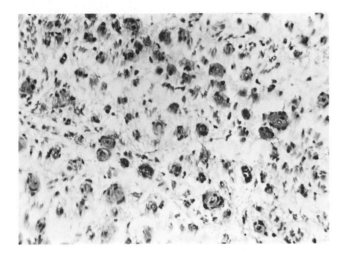

Figure 7–11G. Microscopic section from sural nerve of patient with Dejerine–Sottas disease. Note onion bulbs and enlarged endoneurial space.

8

Neoplasms

8.1   Metastatic Carcinoma

CLINICAL

This 68-year-old man was hospitalized because of respiratory distress. Neurological examination revealed intact cranial nerve function, normal sensation, and intact motor function. Eighteen months previously, he had been diagnosed as having small cell carcinoma of the lung with extension into the pulmonary artery and pericardium. He had been treated with radiation to the chest, chemotherapy, and prophylactic radiation to the brain. The patient died 2 days after admission.

PATHOLOGY

Examination of the exterior of the brain disclosed a nodular metastasis on the undersurface of the right frontal lobe (Fig. 8–1A). Coronal sections of the cerebral hemispheres demonstrated this metastasis to involve cortex and adjacent white matter (Fig. 8–1B). The right frontal lobe was mildly swollen. Sections of the cerebellum revealed a second larger metastasis in the left cerebellar hemisphere (Fig. 8–1C). Histologically, the metastases were composed of relatively small cells with scanty cytoplasm (Fig. 8–1D). Both metastases were partially necrotic.

COMMENT

Metastatic carcinomas account for a large proportion of intracranial neoplasms. Lung and breast carcinomas are by far the most common sources of cerebral metastases, and, in recent years, lung has become the single most common source even among women. Other common sources include the kidney and gastrointestinal tract. Melanomas (Fig. 8–1E) and choriocarcinomas are relatively less common lesions but very frequently metastasize to the central nervous system.

Cerebral metastases are commonly multiple, especially when arising from carcinomas of the lung, breast, and melanoma. Although any area may be involved, most metastases are in the cerebrum in the distribution of the middle cerebral arteries. Cerebellar metastases are less common, roughly in proportion to the smaller volume of the cerebellum. Brain stem metastases (Fig. 8–1F) are distinctly uncommon. Occasionally, multiple cranial nerve deficits can occur in

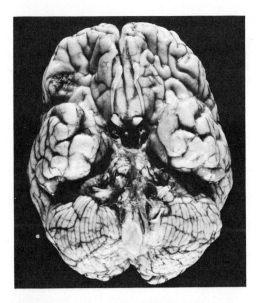

Figure 8–1A. Base of brain showing metastasis on undersurface of right frontal lobe.

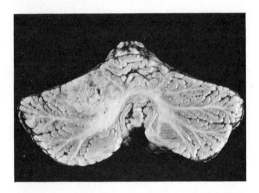

Figure 8–1C. Section of cerebellum showing metastasis in superior portion of left cerebellar hemisphere.

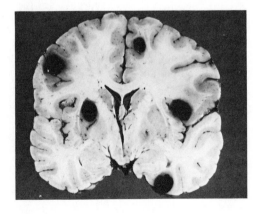

Figure 8–1E. Coronal section showing multiple metastases from a cutaneous melanoma.

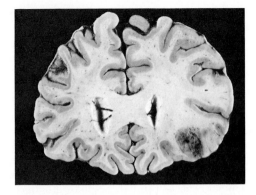

Figure 8–1B. Coronal section showing metastasis in right frontal lobe. Note edema of white matter.

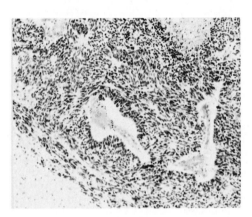

Figure 8–1D. Microscopic section showing the metastasis to be composed of small cells with scanty cytoplasm, consistent with small cell carcinoma of lung.

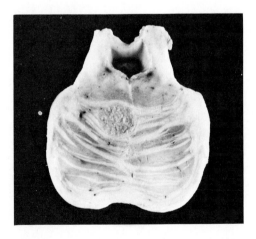

Figure 8–1F. Transverse section of pons with a metastasis.

patients with metastases to the skull with or without associated intracerebral metastases. Figure 8–1G illustrates the base of the skull from a man with nasopharyngeal carcinoma. Despite the extensive bony metastases that produced multiple cranial nerve palsies, he had no intracerebral metastases.

Grossly, the individual metastases are sharply demarcated and frequently located at the junction between cortex and white matter (Fig. 8–1H). The adjacent white matter is often markedly edematous. Metastases are generally firm but may show varying degrees of necrosis. When extensively necrotic, they may mimic abscesses but can be distinguished by the lack of a hyperemic border. Some metastases are hemorrhagic, especially metastatic melanomas and choriocarcinomas.

Histologically, metastases resemble the primary neoplasms from which they are derived, although it is often not possible to determine the origin when the primary is unknown. Among carcinomas of the lung, adenocarcinomas and undifferentiated carcinomas are more apt to metastasize to the brain than are squamous carcinomas. In women, breast was formerly the most common source of metastases; however, in recent years, lung carcinomas have become more frequent. Clear cell carcinomas of the kidney and lung may resemble one another but can generally be distinguished by the presence of abundant glycogen in the metastases from renal cell carcinoma and mucin in the metastases from the lung carcinomas.

Metastases from carcinomas of the gastrointestinal tract are considerably less common and are generally well differentiated adenocarcinomas that resemble the primary neoplasm.

Metastases to the spine are common and cause neurological deficits by spinal cord and root compression. Less commonly, similar deficits are caused by purely epidural metastases. The lesions are found most commonly at lumbosacral and thoracic levels. Major sources for spinal metastases include lung, breast and prostatic carcinomas and lymphomas. Intramedullary spinal metastases are much less common and can produce noncompressive myelopathies.

REFERENCES

Burger PC, Vogel FS: Surgical Pathology of the Nervous System and Its Coverings, 2nd ed. New York, Wiley, 1982, pp 419-433.

Constans JP, de Divitiis E, Donzelli R, et al: Spinal metastases with neurological manifestations: Review of 600 cases. J Neurosurg 1983; 59:111-118.

Greenberg HS, Deck MDF, Vikram B, et al: Metastasis to the base of the skull: Clinical findings in 43 patients. Neurology 1981; 31:530-537.

Winkelman MD, Adelstein DJ, Karlins NL: Intramedullary spinal cord metastasis. Diagnostic and therapeutic considerations. Arch Neurol 1987; 44:526-531.

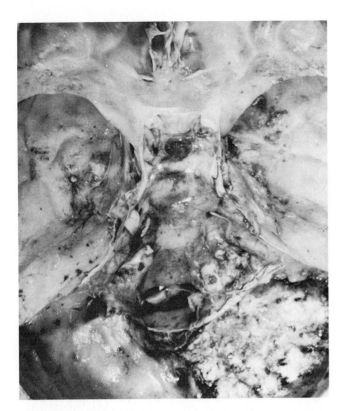

Figure 8–1G. Skull base showing multiple bony metastases. Note the metastasis in the right posterior fossa.

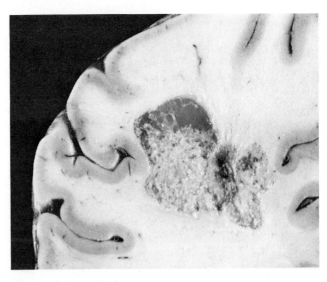

Figure 8–1H. Coronal section showing a sharply demarcated, partially necrotic metastasis with a small area of hemorrhage.

8.2 Leptomeningeal Carcinomatosis

CLINICAL

This 53-year-old woman was diagnosed as having carcinoma of the lung. She received preoperative radiation to the chest, underwent resection of the right upper lobe, and received additional postoperative radiation. In addition, she was treated with chemotherapy. Approximately 15 months later, she developed proximal weakness in the left leg. Electromyography demonstrated findings consistent with a lumbosacral radiculopathy. A lumbar puncture yielded cerebrospinal fluid containing 63 white blood cells, 80 red blood cells, a protein of 68 mg/dL, and a glucose of 56 mg/dL. Cerebrospinal fluid cytology revealed neoplastic cells (Fig. 8–2A). Additional radiation was administered to the lumbosacral region. The patient subsequently developed respiratory distress and died approximately 5 months later.

PATHOLOGY

The brain was unremarkable externally and on multiple sections. There were irregularly thickened, gray-white areas in the leptomeninges on the dorsal surface of the spinal cord and fusiform thickening of some of the spinal roots (Fig. 8–2B). Sections of the spinal cord revealed neoplastic cells in the spinal subarachnoid space. These were most abundant on the ventral surface of the spinal cord in the lumbosacral region (Fig. 8–2C). Additional neoplastic cells extended into the cord along Virchow–Robin spaces. In addition, ventral roots were infiltrated by neoplastic cells. Anterior horn motor neurons displayed central chromatolysis at the levels where the roots were involved by neoplasm.

COMMENT

Leptomeningeal carcinomatosis is the result of metastasis to the leptomeninges and may occur in the absence of intraparenchymal metastases (Fig. 8–2D). Carcinomas of the lung and breast are the most common causes of leptomeningeal carcinomatosis. Less often, the disorder can occur in patients with melanoma or other carcinomas. Leptomeningeal involvement can occur in patients with lymphoma or leukemia but are excluded by definition from this category of disease.

Among the more common clinical manifestations of leptomeningeal carcinomatosis are headache, changes in mental status, multiple cranial nerve palsies, spinal radiculopathies involving especially the legs, and asymmetrical deep tendon reflexes. The resulting neurological deficits may mimic chronic meningitis or multiple cerebral metastases. The diagnosis is established by demonstration of neoplastic cells in the cerebrospinal fluid. Occasionally, multiple lumbar punctures must be performed before the neoplastic cells become evident. The cytological examination can be performed by a variety of sedimentation, cytocentrifuge, and filtration techniques. In general, the filtration techniques recover a larger proportion of cells and can be performed on a relatively large volume of fluid. By contrast, the sedimentation and cytocentrifugation techniques are performed on a smaller volume of fluid but result in better cell preservation. The cerebrospinal fluid protein is often elevated and the glucose may be depressed. Occasionally, myelography will demonstrate the involvement of nerve roots and computerized tomography may show abnormal enhancement of the leptomeninges.

The mechanisms by which the leptomeningeal metastases produce neurological derangements remain controversial. Cranial and spinal nerve roots are often infiltrated by the neoplastic cells; however, the nerves show predominantly segmental demyelination. The neoplasm may also invade the Virchow–Robin spaces but the parenchymal involvement tends to be superficial. Similarly, there may be ischemic involvement of the superficial layers of the cerebral cortex, brain stem, or spinal cord. In some cases the neoplastic infiltrates lead to hydrocephalus by impeding the flow of cerebrospinal fluid. It also has been suggested that the neoplastic cells may compete with the neural parenchyma for essential nutrients.

REFERENCES

Jaeckle KA, Krol G, Posner JB: Evolution of computed tomographic abnormalities in leptomeningeal metastases. Ann Neurol 1985; 17:85-89.

Olson ME, Chernik NL, Posner JB: Infiltration of the leptomeninges by systemic cancer: A clinical and pathologic study. Arch Neurol 1974; 30:122-137.

Theodore WH, Gendelman S: Meningeal carcinomatosis. Arch Neurol 1981; 38:696-699.

Wasserstrom WR, Glass JP, Posner JB: Diagnosis and treatment of leptomeningeal metastases from solid tumors: Experience with 90 patients. Cancer 1982; 49:759-772.

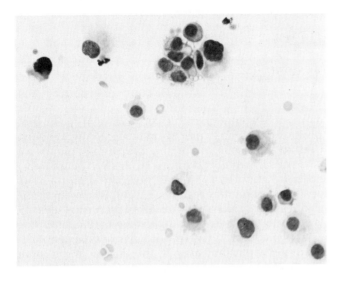

Figure 8–2A. Cerebrospinal fluid sediment showing neoplastic cells.

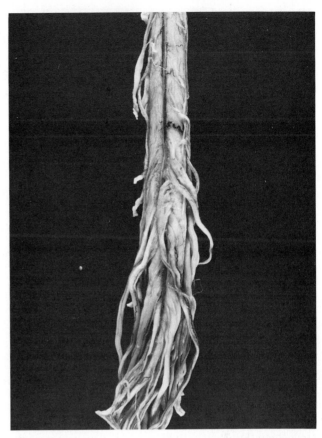

Figure 8–2B. Ventral surface of spinal cord showing irregular thickening of spinal roots by neoplasm.

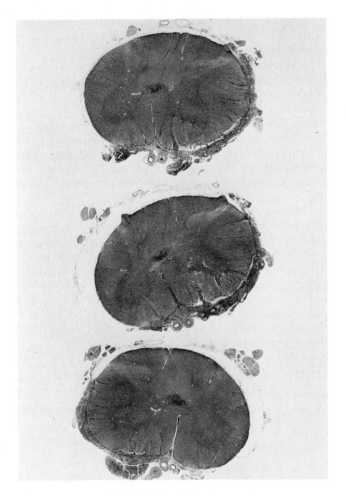

Figure 8–2C. Macrosection of spinal cord showing deposits of neoplasm on ventral and lateral surfaces of lumbosacral spinal cord.

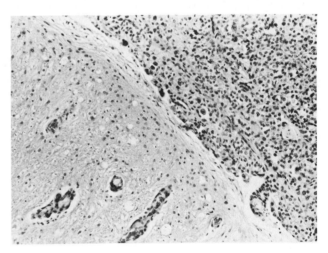

Figure 8–2D. Microscopic section showing neoplasm in the subarachnoid space and extending into the spinal cord within Virchow–Robin spaces.

8.3 Meningiomas

CLINICAL

This 85-year-old woman was hospitalized with severe congestive heart failure and atrial fibrillation. She had a 1-year history of deteriorating mental status, with episodes of lethargy, confusion, and slurred speech. A computerized tomogram revealed a left fronto- temporal enhancing lesion consistent with a meningioma. The patient died 2 days later.

PATHOLOGY

Examination of the brain disclosed a firm hemispheric mass that indented a portion of the left frontal and temporal lobes (Fig. 8–3A). Upon removing the mass, the underlying gyri were noted to be displaced but not invaded by the overlying neoplasm (Fig. 8–3B). Coronal sections confirmed the deformation of the cortex and convolutional white matter but showed no significant shift of the ventricular system or midline structures (Fig. 8–3C). Histological examination of the neoplasm showed interwoven fascicles and whorls composed of slightly elongated cells with poorly defined cytoplasmic margins and vesicular nuclei.

COMMENT

Meningiomas account for about 15 percent of all intracranial neoplasms and about 25 percent of intraspinal neoplasms. They are encountered predominantly in older individuals. Only rarely do meningiomas develop in childhood. The intracranial meningiomas are about twice as common in women as men. The intraspinal lesions show an even more pronounced female predominance. Meningiomas are derived from cells comprising the leptomeninges and can arise in any location where clusters of arachnoid cells are abundant. Among the more common sites are the parasagittal regions (Fig. 8–3D), cerebral convexities, sphenoid ridges, olfactory grooves, and clivus. When they arise in unusual locations, they are more apt to be confused with other types of neoplasms. For example, when they arise in the vicinity of the pineal (Fig. 8–3E), they may be misinterpreted as a germinoma or other pineal region neoplasms. Rarely, they may arise from the invaginations of leptomeninges involved in the formation of the choroid plexi and present as intraventricular masses. These meningiomas may be misinterpreted as ependymomas or choroid plexus papillomas.

Most meningiomas merely indent and deform rather than invade the adjacent cerebral tissue. However, they may penetrate the dura, enter the dural sinuses, or produce hyperostosis in the adjacent bone. Rarely, they may extend through the skull and into the surrounding soft tissues. Although extracranial metastases are rare, meningiomas may recur when they are incompletely resected. An example of a massive, recurrent meningioma is shown in Figure 8–3F.

Meningiomas display a wide variety of histological patterns, most of which are of little biologic significance. Most meningiomas can be classified in one of four major categories designated as syncytial, transitional, fibroblastic, or angioblastic. The neoplastic cells in syncytial meningiomas have moderately abundant cytoplasm, indistinctly demarcated cell margins, and nuclei that are often vacuolated. The fibroblastic meningiomas have elongated or spindle-shaped cells. Transitional meningiomas show a com-

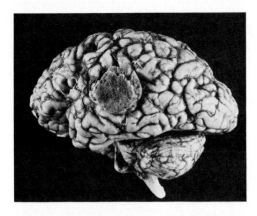

Figure 8–3A. Meningioma in situ on lateral surface of left frontal and temporal lobes.

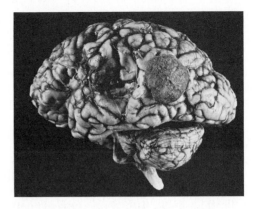

Figure 8–3B. Meningioma moved to show indented area on lateral surface of left frontal and temporal lobes.

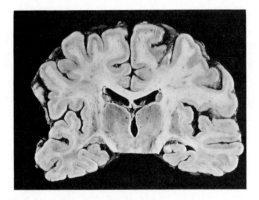

Figure 8–3C. Coronal section to show deformation of underlying brain but no cortical invasion.

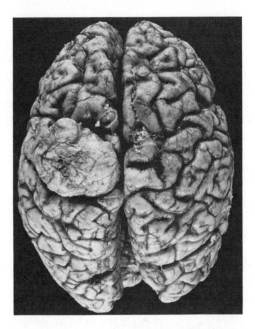

Figure 8–3D. Large parasagittal meningioma.

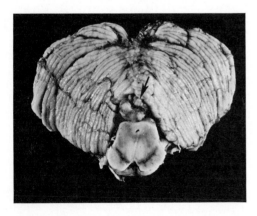

Figure 8–3E. Small meningioma in pineal region (arrow).

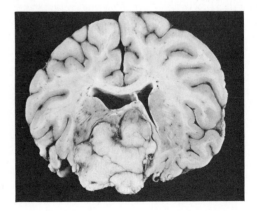

Figure 8–3F. Massive recurrent meningioma.

bination of these features. Almost all meningiomas contain at least a few whorls, a histological feature that is highly characteristic of this group of neoplasms (Fig. 8–3G). Many also contain mineralized concretions, the so-called psammoma bodies. Some meningiomas contain large areas in which there are numerous small cystic spaces (Fig. 8–3H). These so-called microcystic meningiomas show no significant difference in biologic behavior but their unusual appearance may cause difficulty in histological diagnosis. Another pattern that may be confusing is the so-called angiomatous meningioma. These lesions contain myriads of blood vessels often with relatively thick, hyalinized walls (Fig. 8–3I). The more typical features of meningiomas may be confined to small areas within these lesions.

Hemangiopericytomas arising from the meninges are often included as a special category of angioblastic meningiomas. The meningeal hemangiopericytomas are highly cellular neoplasms that scarcely resemble the usual meningiomas (Fig. 8–3J). They are characterized by numerous branched sinusoidal vascular channels that can be more readily delineated with a reticulin stain. These uncommon neoplasms behave in a more aggressive fashion and may metastasize extracranially. Another uncommon group of meningiomas that generally display aggressive behavior are characterized histologically by a papillary pattern. The criteria for malignant behavior among the more usual types of meningiomas are controversial. It has been suggested that high cellularity, large bizarre nuclei, numerous mitotic figures, multiple foci of necrosis, and foci of cortical invasion in otherwise typical meningiomas may portend rapid recurrence and malignant behavior.

REFERENCES

Burger PC, Vogel FS: Surgical Pathology of the Nervous System and Its Coverings, 2nd ed. New York, Wiley, 1982, pp 84-105, 123-130.

Kepes JJ: Meningiomas: Biology, Pathology, and Differential Diagnosis. New York, Masson, 1983.

Michaud J, Gagne F: Microcystic meningioma: Clinico-pathologic report of eight cases. Arch Pathol Lab Med 1983; 107:75-80.

Rutherfoord GS, Marus G: Microcystic meningiomas. Clin Neuropathol 1987; 6:143-148.

Thomas HG, Dolman CL, Berry K: Malignant meningioma: Clinical and pathological features. J Neurosurg 1981; 55:929-934.

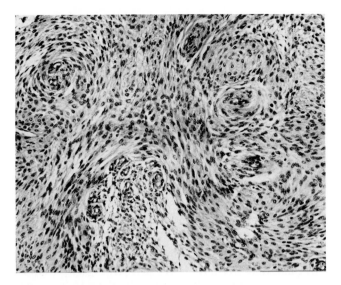

Figure 8–3G. Microscopic section of meningioma showing whorls.

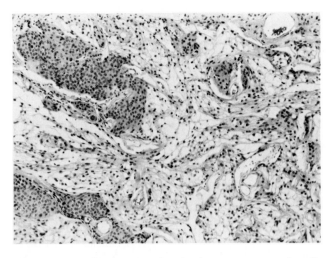

Figure 8–3H. Microscopic section showing numerous small cystic spaces in a microcystic meningioma.

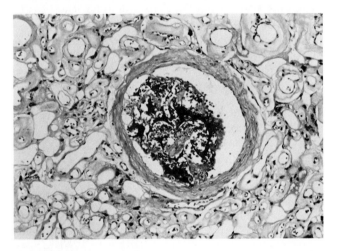

Figure 8–3I. Microscopic section of an angiomatous meningioma. This meningioma was embolized prior to surgery. Note the mass of embolic material in the lumen of the vessels in the center of the illustration.

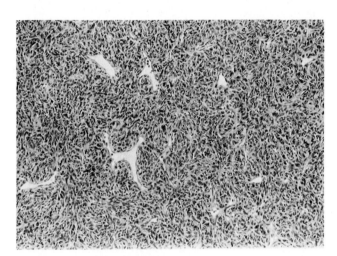

Figure 8–3J. Microscopic section of a meningeal hemangiopericytoma. These highly cellular neoplasms are characterized by branched sinusoidal blood vessels.

8.4   Hemangioblastomas

CLINICAL

This 71-year-old man was hospitalized with a 1-month history of ataxia and loss of balance and a 2-week history of nausea and vomiting. The patient denied headaches or visual symptoms. Neurological examination documented dysmetria and an inability to tandem walk. Computerized tomography disclosed an enhancing posterior fossa mass. Clinical laboratory studies revealed an elevation of the hematocrit and hemoglobin. The patient underwent a suboccipital craniectomy with removal of a cerebellar tumor that consisted of a mural nodule in a smooth walled cyst.

PATHOLOGY

The surgical specimen consisted of a roughly spherical mass of red-brown to yellow tissue measuring approximately 2 cm in diameter. Cross section of the nodule disclosed numerous small cysts and vascular channels (Fig. 8–4A). Histologically, the neoplasm consisted of numerous, thin-walled vascular channels separated by finely vacuolated stromal cells (Fig. 8–4B). Staining with an immunoperoxidase technique for factor VIII accentuated the endothelial cells lining the vascular channels but failed to stain the stromal cells (Fig. 8–4C). The immunoperoxidase technique for anti-GFAP (glial fibrillary acidic protein) stained astrocytes in the accompanying cerebellar tissue but not the stromal cells (Fig. 8–4D).

COMMENT

Hemangioblastomas are relatively uncommon neoplasms accounting for only 1 to 2 percent of all intracranial neoplasms. Most are located in the cerebellum but they also may be found in the brain stem and spinal cord. The tumors may be solid or focally cystic but often form mural nodules in otherwise nonneoplastic cysts. The cysts contain xanthochromic proteinaceous fluid and may be much larger than the mural nodules. In about 7 percent of cases, the tumors are multiple. They are usually discovered in young to middle-aged adults. About 20 percent of patients with hemangioblastomas have the von Hippel–Lindau syndrome. Individuals with this syndrome have hemangioblastomas of the retina and various visceral lesions including adenomas and carcinomas of the kidney, cystadenomas of the epididymis, cysts of the liver and pancreas, and pheochromocytomas.

Hemangioblastomas are composed of thin-walled vascular channels and intervening stromal cells. These two components are quite distinct as seen in the epoxy section shown in Figure 8–4E. The typical yellowish color of the gross specimen is the result of abundant lipid within the stromal cells. The derivation of the stromal cells has been the subject of numerous investigations. Origin from endothelial cells, pericytes, meningothelial cells and even astrocytes has been proposed. An astrocytic origin seems less likely since the neoplasm is often unstained by the anti-GFAP reaction as in the present case. The stromal cells are thought to elaborate erythropoietin. Increased erythropoietin levels result in the polycythemia seen in 10 to 20 percent of patients with these neoplasms.

REFERENCES

Burger PC, Vogel FS: Surgical Pathology of the Nervous System and Its Coverings, 2nd ed. New York, Wiley, 1982, pp 386-398.

Horton WA, Wong V, Eldridge R: Von Hippel–Lindau disease: Clinical and pathological manifestations in nine families with 50 affected members. Arch Intern Med 1976; 136:769-777.

McComb RD, Eastman PJ, Hahn FJ, Bennett DR: Cerebellar hemangioblastoma with prominent stromal astrocytosis: Diagnostic and histogenetic considerations. Clin Neuropathol 1987; 6:149-154.

McComb RD, Jones TR, Pizzo SV, Bigner DD: Localization of factor VIII/von Willebrand factor and glial fibrillary acidic protein in the hemangioblastoma: Implications for stromal cell histogenesis. Acta Neuropathol 1982; 56:207-213.

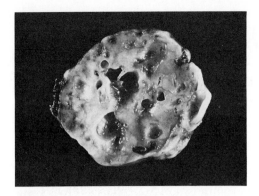

Figure 8–4A. Cross section of a cerebellar hemangioblastoma. Note the numerous small cysts and vascular channels.

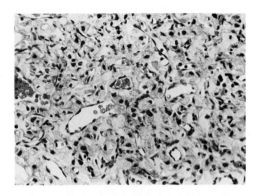

Figure 8–4B. Microscopic section of the hemangioblastoma showing the numerous thin-walled blood vessels and lipidized stromal cells.

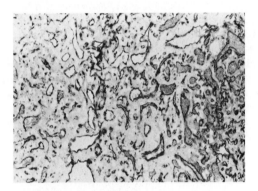

Figure 8–4C. Microscopic section of hemangioblastoma stained by immunoperoxidase technique for factor VIII showing staining of endothelial cells but not the stromal cells.

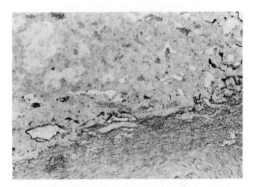

Figure 8–4D. Microscopic section of hemangioblastoma stained by immunoperoxidase technique for GFAP showing staining of surrounding glial tissue but not the stromal cells.

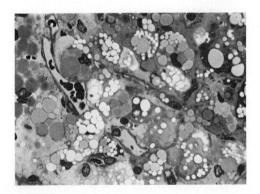

Figure 8–4E. Epoxy section of a hemangioblastoma showing the endothelial cells and lipidized stromal cells.

8.5   Schwann Cell Neoplasms

Acoustic Neurinomas
Schwannomas
Neurofibromas

CLINICAL

This 78-year-old woman had a long history of decreased hearing on the left. She also had a long history of tinnitus. Approximately 2 years previously, she noted the development of numbness on the left side of her face and tongue. Two months prior to admission, she began to have severe but localized headaches, mainly at night. Neurological examination revealed markedly impaired hearing on the left and decreased sensation in all three divisions of the left trigeminal nerve. The patient was also ataxic. A computerized tomogram disclosed an enhancing mass in the left cerebellopontine angle (Fig. 8–5A). A retromastoid craniotomy was performed with resection of the neoplasm.

PATHOLOGY

The surgical specimen consisted of a large mass of firm, gray-white to yellow tissue that measured approximately 3 cm in diameter. The neoplasm displayed two relatively distinct histological patterns (Fig. 8–5B). Part of the specimen was composed of elongated cells arranged in compact interwoven fascicles. In some of the fascicles, the nuclei were in register, producing distinct palisades. Other portions of the neoplasm were composed of loosely aggregated stellate cells with mildly pleomorphic nuclei. The neoplasm was further characterized by the presence of small cysts and thick-walled, hyalinized blood vessels.

COMMENT

Acoustic neurinomas account for about 5 to 10 percent of all intracranial neoplasms and are the most common primary tumors arising in the cerebellopontine angles. They are more common in women than men and are found predominantly in older individuals. However, with increasingly refined diagnostic techniques, small acoustic neurinomas are now being detected in younger patients. Acoustic neurinomas are schwannomas arising from the vestibular branch of the eighth cranial nerve distal to the zone of transition from glial cells to Schwann cells. This transition usually occurs near the internal auditory meatus. The initial intracanalicular growth of these neoplasms results in enlargement of the auditory canal. This can often be demonstrated radiologically, even in patients with relatively small tumors. Computerized tomography, especially with enhancement, can effectively demonstrate the intracranial extension of these tumors.

Hearing loss and tinnitus are the usual early manifestations of these tumors. Further intracranial growth can lead to compression of other cranial nerves, the brain stem, and cerebellum, as seen in Figure 8–5C. Involvement of the trigeminal nerve is common and results in facial pain, paresthesias, and loss of the corneal reflex. The facial nerve is involved in virtually all cases and occasionally leads to loss of taste and pain in the external auditory canal. Compression of the brain stem and cerebellum may lead to long tract signs, ataxia, and nystagmus. Unusually large tumors may impede the flow of cerebrospinal fluid and lead to hydrocephalus. Acoustic neurinomas occur in about 95 percent of patients with central neurofibromatosis and in nearly 5 percent of patients with peripheral neurofibromatosis. Bilateral acoustic neurinomas are virtually diagnostic of neurofibromatosis. Rarely, schwannomas may arise from other intracranial nerves, including the trigeminal, trochlear, oculomotor, and hypoglossal nerves.

Peripheral schwannomas or neurilemmomas commonly arise from spinal roots, especially the dorsal roots. They can occur as isolated lesions or as part of a spectrum of multiple neoplasms in patients with neurofibromatosis. Schwannomas comprise about 30 percent of all intraspinal neoplasms. Like the acoustic neurinoma, the tumors are discrete lobulated masses (Fig. 8–5D) with the nerve of origin incorporated into the capsule of the tumor. The separation into two histological patterns is often more distinct (Fig. 8–5E) than is seen with acoustic neurinomas. The compact fascicles of elongated cells are described as Antoni type A tissue. Discrete aggregates of this tissue are often designated as Verocay bodies. The loosely aggregated stellate cells comprise the Antoni type B tissue.

Peripheral neurofibromas may occur as pedunculated cutaneous lesions or poorly demarcated sub-

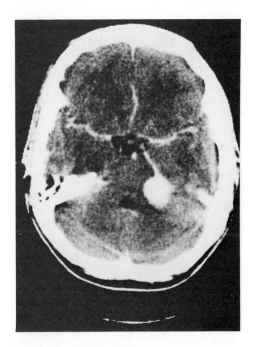

Figure 8–5A. Computerized tomogram showing acoustic neurinoma.

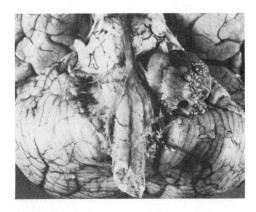

Figure 8–5C. Autopsy specimen showing an acoustic neurinoma in the cerebellopontine angle.

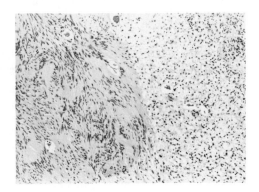

Figure 8–5E. Microscopic section of intraspinal schwannoma showing distinct separation between Antoni type A and Antoni type B tissue components.

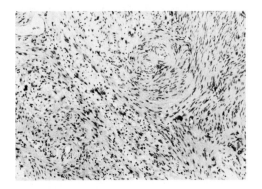

Figure 8–5B. Microscopic section of acoustic neurinoma showing Antoni type A and Antoni type B tissue components.

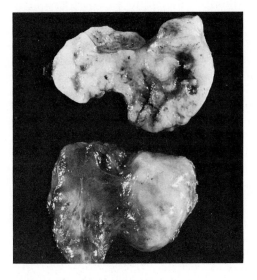

Figure 8–5D. Intraspinal schwannoma.

cutaneous masses. The plexiform neurofibromas enlarge and diffusely infiltrate the nerves from which they arise (Fig. 8–5F). Histologically, the neurofibromas are characterized by an admixture of Schwann cells, fibroblasts, collagenous tissue and a variable quantity of mucoid material (Fig. 8–5G). Occasionally, they may contain compact aggregates of Schwann cells that mimic tactile corpuscles. In contrast to schwannomas, the nerves from which the neurofibromas originate cannot be separated from the neoplasms. Cutaneous neurofibromas may occur as isolated lesions or in association with neurofibromatosis. By contrast, the plexiform neurofibromas, involving major nerve trunks, are virtually diagnostic of neurofibromatosis.

REFERENCES

Burger PC, Vogel FS: Surgical Pathology of the Nervous System and Its Coverings, 2nd ed. New York, Wiley, 1982, pp 602-612, 663-692.

Harner SG, Laws ER Jr: Diagnosis of acoustic neurinoma. Neurosurgery 1981; 9:373-379.

Hart RG, Gardner DP, Howieson J: Acoustic tumors: Atypical features and recent diagnostic tests. Neurology 1983; 33:211-221.

Urich H: Pathology of tumors of cranial nerves, spinal nerve roots and peripheral nerves. In Dyck PJ, Thomas PK, Lambert EH, Bunge R (eds): Peripheral Neuropathy, 2nd ed. Philadelphia, Saunders, 1984, vol II, chap 99, pp 2253-2299.

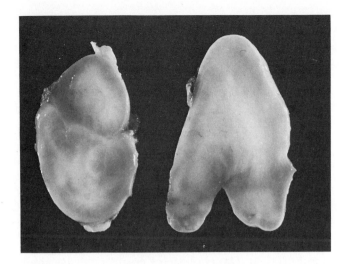

Figure 8–5F. Portions of a plexiform neurofibroma.

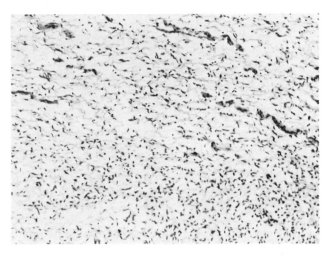

Figure 8–5G. Microscopic section of the neurofibroma showing the Schwann cells and fibroblasts separated by mucoid material.

8.6 Epidermoids

Dermoids

CLINICAL

This 34-year-old woman had a seven year history of seizures. The seizures each lasted 1 to 2 minutes. They were accompanied by complex auras lasting 1 to 2 seconds, followed by tingling sensations in the hands and feet, a feeling of nausea, and an inability to speak. A computerized tomogram had been interpreted as showing a porencephalic cyst in the region of the left sylvian fissure.

For 6 to 8 months prior to the current hospitalization, the patient had difficulty remembering names and saying words. During the same period, she was having daily headaches, impaired use of her right hand, and abnormal sensations upon walking. Neurological examination confirmed the difficulty with naming objects and disclosed weakness of the right upper extremity. She also had decreased pain and position sensation in the right lower extremity. Computerized tomography was repeated and disclosed enlargement of the low density area on the left (Fig. 8–6A). A craniotomy was performed and a large epidermoid tumor was removed.

PATHOLOGY

Much of the surgical specimen consisted of irregular masses of soft gray-white material (Fig 8–6B). Microscopically, this material consisted predominantly of flattened squames that stained darkly with the immunoperoxidase reaction for keratin (Fig. 8–6C). No cutaneous adnexal structures were identified in the surgical specimen.

COMMENT

Epidermoids arise from misplaced rests of epithelial cells and comprise about 1 percent of intracranial tumors. They are encountered predominantly in adults and have a predilection for the cerebellopontine angles, parasellar regions, and ventricles. They also may be found in the spinal canal and skull. Radiologically, they are typically low-density masses but rarely, may appear hyperdense, presumably as the result of bleeding. Grossly, the exterior of the lesion often has a characteristic pearly white appearance. The interior of the cysts contains keratinaceous debris and cholesterol crystals. The cholesterol crystals can be identified in wet mounts, especially when examined with polarized light. The periphery of the cyst is formed by a thin layer of stratified squamous epithelium (Fig. 8–6D). This may be separated from the adjacent neural parenchyma by a thin investment of connective tissue. Leakage or rupture of the cyst may produce a prominent granulomatous meningitis. Rare squamous cell carcinomas have originated from epidermoid cysts.

Dermoids are more commonly encountered in childhood and have a predilection for the spinal canal where they may be associated with various forms of spina bifida. They also may be found in the cerebellum, suprasellar region, and skull. They are distinguished from epidermoids by the presence of cutaneous adnexal structures such as hair follicles and sebaceous glands. The contents of dermoid cysts tend to be softer than epidermoids and may contain strands of hair. Figure 8–6E illustrates a dermoid removed from the skull of a 6-month-old infant.

REFERENCES

Berger MS, Wilson CB: Epidermoid cysts of the posterior fossa. J Neurosurg 1985; 62:214-219.

Dunn RC Jr, Archer CA, Rapport RL II, Looi LM: Unusual CT-dense posterior fossa epidermoid cyst. J Neurosurg 1981; 55:654-656.

Hardman JM: Nonglial tumors of the nervous system. In Rosenberg RN (ed): The Clinical Neurosciences. New York, Churchill Livingstone, 1983, vol 3, chap 4, pp III:162–III:163.

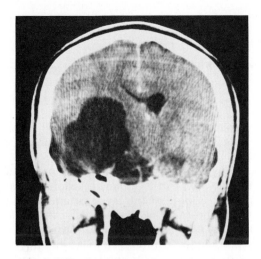

Figure 8–6A. Computerized tomogram showing low-density lesion with displacement of surrounding structures.

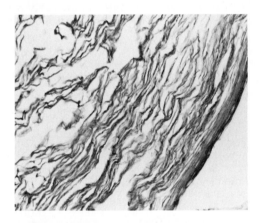

Figure 8–6C. Microscopic section of the surgical specimen stained by immunoperoxidase technique for keratin showing the darkly stained, flattened squames.

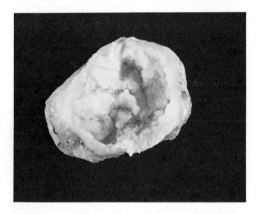

Figure 8–6E. Dermoid from skull of a 6-month-old infant.

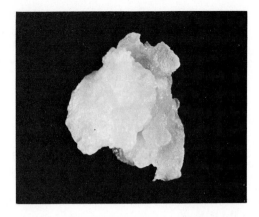

Figure 8–6B. A portion of the surgical specimen that consisted of soft-gray white material.

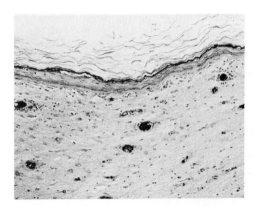

Figure 8–6D. Microscopic section of an epidermoid cyst showing stratified squamous epithelium and adjacent gliotic neural parenchyma.

8.7 Lipomas

CLINICAL

This 34-year-old woman died unexpectedly and was found to have advanced coronary arteriosclerosis.

PATHOLOGY

Examination of the brain revealed a small gray-yellow mass in the left ambient cistern and on the superior surface of the left cerebellar hemisphere (Fig. 8–7A). Histologically, the mass consisted of mature adipose tissue accompanied by a small amount of dense connective tissue and blood vessels (Figs. 8–7B and 8–7C).

COMMENT

Intracranial lipomas are rare lesions comprising less than 1 percent of all intracranial tumors. About one third of intracranial lipomas are found in the interhemispheric fissure. Other sites of predilection include the cisterna ambiens, quadrigeminal plate, and tuber cinereum (Fig. 8–7D). Many are asymptomatic, although nearly half of all patients with callosal lipomas have seizures. The cause of the seizures is controversial. The relatively high incidence of seizures in these individuals has been contrasted with the low incidence of seizures in patients with gliomas of the corpus callosum. Rarely, intracranial lipomas in other locations have been reported to cause diverse neuro-logical manifestations such as aqueductal compression, hydrocephalus, cranial nerve dysfunction, and hypothalamic dysfunction.

Lipomas are also found in the spinal canal both as extradural and intradural mass lesions. Figure 8–7E illustrates a lipoma of the filum terminale in a man with neurofibromatosis. Histologically, this lesion was composed of mature adipose tissue surrounding thick walled blood vessels and nerve twigs (Fig. 8–7F). Other masses of adipose tissue at the caudal end of the spinal canal may be associated with spina bifida and are better described among the lipomeningoceles.

Occasionally the periphery of interhemispheric lipomas undergo mineralization ("eggshell calcification"). As a result, some of these lesions can be visualized in plain skull x-rays. By computerized tomography, lipomas show very low attenuation and must be differentiated from other low-density lesions such as epidermoid tumors. Lipomas are more clearly demonstrated by magnetic resonance imaging.

REFERENCES

Friedman RB, Segal R, Latchaw RE: Computerized tomographic and magnetic resonance imaging of intracranial lipoma. J Neurosurg 1986; 65:407-410.

Gastaut H, Regis H, Gastaut JL, et al: Lipomas of the corpus callosum and epilepsy. Neurology 1980; 30:132-139.

Pierre-Kahn A, Lacombe J, Pichon J, et al: Intraspinal lipomas with spina bifida: Prognosis and treatment in 73 cases. J Neurosurg 1986; 65:756-761.

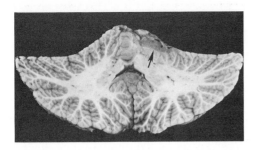

Figure 8–7A. Lipoma on superior surface of cerebellum (arrow).

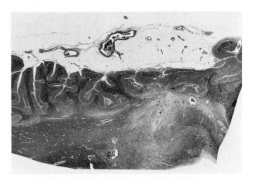

Figure 8–7B. Macrosection of the lipoma.

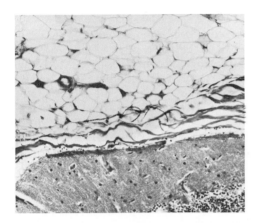

Figure 8–7C. Microscopic section showing the mature adipose tissue.

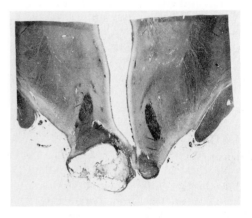

Figure 8–7D. Macrosection of a lipoma involving the mammillary body.

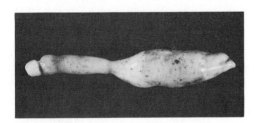

Figure 8–7E. Lipoma of filum terminale.

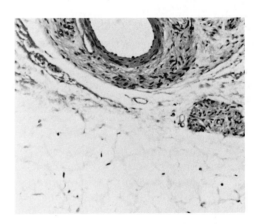

Figure 8–7F. Microscopic section of lipoma of filum terminale showing aberrant blood vessels, nerve twigs, and adipose tissue.

8.8 Cerebral Lymphoma

CLINICAL

This 63-year-old man developed confusion, slurred speech, and right-sided weakness over a 4-month period. Neurological examination disclosed a partial right third nerve palsy, mild right-sided weakness, increased deep tendon reflexes, and an equivocal right Babinski sign. He had marked ataxia on finger to nose testing and fell to the left when he attempted to walk. Computerized tomography disclosed a low-density area in the right thalamus and slight shift of the third ventricle. Magnetic resonance imaging disclosed a lesion involving the medial aspect of the right temporal lobe, thalamus, mesencephalon, and rostral pons. Before a definitive diagnosis could be established, the patient died of pulmonary emboli.

PATHOLOGY

The brain showed diffuse swelling that was more marked in the right temporal lobe. Upon removing the cerebellum and caudal brain stem, infiltrative, gray-white neoplasm was evident in the right half of the mesencephalon (Fig. 8–8A). Horizontal sections of the cerebral hemispheres, viewed from below, revealed poorly demarcated, gray-white neoplasm infiltrating the right hypothalamus and thalamus with massive swelling of the right temporal lobe (Fig. 8–8B). Histological examination showed a highly cellular neoplasm composed of poorly cohesive, moderately pleomorphic cells (Fig. 8–8C). In areas, the neoplastic cells were arranged in concentric layers around blood vessels (Fig. 8–8D).

COMMENT

Primary cerebral lymphomas, formerly designated as microgliomas, are generally considered to account for less than 1 percent of all intracranial neoplasms. However, these neoplasms occur more often in patients with immunologic abnormalities. They will probably become more prevalent in view of the growing population of immunocompromised patients including organ transplant recipients and individuals with the acquired immune deficiency syndrome. The neoplasms usually become manifest during the fifth to seventh decades and are more common in men than women. The clinical manifestations are protean. Some of the cases present as space-occupying masses while others mimic infectious, demyelinating, or psychiatric illnesses. By computerized tomography, the lesions show variable densities and variable degrees of contrast enhancement. Magnetic resonance imaging may prove to be a more effective means of demonstrating these neoplasms.

Grossly, cerebral lymphomas generally appear as poorly demarcated, infiltrative lesions with a slightly granular texture and a gray-white to tan color. Virtually any part of the nervous system can be involved and in some cases, the neoplasms are multifocal. Histologically, they are highly cellular, moderately pleomorphic neoplasms. In areas, they infiltrate the walls of blood vessels and may elicit proliferation of concentric lamellae of reticulin (Fig. 8–8E). Staining by immunoperoxidase techniques and flow cytometry studies have demonstrated the majority of the primary cerebral lymphomas to be derived from B cells.

The nervous system can also be involved by systemic lymphomas. However, in these cases, the leptomeninges and nerve roots are more apt to be involved than the parenchyma of the central nervous system. Hodgkin's disease and other systemic lymphomas frequently cause spinal cord compression from epidural neoplastic infiltrates. Myeloma also commonly causes spinal cord compression from epidural infiltrates and from collapse of involved vertebral bodies. In addition, myeloma, especially osteosclerotic myeloma, is an important cause of peripheral neuropathy. In rare instances, myeloproliferative diseases will be complicated by spinal cord or cerebral compression from mass lesions. These masses are either composed of neoplastic cells (so-called chloroma or granulocytic sarcoma) or result from exuberant extramedullary hematopoiesis. Figure 8–8F illustrates subdural masses of granulocytic sarcoma in a man who had originally presented with polycythemia vera.

REFERENCES

Jiddane M, Nicoli F, Diaz P, et al: Intracranial malignant lymphoma: Report based on 30 cases and review of the literature. J Neurosurg 1986; 65:592-599.

Kawakami Y, Tabuchi K, Ohnishi R, et al: Primary central nervous system lymphoma. J Neurosurg 1985; 62:522-527.

Lysy J, Globus M, Okon E, et al: Solitary intracranial chloroma in a patient with chronic granulocytic leukemia. Neurology 1983; 33:1089-1091.

O'Neill BP, Kelly PJ, Earle JD, et al: Computer-assisted stereotaxic biopsy for the diagnosis of primary central nervous system lymphoma. Neurology 1987; 37:1160-1164.

So YT, Beckstead JH, Davis RL: Primary central nervous system lymphoma in acquired immune deficiency syndrome: A clinical and pathological study. Ann Neurol 1986; 20:566-572.

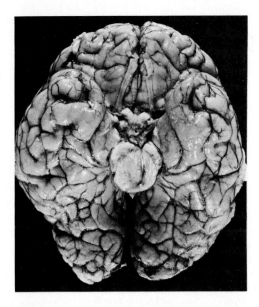

Figure 8–8A. Base of brain with brain stem removed showing swelling of the right temporal lobe and neoplasm infiltrating the mesencephalon.

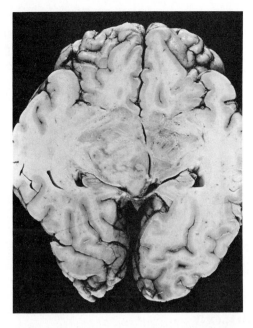

Figure 8–8B. Horizontal section of brain showing poorly demarcated neoplasm infiltrating thalamus and hypothalamus.

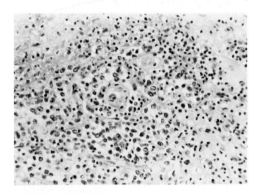

Figure 8–8C. Microscopic section of the highly cellular neoplasm showing poorly cohesive cells, consistent with lymphoma.

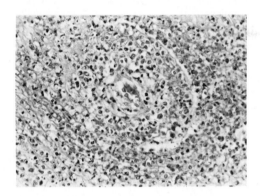

Figure 8–8D. Microscopic section showing neoplastic cells aggregated about blood vessel.

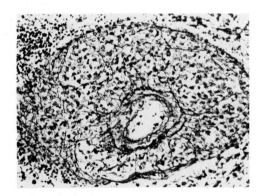

Figure 8–8E. Microscopic section showing the characteristic concentric lamellae that can be demonstrated with the reticulin stain.

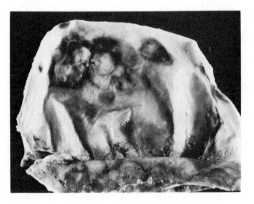

Figure 8–8F. Inner surface of dura studded with nodular masses of granulocytic sarcoma.

8.9   Intraspinal Epithelial Cyst

CLINICAL

This 50-year-old man had a 4- to 5-month history of back pain accompanied by left hand weakness, bilateral leg weakness, and paresthesias in both legs. Myelography and magnetic resonance imaging showed an intradural, extramedullary lesion, ventral to the spinal cord, extending from C5 to T2. No defects were evident in the adjacent vertebral bodies. A laminectomy was performed, with removal of a thin-walled cyst that contained opalescent fluid.

PATHOLOGY

The partially collapsed cyst measured 2.0 × 0.5 × 0.3 cm (Fig. 8–9A). A macrosection showed the walls to be very thin, consisting of an epithelial lining covered by a thin layer of fibrous tissue (Fig. 8–9B). The lining epithelium varied from cuboidal to columnar and included both mucus-secreting cells and ciliated cells (Fig. 8–9C).

COMMENT

There are a wide variety of cystic intraspinal lesions, including dermoids, epidermoids, meningeal cysts, ependymal cysts, and enterogenous cysts. Enterogenous cysts are rare lesions and usually become manifest clinically during childhood. They are typically located ventral to the spinal cord although a few examples are at least partially intramedullary. They are presumed to be derived from displaced remnants of the gastrointestinal anlage and are often accompanied by defects in the underlying vertebral bodies. These cysts have also been interpreted as teratomatous lesions. By contrast, ependymal cysts more often become manifest during adult life and are not accompanied by defects in the vertebral bodies. The lining of enterogenous and ependymal cysts are cuboidal to columnar epithelium and both may contain at least some mucus-secreting cells. In contrast to the enterogenous cysts the ependymal cysts usually contain ciliated epithelial cells.

REFERENCES

Burger PC, Vogel FS: Surgical Pathology of the Nervous System and Its Coverings, 2nd ed. New York, Wiley, 1982, pp 598-600.

Kwok DMF, Jeffreys RV: Intramedullary enterogenous cyst of the spinal cord: Case report. J Neurosurg 1982; 56:270-274.

Leech RW, Olafson RA: Epithelial cysts of the neuraxis: Presentation of three cases and a review of the origins and classification. Arch Pathol Lab Med 1977; 101:196-202.

Miyagi K, Mukawa J, Mekaru S, et al: Enterogenous cyst in the cervical spinal canal: Case Report. J Neurosurg 1988; 68:292-296.

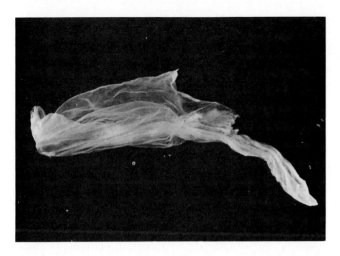

Figure 8–9A. Partially collapsed thin-walled intraspinal epithelial cyst.

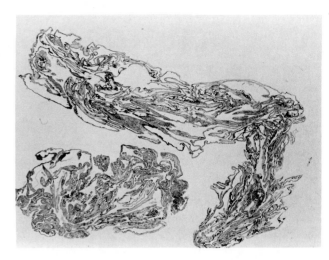

Figure 8–9B. Macrosection of collapsed intraspinal epithelial cyst.

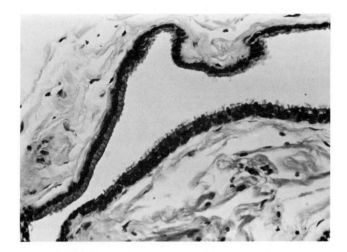

Figure 8–9C. Microscopic section of the intraspinal epithelial cyst showing the lining composed of cuboidal cells. Some of the cells are ciliated while others are goblet cells and contain droplets of mucin.

8.10   Glioblastoma Multiforme

CLINICAL

This 80-year-old woman had a long history of Alzheimer's disease. Approximately 1 year prior to her death, she suddenly lost the ability to feed herself and began to talk in only brief phrases. Within a short period of time she became bedridden and developed generalized seizures.

PATHOLOGY

The brain weighed 1159 grams. The frontal lobes were moderately swollen and neoplastic tissue extended into the subarachnoid space from the undersurface of the right gyrus rectus (Fig. 8–10A). Coronal sections of the cerebral hemispheres revealed a massive, extensively necrotic neoplasm (Fig. 8–10B). The tumor extended across the corpus callosum to involve both frontal lobes (Fig. 8–10C). The lateral margins of the neoplasm blended into the surrounding edematous white matter. Additional nodules of neoplastic tissue protruded from the ependymal surfaces into the cavities of the lateral ventricles. Histologically, the lesion was a highly cellular glial neoplasm with irregular geographic areas of necrosis surrounded by pseudopalisades. In addition, the hippocampi and isocortex contained numerous senile plaques and neurofibrillary tangles, consistent with the clinical diagnosis of Alzheimer's disease.

COMMENT

Glioblastoma multiforme is the most common glial neoplasm and accounts for more than one half of all gliomas. These neoplasms have a peak incidence in the fifth and sixth decades and occur somewhat more commonly in men than women. The clinical manifestations reflect both rapidly evolving mass effect and features specific to the site of involvement. Glioblastomas develop most often in the white matter of the frontal or temporal lobes (Fig. 8–10D) but are also found frequently in the basal ganglia and thalamus. Nearly one fourth extend across the corpus callosum to involve the opposite hemisphere. They may arise in the caudal brain stem at an early age in individuals with preexisting pontine gliomas. The cerebellum is rarely involved by glioblastoma multiforme.

Grossly, glioblastomas have a variegated appearance that is produced by areas of cystic degeneration, necrosis, and hemorrhage. Although some of these tumors appear deceptively well demarcated, they extensively infiltrate the surrounding edematous neural parenchyma. As in the present case, they may also extend into the subarachnoid space and ventricular system. Nevertheless, they rarely metastasize outside of the nervous system.

Glioblastomas have a wide variety of appearances histologically. They are highly cellular glial neoplasms with varying degrees of cellular pleomorphism. Some may contain numerous, large grotesque cells and can be further designated as giant cell glioblastomas (Fig. 8–10E). Others are composed mainly of small cells. Most often, they contain an admixture of both large and small cells. Mitoses may be abundant, and in some cases are atypical. In other specimens, they are remarkably scanty. Another histological feature, encountered frequently in glioblastomas, is the presence of glomeruloids (Fig. 8–10F). Previously, these complex vascular structures were thought to be derived from endothelial proliferation. However, recent immunohistochemical studies have suggested that they are composed predominantly of smooth muscle cells and

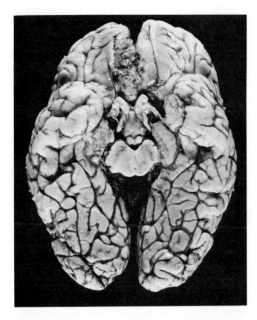

Figure 8–10A. Base of brain showing neoplasm extending to the ventral surface of the right frontal lobe.

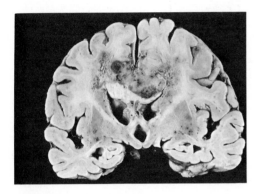

Figure 8–10C. Coronal section showing extension of the neoplasm across the corpus callosum.

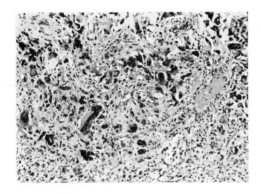

Figure 8–10E. Microscopic section of a glioblastoma in which there were numerous giant cells.

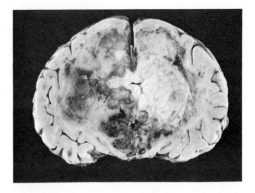

Figure 8–10B. Coronal section showing a massive glioblastoma involving both frontal lobes.

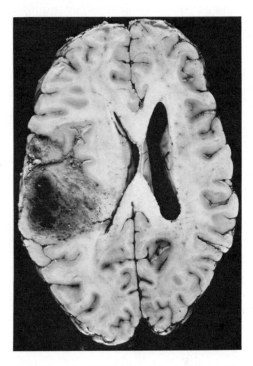

Figure 8–10D. Horizontal section showing a glioblastoma involving the temporal lobe.

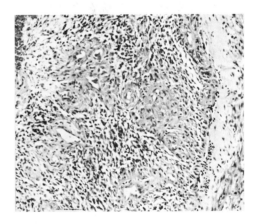

Figure 8–10F. Microscopic section of a glioblastoma showing vascular proliferation and glomeruloid formations.

pericytes. Nevertheless, the most characteristic and histologically diagnostic feature of glioblastoma multiforme is the presence of foci of necrosis surrounded by pseudopalisades (Fig. 8–10G). Neoplasms similar in other respects, but, lacking the characteristic areas of necrosis surrounded by pseudopalisades, are better designated as anaplastic astrocytomas. These gliomas may pursue a somewhat less pernicious course than the glioblastoma. However, predicting prognosis in individual cases on the basis of biopsy specimens, especially needle biopsy specimens, is subject to sampling error. Occasionally, neoplastic transformation of mesenchymal elements from blood vessels and the adjacent meninges gives rise to sarcomas. These composite neoplasms are usually designated as gliosarcomas and pursue a course similar to that of glioblastoma multiforme.

REFERENCES

Burger PC, Vogel FS: Surgical Pathology of the Nervous System and Its Coverings, 2nd ed. New York, Wiley, 1982, pp 242-266.

Hoshino T: A commentary on the biology and growth kinetics of low-grade and high-grade gliomas. J Neurosurg 1984; 61:895-900.

Klinken LH, Kiemer NH, Gjerris F: Automated image analysis, histologic malignancy grading, and survival in patients with astrocytic gliomas. Clin Neuropathol 1984; 3:107-112.

McComb RD, Jones TR, Pizzo SV, Bigner DD: Immunohistochemical detection of factor VIII/von Willebrand factor in hyperplastic endothelial cells in glioblastoma and mixed glioma-sarcoma. J Neuropathol Exp Neurol 1982; 41:479-489.

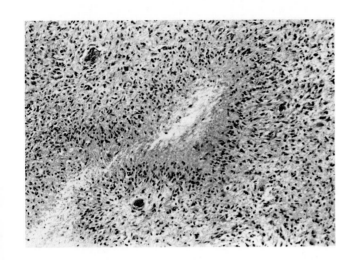

Figure 8–10G. Microscopic section of a glioblastoma showing an area of necrosis surrounded by a pseudopalisade.

8.11 Fibrillary Astrocytomas

Cerebral
Brain Stem

CLINICAL

This 64-year-old man, with long-standing diabetes and coronary arteriosclerosis, gradually developed difficulty walking, left-sided weakness, and urinary incontinence. Neurological examination disclosed mild left hemiparesis. The patient died of his cardiac disease before neuro-diagnostic studies could be undertaken.

PATHOLOGY

The cerebral hemispheres were slightly asymmetrical due to fullness of the right cerebral hemisphere. The right uncus was deeply grooved approximately 0.7 cm lateral to its medial surface and the mammillary bodies were displaced ventrally. Coronal sections of the cerebral hemispheres revealed expansion of the white matter of the right frontal lobe, the right basal ganglia and the right thalamus (Figs. 8–11A and 8–11B). These areas had an abnormally firm consistency. The right lateral ventricle and third ventricle were compressed and distorted. Histologically, the neoplasm was composed of relatively uniform, heavily fibrillated astrocytes (Fig. 8–11C). There were no areas of hemorrhage, necrosis, or vascular proliferation.

COMMENT

Grossly and microscopically, this lesion was consistent with a diffuse, fibrillary astrocytoma. In the cere-bral hemispheres of adults, this type of neoplasm is encountered much less commonly than the more malignant anaplastic astrocytomas or glioblastomas. Occasionally, fibrillary astrocytomas occur in the brain stem of children, where they are often designated as "pontine gliomas." In this location, the neoplasms are also relatively slow growing and produce progressive cranial nerve deficits and long tract signs. The neoplasms diffusely but irregularly expand the brain stem. Ventral enlargement may cause the basilar artery to become partially surrounded by neoplasm. Sections of the infiltrated brain stem show obliteration of normal architectural features (Fig. 8–11D). The astrocytes comprising these tumors may be markedly elongated. Occasionally, these tumors evolve into glioblastomas before leading to the death of the individual.

REFERENCES

Burger PC, Vogel FS: Surgical Pathology of the Nervous System and Its Coverings, 2nd ed. New York, Wiley, 1982, pp 226-240, 288-292.

Stroink AR, Hoffman HJ, Hendrick EB, Humphreys RP: Diagnosis and management of pediatric brain-stem gliomas. J Neurosurg 1986; 65:745-750.

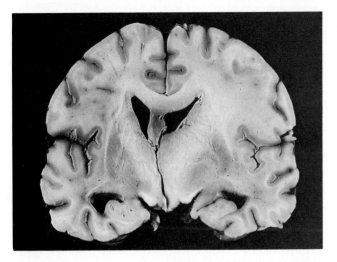

Figure 8–11A. Coronal section showing enlargement of the white matter of the right frontal lobe and basal ganglia.

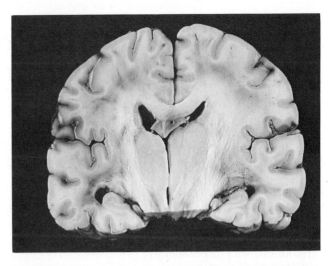

Figure 8–11B. Coronal section showing enlargement of the white matter of the right frontal lobe and thalamus.

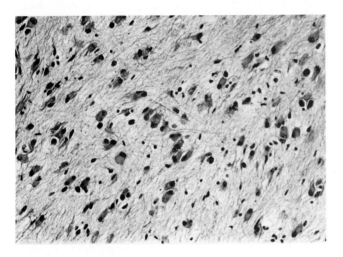

Figure 8–11C. Microscopic section showing fibrillary astrocytoma.

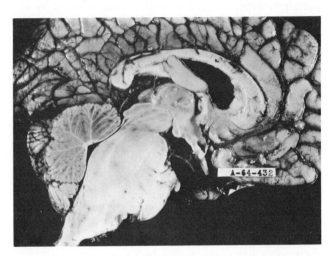

Figure 8–11D. Diffuse enlargement of pons secondary to infiltration by brain stem glioma.

8.12 Juvenile Pilocytic Astrocytoma

Cerebellar Astrocytoma
Optic Glioma
Diencephalic Astrocytoma

CLINICAL

This 16-year-old girl was found to have bilateral papilledema during a physical examination following a minor automobile accident. No other neurological abnormalities were evident. Computerized tomography demonstrated a large cystic lesion in the midline of the posterior fossa. A craniotomy was performed.

PATHOLOGY

The surgical specimen consisted of part of the cyst wall on which there was a mural nodule (Fig. 8–12A). Histologically, the neoplasm had a distinctive pattern that resulted from the presence of compact, elongated glial cells around blood vessels and stellate cells with extensive microcystic degeneration in the areas between blood vessels (Fig. 8–12B). The tissue comprising the cyst wall was densely gliotic and contained numerous Rosenthal fibers.

COMMENT

The gross and microscopic features of this neoplasm are typical of the usual cerebellar astrocytoma. These tumors are generally encountered in the first or second decades and are usually at least partially cystic. Often, as in the present case, the neoplasm consists of a mural nodule in a larger, nonneoplastic glial cyst. The tumors are found most often in the cerebellar hemispheres but also commonly involve the cerebellar vermis. The distinctive histological pattern includes features associated with both fibrillary and protoplasmic astrocytomas. In addition, some of the cells resemble oligodendrocytes. These tumors may contain numerous Rosenthal fibers, especially in the compact neoplastic tissue around blood vessels and in the glial tissue surrounding the accompanying

cyst. Some of these tumors show prominent vascular proliferation. The classification of these tumors is controversial. Some authors consider the neoplasms to be spongioblastomas or derived from tanycytes, rather than true astrocytomas. Cerebellar astrocytomas generally have a favorable prognosis, even when incompletely resected. However, in some cases, the recurrences develop many years later. Generally, the outcome is less favorable when the brain stem is involved.

Histologically similar lesions (Fig. 8–12C) may occur around the third ventricle in the diencephalon of children. These tumors generally have a worse prognosis if for no other reason than their location. Some authors regard the optic gliomas of childhood as juvenile pilocytic astrocytomas. These lesions typically cause massive enlargement of the optic nerve and may infiltrate the surrounding subarachnoid space and leptomeninges (Fig. 8–12D). Nevertheless, these lesions usually have a favorable prognosis when the chiasm is spared. They are more apt to be bilateral when they occur in patients with neurofibromatosis.

REFERENCES

Alvord EC Jr, Lofton S: Gliomas of the optic nerve or chiasm: Outcome by patients' age, tumor site, and treatment. J Neurosurg 1988; 68:85-98.

Austin EJ, Alvord EC Jr: Recurrence of cerebellar astrocytomas: A violation of Collins' law. J Neurosurg 1988; 68:41-47.

Burger PC, Vogel FS: Surgical Pathology of the Nervous System and Its Coverings, 2nd ed. New York, Wiley, 1982, pp 269-288.

Ilgren EB, Stiller CA: Cerebellar astrocytomas: Part I. Macroscopic and microscopic features. Clin Neuropathol 1987; 6:185-200.

Ilgren EB, Stiller CA: Cerebellar astrocytomas: Part II. Pathologic features indicative of malignancy. Clin Neuropathol 1987; 6:210-214.

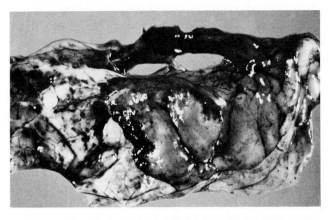

Figure 8–12A. Cerebellar astrocytoma showing mural nodule (bisected in center of illustration) and accompanying cyst.

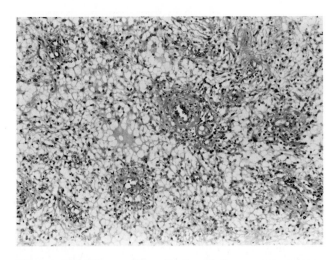

Figure 8–12B. Microscopic section of cerebellar astrocytoma showing compact aggregation about blood vessels and microcystic areas between vessels.

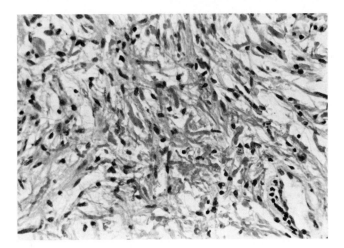

Figure 8–12C. Microscopic section showing similar appearing pilocytic astrocytoma of diencephalon.

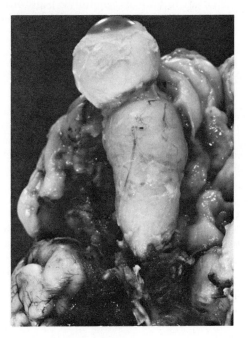

Figure 8–12D. Optic nerve glioma in an infant with neurofibromatosis.

8.13 Intracranial Ependymoma

CLINICAL

This 11-month-old child was hospitalized because of vomiting. Examination disclosed an enlarged head with a tense, bulging fontanelle. The cranial nerves were intact. The child had gross truncal ataxia and tremor of the upper extremities. The deep tendon reflexes were hyperactive, and he had sustained clonus bilaterally. Plain skull x-rays showed all sutures to be widely separated. A ventriculogram revealed hydrocephalus, occlusion of the aqueduct, and tumor in the fourth ventricle. Following placement of a ventriculoperitoneal shunt, subtotal removal of neoplasm was performed. Post-operative radiation was administered and a shunt revision was performed. The child died approximately 6 weeks later.

PATHOLOGY

Parasagittal sections of the brain revealed massive hydrocephalus and a neoplasm that completely filled the fourth ventricle (Fig. 8–13A). The tumor compressed and distorted the brain stem and cerebellum but did not invade these structures. There were foci of necrosis and hemosiderin staining at the site of previous surgery. Additional neoplasm had extended through the outlet foramina of the fourth ventricle and was present on the ventral surface of the pons and medulla. Histologically, the original surgical specimen and autopsy material were similar. The neoplasm was moderately cellular, with many of the cells arranged to form anuclear zones around blood vessels (Fig. 8–13B).

COMMENT

Intracranial ependymomas account for only 5 to 6 percent of cerebral gliomas and are found predominantly during the first or second decades. They may arise in any of the ventricular cavities and even within the cerebral hemispheres. However, the majority are found in the fourth ventricle, where they comprise the third most common glioma of childhood. These tumors show relatively little tendency to infiltrate the surrounding neural parenchyma but readily extend into the subarachnoid space, as in the present case. Histologically, ependymomas are most readily recognized by the formation of anuclear, perivascular pseudorosettes. In addition, some recapitulate the ventricular system by forming ependymal-lined rosettes and canals (Fig. 8–13C). These tumors show limited responsiveness to radiation and generally have a relatively poor prognosis.

REFERENCES

Burger PC, Vogel FS: Surgical Pathology of the Nervous System and Its Coverings, 2nd ed. New York, Wiley, 1982, pp 302-315.

Ilgren EB, Stiller CA, Hughes JT, et al: Ependymomas: A clinical and pathologic study. Part I — Biologic features. Clin Neuropathol 1984; 3:113-121.

Ilgren EB, Stiller CA, Hughes JT, et al: Ependymomas: A clinical and pathologic study. Part II — Survival features. Clin Neuropathol 1984; 3:122-127.

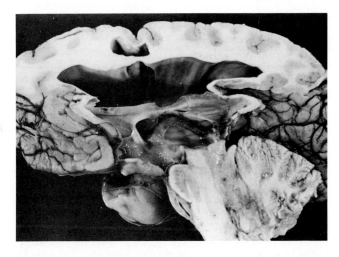

Figure 8–13A. Sagittal section showing hydrocephalus secondary to an ependymoma in the fourth ventricle. Note the extension of the tumor into the subarachnoid space beneath the brain stem.

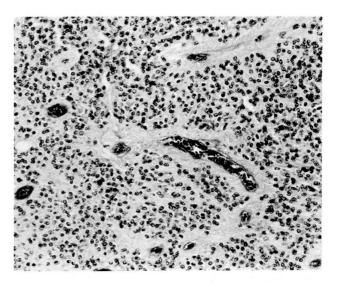

Figure 8–13B. Microscopic section showing perivascular pseudo-rosettes, typical of ependymoma.

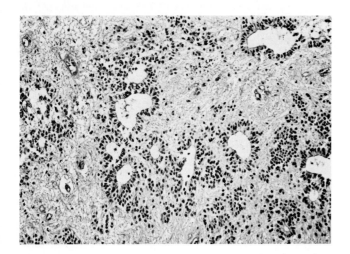

Figure 8–13C. Microscopic section of an ependymoma showing small ependymal-lined canals and perivascular pseudorosettes.

8.14 Spinal Ependymoma

CLINICAL

This 30-year-old man complained of progressive weakness of his right leg for 1 year and weakness of his left leg for 2 months. On examination he was found to have intact cranial nerves. His sensory examination was described as normal. The deep tendon reflexes were increased at the knees and ankles, and he had ankle clonus. The patient had difficulty walking on his toes and circumducted his right leg. He denied any bowel or bladder problems. Magnetic resonance imaging disclosed a cervical cord lesion.

PATHOLOGY

The surgical specimen consisted of a partially cystic mass measuring approximately 2.5 × 1.0 × 1.0 cm (Fig. 8–14A). Histological examination demonstrated anuclear zones around blood vessels forming perivascular pseudorosettes and small canals lined by cuboidal ependymal cells (Fig. 8–14B).

COMMENT

In contrast to their intracranial counterparts, ependymomas are the most common spinal glioma and account for about 60 percent of all primary spinal cord neoplasms. They may occur at any age but the majority are encountered in adults. Ependymomas may arise from any level of the spinal cord or from the cauda equina. The intramedullary lesions often form a discrete mass that can be partially separated from the remainder of the spinal cord. The tumors are usually solid but may be partially cystic. Even solid intramedullary ependymomas may be accompanied by a syrinx. Ependymomas arising from the filum terminale and conus medullaris often have a distinctive histological appearance. This is due to the presence of abundant mucoid material about blood vessels and in microcystic areas (Fig. 8–14C). These lesions are described as myxopapillary ependymomas. Although most of the myxopapillary ependymomas are slow growing, they may be insinuated among the nerve roots and difficult to remove. Some may recur locally or even spread within the subarachnoid space.

REFERENCES

Burger PC, Vogel FS: Surgical Pathology of the Nervous System and Its Coverings, 2nd ed. New York, Wiley, 1982, pp 620-633.
Davis C, Barnard RO: Malignant behavior of myxopapillary ependymoma: Report of three cases. J Neurosurg 1985; 62:925-929.

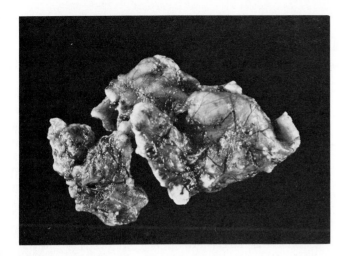

Figure 8–14A. Partially cystic ependymoma removed from cervical spinal cord.

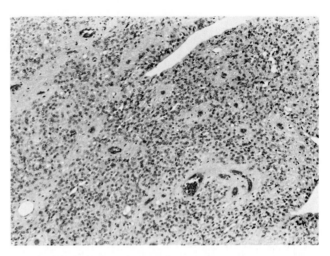

Figure 8–14B. Microscopic section showing perivascular pseudo-rosettes and ependymal-lined canals.

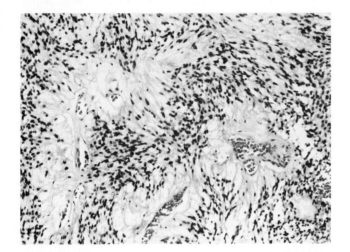

Figure 8–14C. Microscopic section of a myxopapillary ependymoma from the filum terminale. Note the mucoid material about vessels.

8.15   Subependymoma

CLINICAL

This 55-year-old woman was found dead in bed.

PATHOLOGY

Examination of the exterior of the brain disclosed a firm, gray-white mass protruding from the foramen of Magendie onto the dorsal surface of the upper cervical spinal cord. Sagittal sections of the brain demonstrated a gray-white neoplasm within the cavity of the fourth ventricle (Fig. 8–15A). The mass was loosely attached to the floor of the fourth ventricle at the obex. The brain showed no hydrocephalus. Histologically, the neoplasm was sparsely cellular. The neoplastic cells aggregated in small groups that were widely separated by broad expanses of densely fibrillary cell processes (Fig. 8–15B). The vessels within the tumor had thick walls and were hyalinized. The neoplasm also contained small foci of mineralization.

COMMENT

The gross and histological features of this neoplasm are consistent with a subependymoma. Small subependymomas are relatively common incidental findings at the time of autopsy in elderly individuals. The incidental lesions occur most often in the fourth ventricle but also may arise from the septum pellucidum or roof of the lateral ventricles (Fig. 8–15C). Larger, symptomatic lesions are much less common and are generally found in younger patients. Subependymomas have been variously interpreted as astrocytomas, ependymomas or a mixture of these two neoplasms. In contrast to the small, incidental lesions, the larger subependymomas may contain areas that are histologically similar to cellular ependymomas. Symptoms generally result from obstruction of the cerebrospinal fluid pathways, although rare cases of hemorrhage and spinal cord compression have been reported.

REFERENCES

Shangaris DG, Powers JM, Perot PL Jr, et al: Subependymoma presenting as subarachnoid hemorrhage: Case report. J Neurosurg 1981; 55:643-645.

Jooma R, Torrens MJ, Bradshaw J, Brownell B: Subependymomas of the fourth ventricle: Surgical treatment in 12 cases. J Neurosurg 1985; 62:508-512.

Lee KS, Angelo JN, McWhorter JM, Davis CH Jr: Symptomatic subependymoma of the cervical spinal cord: Report of two cases. J Neurosurg 1987; 67:128-131.

Scheithauer BW: Symptomatic subependymoma: Report of 21 cases with review of the literature. J Neurosurg 1978; 49:689-696.

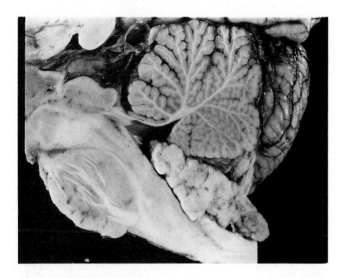

Figure 8–15A. Sagittal section of brain showing a subependymoma within the fourth ventricle.

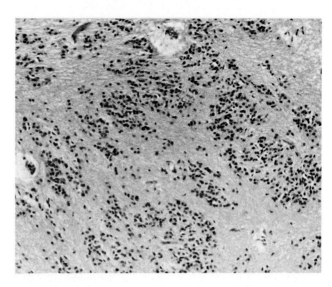

Figure 8–15B. Microscopic section of the subependymoma showing nests of cells separated by wide expanses of fibrillated cytoplasm.

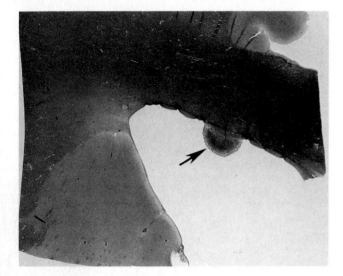

Figure 8–15C. Macrosection showing a small subependymoma attached to the roof of the lateral ventricle (arrow).

8.16   Choroid Plexus Papilloma

CLINICAL

This 13-year-old girl had a 2-month history of dizziness and a 2-week history of blurred vision. She denied having headaches, nausea, or vomiting. Physical examination revealed bilateral papilledema, normal pupillary responses, and nystagmus on right lateral gaze. She also had a slight intention tremor and difficulty with rapid alternating movements. Computerized tomography revealed a markedly enhancing, midline posterior fossa lesion (Fig. 8–16A). Tumor resection was performed following the placement of a ventriculostomy.

PATHOLOGY

The surgical specimen consisted of a moderately cellular, papillary neoplasm (Fig. 8–16B). The individual neoplastic cells ranged from cuboidal to columnar. Some contained vacuoles in their cytoplasm. A single layer of neoplastic cells were applied to fibrovascular cores comprising the papillae. The nuclei of the neoplastic cells were relatively uniform and free of mitotic activity. In areas, there were small, laminated mineralized concretions.

COMMENT

Choroid plexus papillomas are relatively uncommon lesions and account for less than 1 percent of all primary intracranial neoplasms. They occur in all age groups but are encountered most frequently in childhood. In children, the tumors are found more often in the lateral ventricles, while in adults the tumors are found predominantly in the fourth ventricle (Figs. 8–16C and 8–16D). Choroid plexus papillomas produce hydrocephalus by obstructing the flow of cerebrospinal fluid. These tumors can be a source of hemorrhage. The neoplasms are generally composed of relatively uniform cuboidal to columnar cells that mimic the normal choroid plexus. In contrast to papillary ependymomas, the papillae of the choroid plexus papillomas have fibrovascular cores. Malignant choroid plexus tumors or choroid plexus carcinomas show less orderly papillae, scattered mitotic figures, and foci of necrosis. These malignant neoplasms tend to invade the adjacent neural tissue and may even metastasize outside of the nervous system.

REFERENCES

Boyd MC, Steinbok P: Choroid plexus tumors: Problems in diagnosis and management. J Neurosurg 1987; 66:800-805.
Carpenter DB, Michelsen WJ, Hays AP: Carcinoma of the choroid plexus. J Neurosurg 1982; 56:722-727.

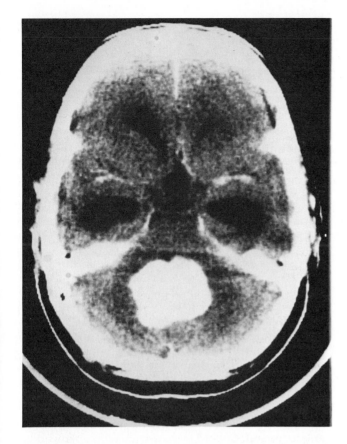

Figure 8–16A. Computerized tomogram showing markedly enhancing choroid plexus papilloma in the fourth ventricle.

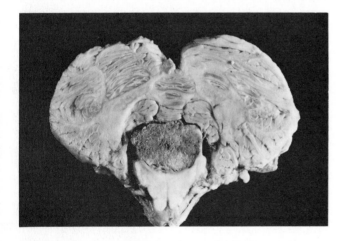

Figure 8–16C. Choroid plexus papilloma in the fourth ventricle of an adult.

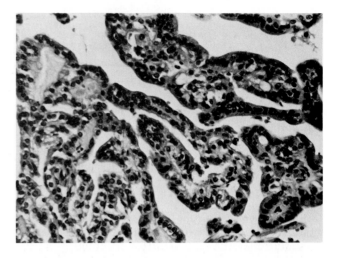

Figure 8–16B. Microscopic section of the choroid plexus papilloma.

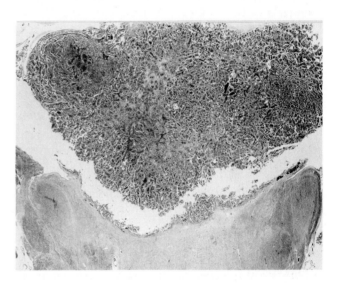

Figure 8–16D. Macrosection of the choroid plexus papilloma.

8.17   Colloid Cyst

CLINICAL

This 23-year-old man had been followed at a mental health clinic for rage attacks and headaches. He developed malaise and nausea followed by vomiting. Subsequently, he had a generalized tonic–clonic seizure. He was taken to a hospital where it was noted that he had disconjugate eye movements. He subsequently suffered a cardiac arrest and died.

PATHOLOGY

Externally, the brain appeared diffusely swollen with widened gyri and narrowed sulci. Both unci were grooved and there was mild parahippocampal herniation. Coronal sections demonstrated marked enlargement of the lateral ventricles with rounding of the lateral angles (Fig. 8–17A). The third ventricle was not enlarged and contained a colloid cyst, measuring approximately 1.4 cm in diameter, at the foramina of Monro (Fig. 8–17B). The contents of the cyst were firm and had a tan color. Histologically, the cyst was composed of a single layer of cuboidal to columnar epithelium surrounded by a thin layer of fibrovascular connective tissue (Fig. 8–17C).

COMMENT

Colloid cysts are uncommon lesions accounting for less than 1 percent of intracranial tumors in adults. They are typically found in the rostral portion of the third ventricle where they may obstruct the foramina of Monro. They may be adherent to the walls or roof of the third ventricle or to the fornices. The cyst contents are usually a glairy mucinous fluid when approached surgically. This fluid tends to harden with formalin fixation. In addition, debris from desquamated cells may be scattered in the cyst contents. The epithelium lining the cyst varies from cuboidal to columnar. Some of the cells may be ciliated while others may contain intracellular vacuoles. The vacuoles, like the cyst contents, stain variably with the mucicarmine and periodic acid–Schiff stains. The derivation of colloid cysts is controversial. Among the proposed sources are ependyma, choroid plexi, endoderm, neuroepithelium, and vestigial structures like the paraphysis. Occasionally, similar cystic lesions have been encountered in other parts of the ventricular system.

Clinically, colloid cysts may cause headaches that are attributed to obstruction of the flow of cerebrospinal fluid. Occasionally, the headaches are claimed to be exacerbated and relieved by movement of the colloid cyst when the position of the head is changed. By computerized tomography, the cysts may appear as hypodense, isodense, or hyperdense lesions. They also show a variable degree of contrast enhancement. Colloid cysts are a well recognized but rare cause of sudden, unexpected death. In other individuals, they may be an incidental finding at autopsy.

REFERENCES

Hall WA, Lunsford LD: Changing concepts in the treatment of colloid cysts: An 11-year experience in the CT era. J Neurosurg 1987; 66:186-191.

Michels LG, Rutz D: Colloid cysts of the third ventricle: A radiologic–pathologic correlation. Arch Neurol 1982; 39:640-643.

Ryder JW, Kleinschmidt-DeMasters BK, Keller TS: Sudden deterioration and death in patients with benign tumors of the third ventricle area. J Neurosurg 1986; 64:216-233.

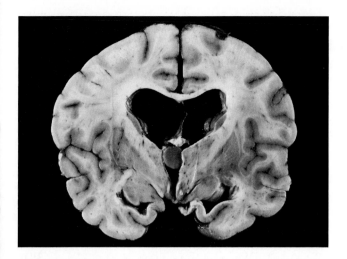

Figure 8–17A. Coronal section showing hydrocephalus due to colloid cyst.

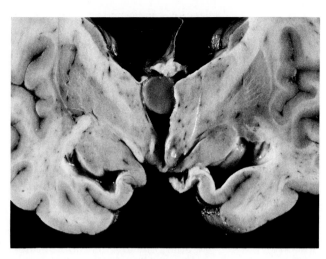

Figure 8–17B. Coronal section showing the colloid cyst located at the foramen of Monro.

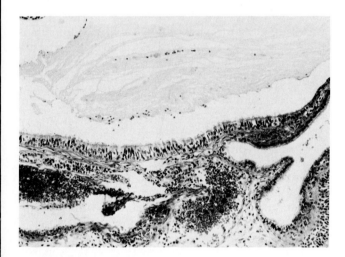

Figure 8–17C. Microscopic section showing the mucoid contents and columnar epithelial lining of the colloid cyst.

8.18 Oligodendroglioma

CLINICAL

This 44-year-old woman presented with a 2-week history of tingling in the left arm and leg. One week previously, she had noted an episode of left leg twitching. Physical examination revealed only hypesthesia in the left leg. A computerized tomogram showed an enhancing mass lesion in the right parietal lobe (Fig. 8–18A). A craniotomy and resection of neoplasm were performed.

PATHOLOGY

The surgical specimen revealed a moderately cellular glial neoplasm consistent with an oligodendroglioma. The neoplastic cells were relatively uniform and polyhedral with spherical, vesicular nuclei. Mitotic figures were scanty. The cytoplasm of many of the neoplastic cells was vacuolated forming perinuclear halos (Fig. 8–18B). The neoplasm was traversed and compartmentalized by thin-walled blood vessels. Foci of mineralization were encountered predominantly at the periphery of the neoplasm.

COMMENT

Oligodendrogliomas account for about 5 percent of primary intracranial neoplasms. They occur predominantly in adults and usually become manifest during the fifth or sixth decades. Most are supratentorial in location. In many cases, seizures are the initial clinical manifestation. About one fourth of these tumors are sufficiently mineralized to be detectable with plain skull x-rays. Occasionally, oligodendrogliomas may undergo spontaneous hemorrhage and present as a stroke.

Histologically, oligodendrogliomas characteristically appear as sheets of relatively uniform round to polygonal cells with spherical, vesicular nuclei. The cytoplasm often becomes vacuolated forming a perinuclear halo. This alteration is generally considered to be a fixation artifact and is usually more pronounced in autopsy specimens than surgical material. Another highly characteristic feature is the compartmentalization of the neoplasm by relatively thin-walled blood vessels (Fig. 8–18C). Laminated mineralized concretions are commonly present and are often most numerous at the periphery of the neoplasm. Spread of the neoplasm through the cerebral cortex often leads to development of very prominent secondary structuring including perineuronal satellitosis. Further spread to the surface may lead to subpial and subarachnoid deposits of neoplastic cells. Occasionally, subarachnoid spread is so pronounced that much of the neoplasm presents as an extra-axial mass.

Oligodendrogliomas are generally regarded as relatively slow growing gliomas with unpredictable biologic behavior. Recently, the histological features in several large series have been analyzed in an attempt to provide better prognostic information. Although the studies yielded somewhat conflicting conclusions, features that may portend a less favorable prognosis include high cellularity, cellular pleomorphism, nuclear pleomorphism, numerous mitoses, extensive necrosis, and prominent endothelial proliferation. Features that may support a more favorable prognosis include low cellularity, microcyst formation, and prominent mineralization. Many mixed gliomas have a prominent oligodendroglial component. This further complicates estimation of prognosis from small surgical specimens.

REFERENCES

Ludwig CL, Smith MT, Godfrey AD, Armbrustmacher VW: A clinicopathological study of 323 patients with oligodendrogliomas. Ann Neurol 1986; 19:15-21.

Mork SJ, Halvorsen TB, Lindegaard K-F, Eide GE: Oligodendroglioma: Histologic evaluation and prognosis. J Neuropathol Exp Neurol 1986; 45:65-78.

Mork SJ, Lindegaard K-F, Halvorsen TB, et al: Oligodendroglioma: Incidence and biological behavior in a defined population. J Neurosurg 1985; 63:881-889.

Scarpelli M, Montironi R, Ansuini G, et al: The value of morphometry in prediction of survival in oligodendrogliomas. Clin Neuropathol 1987; 6:155-159.

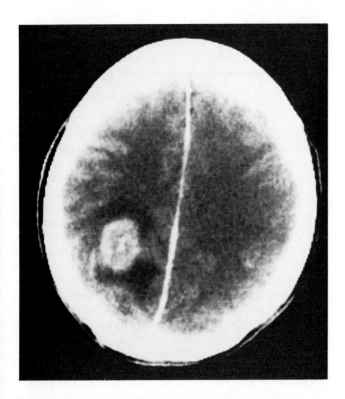

Figure 8–18A. Computerized tomogram showing dense mass lesion with surrounding edema in the right parietal lobe.

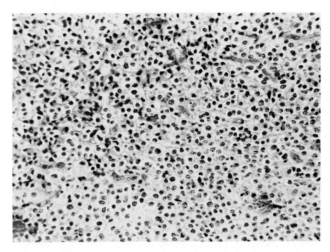

Figure 8–18B. Microscopic section of the oligodendroglioma showing vacuolization of the perinuclear cytoplasm.

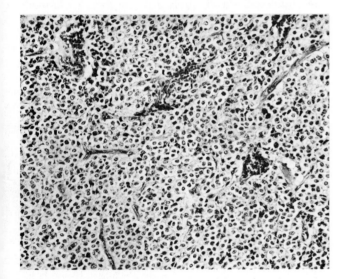

Figure 8–18C. Microscopic section of an oligodendroglioma showing the compartmentalization of the neoplasm by thin-walled blood vessels.

8.19   Medulloblastoma

CLINICAL

This 7-year-old boy had a 3-week history of lethargy, occipital headaches, and vomiting. When examined, he was found to resist neck movements. He had spontaneous nystagmus in the primary position that was exacerbated by gaze in any direction. Funduscopic examination revealed bilateral papilledema. He had an ataxic gait and dysmetria in the upper extremities. His deep tendon reflexes were symmetrically hyperactive. A computerized tomogram demonstrated hydrocephalus and a midline posterior fossa mass with moderate contrast enhancement (Fig. 8–19A). At surgery, the tumor was found to fill and extend to the floor of the fourth ventricle.

PATHOLOGY

Histological examination revealed a highly cellular neoplasm composed of relatively small cells that generally had scanty cytoplasm (Fig. 8–19B). The neoplastic cell nuclei varied from spherical to vesicular to angular and were hyperchromatic. Numerous mitoses were present. Pycnotic nuclei in individual degenerating cells were scattered throughout the tumor and were more numerous around obvious foci of necrosis. In a few areas, there were distinct Homer Wright rosettes (Fig. 8–19C). These were formed by a collar of neoplastic cells surrounding a central area containing fibrillary cell processes (curved arrow).

COMMENT

Medulloblastomas are relatively common tumors and are encountered predominantly in the first two decades of life. Rarely, they may occur in young adults. In children, they are only slightly less common than cerebellar astrocytomas. They are generally thought to arise from primitive, multipotential cells that normally give rise to the external granular layer of the cerebellum. They have also been interpreted as neuroblastomas of the cerebellum. More recently, Rorke has suggested that medulloblastomas should be regarded simply as part of the spectrum of primitive neuroectodermal tumors.

In young children, medulloblastomas usually arise in the vermis of the cerebellum whereas in older individuals, the tumors are more apt to develop in the cerebellar hemispheres. The tumors in older patients may contain more connective tissue and were often described erroneously as "cerebellar sarcomas." Histologically, medulloblastomas are generally composed of small undifferentiated cells, although some examples show evidence of spongioblastic or neuroblastic differentiation. The characteristic Homer Wright rosettes, that are found in only some medulloblastomas, are regarded as a manifestation of neuroblastic differentiation. This line of differentiation has also been supported by ultrastructural and immunocytochemical studies. Spongioblastic differentiation is manifested by areas of palisading that resemble the so-called polar spongioblastoma and by immunocytochemical studies. Rare tumors, which otherwise resemble medulloblastomas, may contain striated muscle. These lesions, designated as medullomyoblastomas, have also been interpreted as teratomas.

Medulloblastomas are treated by various combinations of surgery, radiation, and chemotherapy. The tumors often spread widely throughout the subarachnoid space and, rarely, may metastasize outside of the central nervous system. Because of the propensity to disseminate, radiation is administered to the entire neuraxis. The neoplasm is highly radiosensitive, and over the years, the 5-year survival rate has been increasing. Attempts to predict the outcome on the basis of histological appearance and apparent degree of differentiation have yielded conflicting data.

REFERENCES

Caputy AJ, McCullough DC, Manz HJ, et al: A review of the factors influencing the prognosis of medulloblastoma: The importance of cell differentiation. J Neurosurg 1987; 66:80-87.

Dickson DW, Hart MN, Menezes A, Cancilla PA: Medulloblastoma with glial and rhabdomyoblastic differentiation. A myoglobin and glial fibrillary acidic protein immunohistochemical and ultrastructural study. J Neuropathol Exp Neurol 1983; 42:639-647.

Packer RJ, Sutton LN, Rorke LB, et al: Prognostic importance of cellular differentiation on medulloblastoma of childhood. J Neurosurg 1984; 61:296-301.

Park TS, Hoffman HJ, Hendrick EB, et al: Medulloblastoma: Clinical presentation and management. Experience at the Hospital for Sick Children, Toronto, 1950-1980. J Neurosurg 1983; 58:543-552.

Rorke LB: The cerebellar medulloblastoma and its relationship to primitive neuroectodermal tumors. J Neuropathol Exp Neurol 1983; 42:1-15.

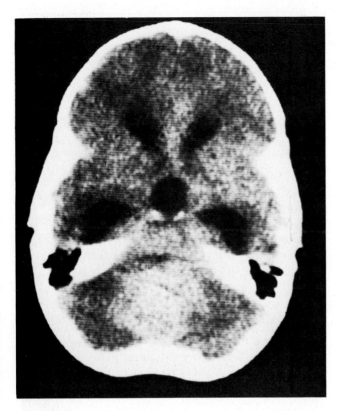

Figure 8–19A. Computerized tomogram showing a moderately enhancing posterior fossa tumor.

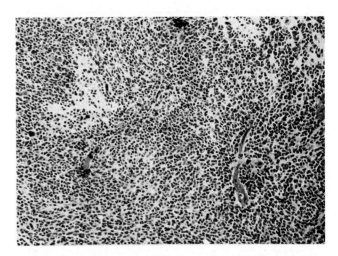

Figure 8–19B. Microscopic section showing a highly cellular neoplasm composed of small cells with scanty cytoplasm, consistent with a medulloblastoma.

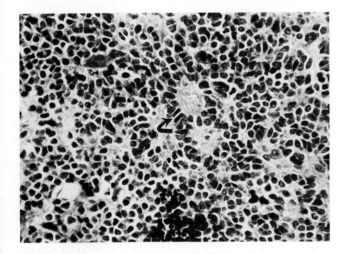

Figure 8–19C. Microscopic section showing Homer Wright rosettes (curved arrow).

8.20   Ganglioglioma

CLINICAL

This 5-year-old boy suddenly gasped, stopped breathing, and died while being bathed under the supervision of his mother. No seizure activity was evident; however, the child had a history of developmental delay, intermittent focal seizures, and apneic episodes.

PATHOLOGY

The brain weighed 1302 grams and appeared diffusely swollen. The medulla and the rostral portion of the cervical spinal cord were irregularly enlarged and infiltrated by neoplasm. The neoplasm extended into the cavity of the fourth ventricle but did not invade the cerebellum (Fig. 8–20A). The aqueduct, third ventricle, and lateral ventricles were not significantly enlarged. The cerebral cortex, including the hippocampi, basal ganglia, and rostral brain stem, were unremarkable. Histologically, the neoplasm was moderately cellular and contained a mixture of astrocytic and oligodendroglial components along with atypical neuronal elements (Fig. 8–20B). The neoplastic neurons varied in size and shape and, rarely, were binucleated (Fig. 8–20C). Axonal spheroids, Rosenthal fibers, and foci of mineralization were scattered throughout the neoplasm. The neoplasm, including the neoplastic ganglion cells, extended into the meninges around the medulla (Fig. 8–20D).

COMMENT

Gangliogliomas are uncommon tumors that are composed of both neoplastic glial cells, predominantly astrocytes, and neoplastic ganglion cells. They were formerly regarded as very rare or even nonexistent but are now being diagnosed with increasing frequency. They are encountered most often in children and young adults but may occur at all ages. Gangliogliomas can be found anywhere in the central nervous system but arise most often from the frontal and temporal lobes, and from the diencephalon. They also may involve the caudal brain stem, cerebellum, and fourth ventricle as in the present case. Patients harboring these tumors present most often with seizures. The neoplasms usually appear as low-density lesions when demonstrated by computerized tomography. Foci of mineralization may be present. Gangliogliomas are slow-growing neoplasms and generally have a favorable prognosis when surgically accessible.

The critical issue in establishing the correct histopathological diagnosis is recognition of the neoplastic ganglion cells. The cells in question must be indisputably neuronal and an integral part of the neoplasm rather than preexisting neurons that have been entrapped by a glial neoplasm. Evidence for the neoplastic nature of the neurons is provided by heterotopic location, and, even more, by the presence of atypical cytological features. These include excessive variation in size and shape, disorientation, and binucleation. In addition, dystrophic axonal swellings may be associated with some of the neoplastic neurons.

REFERENCES

Demierre B, Stichnoth FA, Hori A, Spoerri O: Intracerebral ganglioglioma. J Neurosurg 1986; 65:177-182.

Garcia CA, McGarry PA, Collada M: Ganglioglioma of the brain stem: Case report. J Neurosurg 1984; 60:431-434.

Johannsson JH, Rekate HL, Roessmann U: Gangliogliomas: Pathological and clinical correlation. J Neurosurg 1981; 54:58-63.

Nelson J, Frost JL, Schochet SS Jr: Sudden, unexpected death in a 5-year-old boy with an unusual primary intracranial neoplasm: Ganglioglioma of the medulla. Am J Forensic Med Pathol 1987; 8:148-152.

Sutton LN, Packer RJ, Rorke LB, et al: Cerebral gangliogliomas during childhood. Neurosurgery 1983; 13:124-128.

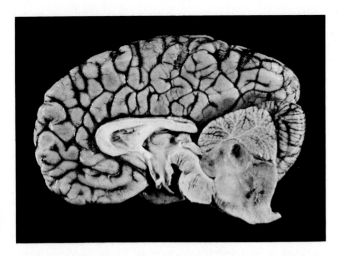

Figure 8–20A. Sagittal section showing a neoplasm arising from the medulla and extending into the fourth ventricle.

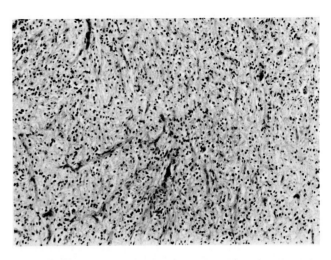

Figure 8–20B. Microscopic section of the neoplasm showing a mixture of oligodendroglial and astrocytic components along with neoplastic neuronal elements.

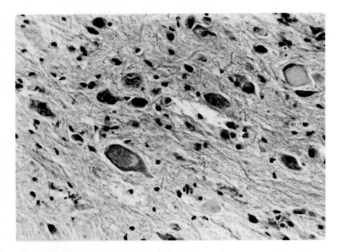

Figure 8–20C. Microscopic section at higher magnification showing some of the neoplastic neurons and axonal swellings.

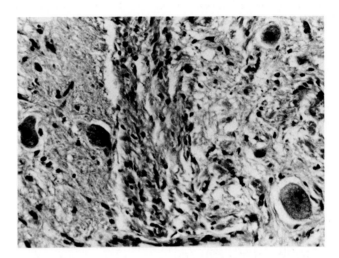

Figure 8–20D. Microscopic section showing extension of the neoplasm with neoplastic neurons into the surrounding leptomeninges (right side of illustration).

8.21 Germinoma

Pineal
Suprasellar

CLINICAL

This 15-year-old boy had "problems with his vision" for 3 to 4 months. He denied headaches, nausea, or vomiting. On examination, he was found to have restriction of upward gaze, vertical nystagmus, and an afferent pupillary defect. There was no papilledema. A computerized tomogram showed a mildly enhancing pineal region mass but no hydrocephalus. A craniotomy was performed.

PATHOLOGY

The surgical specimen consisted of fragments of a neoplasm that was characterized by the presence of two types of cells (Fig. 8–21A). Some of the cells were large, with vesicular nuclei and prominent nucleoli, while others were small with pycnotic nuclei, resembling lymphocytes.

COMMENT

Pineal neoplasms are rare; however, they have been reported somewhat more commonly in Japan than in the Western hemisphere. Germinomas are the most common neoplasm in the pineal region. They are germ cell neoplasms and are histologically identical to the germinomas of the testis, ovary, mediastinum, and hypothalamus. The pineal germinomas are more common in males than females and occur predominantly during the first three decades of life. Pineal germinomas compress and infiltrate the mesencephalic tectum. They may cause preferential impairment of upward gaze. In some patients, this is accompanied by pupils that fail to react to light but constrict on accommodation. Pineal tumors also cause obstructive hydrocephalus and manifestations of increased intracranial pressure are among their most common signs and symptoms. The morphologically identical tumors that arise in the hypothalamus and suprasellar region (Fig. 8–21B) show a less pronounced male predominance and may produce precocious puberty. Germinomas are radiosensitive but may metastasize to the subarachnoid space and ependymal surfaces of the ventricular system (Fig. 8–21C). For this reason, radiation therapy is often administered to the entire neuraxis.

Other less common pineal neoplasms that are also derived from germ cell lines include embryonal carcinomas, teratomas, endodermal sinus tumors, and choriocarcinomas. The pineal also gives rise to small cell tumors designated as pineoblastomas and pineocytomas. These very rare tumors are thought to be derived from the pineal parenchyma and may be similar to primitive neuroectodermal tumors.

REFERENCES

Bjornsson J, Scheithauer BW, Okazaki H, Leech RW: Intracranial germ cell tumors: Pathobiological and immunohistochemical aspects of 70 cases. J Neuropathol Exp Neurol 1985; 44:32-46.

Jennings MT, Gelman R, Hochberg F: Intracranial germ-cell tumors: Natural history and pathogenesis. J Neurosurg 1985; 63:155-167.

Jooma R, Kendall BE: Diagnosis and management of pineal tumors. J Neurosurg 1983; 58:654-665.

Shokry A, Janzer RC, Von Hochstetter AR, et al: Primary intracranial germ-cell tumors: A clinicopathological study of 14 cases. J Neurosurg 1985; 62:826-830.

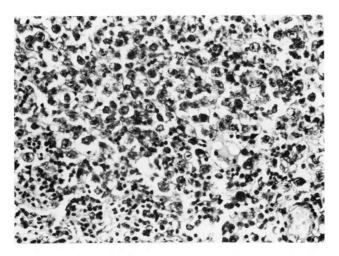

Figure 8–21A. Microscopic section showing the two types of cells in the pineal germinoma, large neoplastic cells with vesicular nuclei and prominent nucleoli (center) and small cells resembling lymphocytes (lower left).

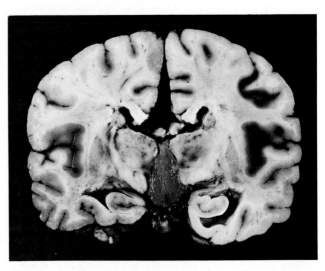

Figure 8–21B. Extensively necrotic hypothalamic germinoma filling the third ventricle.

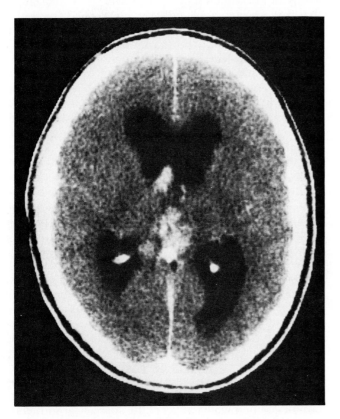

Figure 8–21C. Computerized tomogram from a patient with hydrocephalus and intraventricular seeding from a pineal germinoma.

8.22   Pituitary Adenomas

Prolactinomas
Acromegaly
Null-cell Adenomas

CLINICAL

This 41-year-old man had a 1-year history of impotence and a 2-month history of left-sided frontal and parietal headaches. He also complained of impaired vision in his left eye. On physical examination, he was found to have mild gynecomastia, decreased corneal reflex in the left eye, and impaired sensation over the maxillary division of the left trigeminal nerve. The serum prolactin level was 1190 ng/mL (normal up to 20 ng/mL). A computerized tomogram showed an enhancing mass lesion arising from an enlarged sella (Fig. 8–22A). An angiogram showed displacement of the cavernous portion of the left carotid artery. A transsphenoidal hypophysectomy was performed.

PATHOLOGY

A smear prepared from a portion of the specimen submitted for frozen section revealed relatively uniform neoplastic cells with faintly granular cytoplasm and vesicular nuclei. Permanent sections of the surgical specimen demonstrated the neoplastic cells to be arranged in sheets and sinusoidal arrays. The individual neoplastic cells were relatively uniform in size and had a polygonal configuration (Fig. 8–22B). The cytoplasm was finely granular and the nuclei showed only mild pleomorphism. Fibrovascular trabecula transversed and compartmentalized the tumor. Occasional mineralized concretions were present (Fig. 8–22C). Immunohistochemical stains confirmed the presence of prolactin in the neoplasm.

COMMENT

Pituitary adenomas are common neoplasms that are found almost exclusively in adults. Small, asymptomatic pituitary adenomas have been reported as incidental findings in 2.7 to 27 percent of individuals at the time of autopsy. Symptomatic adenomas account for about 10 percent of all primary intracranial neoplasms. The symptoms are predominantly of two types, those that result from excess hormone production and those that result from mass effects. Rarely,

pituitary adenomas can become manifest by apoplectic hemorrhage.

About three fourths of symptomatic pituitary adenomas are hormonally active and a large proportion of these tumors are so-called microadenomas. By definition, the microadenomas are less than 1 cm in diameter. Pituitary tumors are being diagnosed more frequently, often while still quite small, as a result of improvements in radiological techniques and availability of hormone assays. It has also been suggested that the prevalence of pituitary adenomas is actually increasing, especially among young women.

The majority of the hormonally active pituitary tumors are prolactin-secreting adenomas, otherwise known as prolactinomas. In women, these lesions classically produce the amenorrhea–galactorrhea syndrome. In men, they may cause decreased libido, impotence, and sterility. The presence of this type of tumor is usually reflected by a markedly increased serum prolactin level. It should be noted that modest elevations of serum prolactin can accompany other types of pituitary adenomas and even nonendocrine lesions of the pituitary and hypothalamus. The definitive morphological diagnosis of these lesions is accompanied by immunocytochemical demonstration of prolactin in the neoplastic cells. The immunologic techniques have largely superseded the use of histochemical stains and electron microscopy for diagnosing the various types of pituitary adenomas. Among the various types of pituitary adenomas, prolactinomas are the most likely to contain mineralized concretions. These were readily seen in the smears and permanent sections from the present case.

Adenomas that secrete excessive amounts of growth hormone may cause acromegaly. In addition to growth hormone that can be demonstrated immunocytochemically, many of the sparsely granulated growth hormone-secreting adenomas contain intracytoplasmic spheroids. These can occasionally be seen in smears (Fig. 8–22D) and permanent sections. By electron microscopy, these spheroids are composed of compact aggregates of microfilaments.

Cushing's syndrome may result from adenomas composed of cells that can be demonstrated immunocytochemically to contain ACTH/MSH (Fig. 8–22E). These cells may stain relatively basophilic with

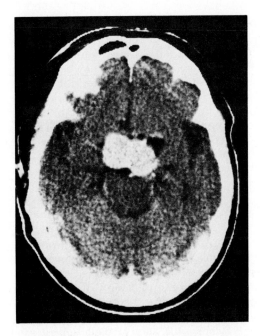

Figure 8–22A. Computerized tomogram showing a pituitary prolactinoma with suprasellar extension.

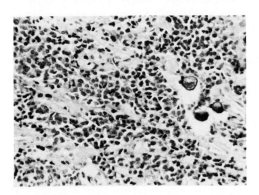

Figure 8–22C. Microscopic section of the pituitary prolactinoma showing the presence of occasional mineralized concretions (right side of illustration).

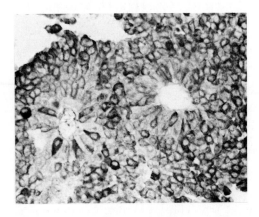

Figure 8–22E. Microscopic section of a pituitary microadenoma from a patient with Cushing's disease stained by an immunoperoxidase technique for ACTH.

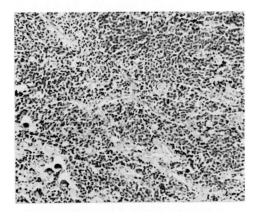

Figure 8–22B. Microscopic section of the prolactinoma showing the relatively uniform appearance of the neoplastic cells.

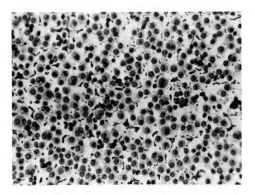

Figure 8–22D. Smear preparation from a sparsely granulated growth hormone-secreting adenoma. Some of the neoplastic cells contained intracytoplasmic spheroids composed of microfilaments.

hematoxylin–eosin and are also stained red by the periodic acid–Schiff technique. Some of the adenomas causing Cushing's disease may be located in the neurohypophysis. These tumors presumably arise from ACTH/MSH cells that are normally located in the neurohypophysis, so-called basophilic invasion of the posterior lobe. The ACTH/MSH cells in nonneoplastic portions of a pituitary harboring an ACTH/MSH adenoma may display the so-called Crooke cell change. The Crooke cells contain skeins of intermediate filaments that impart a hyaline appearance to their cytoplasm. This cellular alteration can be seen in any condition where corticosteroid levels are elevated.

Still other hormone secreting adenomas are composed of mixtures of various cell types including especially prolactin and growth hormone secreting cells. Adenomas derived from cells producing thyroid-stimulating hormone, follicle-stimulating hormone, and luteinizing hormone are extremely rare.

About one fourth of symptomatic pituitary adenomas are composed of so-called null cells. These are undifferentiated cells that do not secrete the usual pituitary hormones. These tumors and some of the larger hormone-secreting adenomas may produce symptoms by mass effect. As the tumors enlarge, they compress the chiasm and optic tracts. This can produce superior temporal quadrantanopsia and, eventually, bitemporal hemianopsia.

Figure 8–22F illustrates a pituitary adenoma extending dorsally out of the sella. The neoplasm contained areas of hemorrhagic necrosis. This is a relatively uncommon complication described as pituitary apoplexy. When extensive, it may produce an abrupt onset of symptoms, including visual impairment, loss of consciousness, and even death. However, smaller areas of hemorrhagic necrosis may be encountered in other cases with minimal or no additional symptoms. Although pituitary adenomas are histologically benign neoplasms, the frequent occurrence of dural invasion has been emphasized in recent years. This feature is especially common in patients with large tumors that show suprasellar extension.

REFERENCES

Black P McL, Hsu DW, Dlibanski A, et al: Hormone production in clinically nonfunctioning pituitary adenomas. J Neurosurg 1987; 66:244-250.

Hardman JM: Nonglial tumors of the nervous system. In Rosenberg RN (ed): The Clinical Neurosciences. New York, Churchill Livingstone, 1983, vol 3, chap 4, pp III:126–III:145.

Lipper S, Isenberg HD, Kahn LB: Calcospherites in pituitary prolactinomas: A hypothesis for their formation. Arch Pathol Lab Med 1984; 108:31-34.

Scheithauer BW, Kovacs KT, Laws ER Jr, Randall RV: Pathology of invasive pituitary tumors with special reference to functional classification. J Neurosurg 1986; 65:733-744.

Wakai S, Fukushima T, Teramoto A, Sano K: Pituitary apoplexy: Its incidence and clinical significance. J Neurosurg 1981; 55:187-193.

Wilson CB: A decade of pituitary microsurgery: The Herbert Olivecrona lecture. J Neurosurg 1984; 61:814-833.

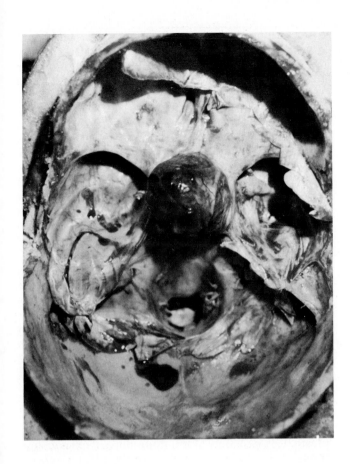

Figure 8–22F. Large, partially necrotic null cell adenoma.

8.23 Craniopharyngioma

CLINICAL

This 33-year-old man had a 2-month history of headaches. These were accompanied by blurred vision, however, he denied any nausea or vomiting. In addition, the patient was described by his family as becoming more somnolent and forgetful. His neurological examination was described as normal except for a slightly flattened affect. An unenhanced computerized tomogram revealed a large cystic lesion that was partially obstructing the third ventricle (Fig. 8–23A). A frontoparietal craniotomy was performed.

PATHOLOGY

The surgical specimen was composed of multiple fragments of firm gray-white tissue with foci of mineralization. Histologically, much of the specimen consisted of irregular masses of squamous epithelium (Fig. 8-23B). Many of the aggregates of squamous epithelium were bordered by a basal layer of columnar epithelium that gradually merged into expanses of less compact stellate cells. There were multiple foci of cystic degeneration among the stellate cells. Some of the squamous epithelium contained nests of keratinized epithelial cells (Fig. 8–23C). Foci of mineralization were found predominantly in these keratinized areas. Some of the epithelial cells adjacent to the foci of keratin contained basophilic keratohyalin granules. The basal layer was surrounded by a layer of connective tissue. The adherent fragments of neuroglial tissue showed gliosis and contained scattered Rosenthal fibers. In some areas, there were collections of macrophages, cholesterol clefts, and even rare foreign body giant cells.

COMMENT

Craniopharyngiomas comprise less than 5 percent of all intracranial neoplasms. They occur in individuals of all ages and are one of the most common supratentorial tumors in children. Craniopharyngiomas are generally regarded as arising from squamous epithelial cells that are remnants of Rathke's pouch or derived from the metaplasia of adenohypophyseal cells. Small nests of squamous epithelium, otherwise known as Erdheim's rests, are occasionally found on the surface of the infundibular stalk (Fig. 8–23D). These rests are encountered more commonly in adults than children.

Grossly, craniopharyngiomas are partially cystic, multilobular masses that compress and distort the adjacent brain (Fig. 8–23E). The fluid within the cysts is sometimes greenish-brown and described as resembling "machine oil." Small glittering cholesterol crystals are often suspended in the dark fluid. Craniopharyngiomas are more commonly mineralized when they occur in children rather than in adults. Radiological demonstration of suprasellar mineralization in a child is considered virtually diagnostic of a craniopharyngioma. Visual field abnormalities are common in both children and adults with this neoplasm. Compression of the optic nerves, chiasm, and tracts may produce unilateral blindness, bitemporal scotomas, or incongruous hemianopsias as well as the classical bitemporal hemianopsia. Distortion of the overlying third ventricle may produce hydrocephalus; however, papilledema is more commonly observed in children rather than adults with these tumors. Growth retardation is common in children, and adults often display some degree of hypopituitarism.

The lesions are generally treated surgically; however, total removal is often not possible. Some authors recommend postoperative radiation.

REFERENCES

Baskin DS, Wilson CB: Surgical management of craniopharyngiomas: A review of 74 cases. J Neurosurg 1986; 65:22-27.

Petito CK, DeGirolami U, Earle KM: Craniopharyngiomas: A clinical and pathological review. Cancer 1976; 37:1944-1952.

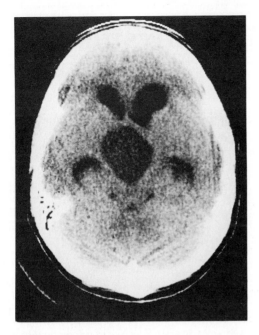

Figure 8–23A. Computerized tomogram showing cystic suprasellar extension of a craniopharyngioma.

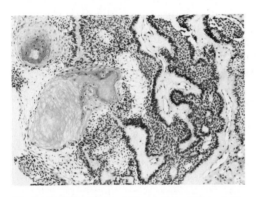

Figure 8–23C. Microscopic section of the craniopharyngioma showing foci of keratinization.

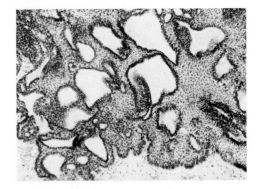

Figure 8–23B. Microscopic section of the craniopharyngioma showing irregular masses of squamous epithelium.

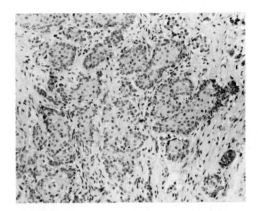

Figure 8–23D. Microscopic section showing foci of squamous epithelium, so-called Erdheim's rests, on the surface of the infundibular stalk.

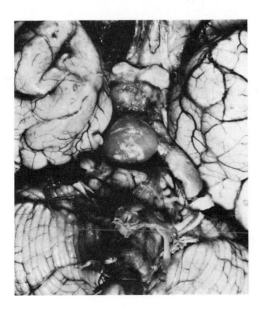

Figure 8–23E. Base of a brain with a multilobulated craniopharyngioma.

8.24   Lymphoid Hypophysitis

CLINICAL

This 19-year-old woman was evaluated for pan-hypopituitarism and headaches approximately 8 months after she had delivered a baby. A computerized tomogram demonstrated a sellar mass. A tissue specimen was obtained by transsphenoidal hypophysectomy.

PATHOLOGY

The specimen consisted of fragments of adenohypophysis that were markedly fibrotic and heavily infiltrated by mononuclear cells. These were predominantly lymphocytes but were accompanied by occasional plasma cells (Fig. 8–24A). In areas, the lymphoid cells were aggregated into small lymphoid nodules. No granulomas or giant cells were present. The residual adenohypophyseal glandular tissue was confined to small nests and follicles (Fig. 8–24B).

COMMENT

This case illustrates an unusual entity, lymphoid hypophysitis. This lesion is typically encountered in women who are pregnant or during the first year postpartum. Clinically, the lesion mimics a pituitary neoplasm and can produce both hypopituitarism and mass effects. The etiology of the process is uncertain but an autoimmune mechanism has been suggested. About one third of the patients have evidence of preexisting endocrine disorders. In some of the patients, other endocrine organs are similarly infiltrated by lymphoid cells.

REFERENCES

Asa SL, Bilbao JM, Kovacs K, et al: Lymphocytic hypophysitis of pregnancy resulting in hypopituitarism: A distinct clinicopathological entity. Ann Intern Med 1981; 95: 166-171.

Baskin DS, Townsend JJ, Wilson CB: Lymphocytic adenohypophysitis of pregnancy simulating a pituitary adenoma: A distinct pathological entity. J Neurosurg 1982; 56:148-153.

Meichner RH, Riggio S, Manz HJ, Earll JM: Lymphocytic adenohypophysitis causing pituitary mass. Neurology 1987; 37:158-161.

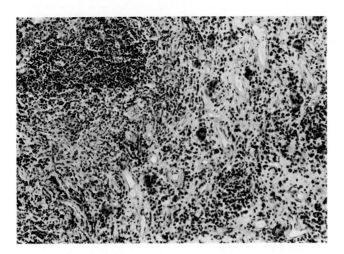

Figure 8–24A. Microscopic section showing lymphoid hypophysitis.

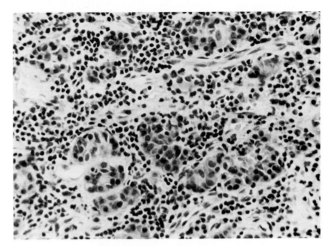

Figure 8–24B. Microscopic section at higher magnification showing the nests of adenohypophyseal cells and the interstitial mononuclear cell infiltrate.

INDEX

A68 protein, 284
Abscess
  brain, 72, 96
  causative organisms, 72, 74, 76, 96
  complications, 72
  distinction from metastasis, 324
  due to *Nocardia asteroides*, 74
  due to toxoplasmosis, 96
  epidural, 76
  predisposing factors, 72, 74
  subdural, 70
Acanthamoeba, 100
Acoustic neurinomas, 336
Acquired immune deficiency syndrome. (*See* AIDS)
Acromegaly, 374
Adenoma sebacea, 32
Adenomas
  ACTH/MSH secreting, 374
  growth hormone, 374
  null–cell, 374
  pituitary, 374
  prolactinomas, 374
Adrenoleukodystrophy, 272
Adrenomyeloneuropathy, 272
Agenesis of corpus callosum, 18, 342
  and lipomas, 342
Agenesis of olfactory bulbs, 22
Agyria, 24
AIDS
  brain abscesses in, 72, 96
  candidiasis in, 86
  cerebral lymphoma in, 344
  cryptococcal meningitis in, 84
  cytomegalovirus in, 110
  progressive multifocal
    leukoencephalopathy in, 114
  toxoplasmosis in, 96
Alcoholism, complications of, 64, 196,
    234, 238, 240

Alexander's disease, 278
ALS. *See* Amyotrophic lateral sclerosis
Alzheimer type I astrocytes, 302
Alzheimer type II astrocytes, 302
Alzheimer's disease, 284
Amebiasis
    Acanthamoeba, 100
    Naegleria, 100
Amphetamines, 148
Amyloid angiopathy, 162
  in Alzheimer's disease, 284
Amyloidosis, 162
Amyotrophic lateral sclerosis, 314
Anencephaly, 2
Aneurysm
  arteriosclerotic, 188
  berry, 180, 184
  Charcot–Bouchard, 152
  complications, 184
  infectious, 188
  "mycotic," 188
  prevalence, 180
  ruptured, 184
  saccular, 180, 184
  unruptured, 180
  vein of Galen, 172
Angiitis, granulomatous, 148
Angioma
  cavernous, 168, 174, 176
  venous, 168, 178
Angiomyolipomas, 32
Angiopathy
  amyloid, 162
  amyloid in Alzheimer's disease, 284
Anoxia
  acute effects, 226
  delayed effects, 228
Antoni type A tissue, 336
Antoni type B tissue, 336
Aphasia, 126

Apoplexy, pituitary, 374
Aqueductal stenosis, 12, 36
Area cerebrovasculosa, 2
Arnold–Chiari malformation, 12
Arnold–Chiari malformation, adult
    type, 12
Arteriovenous malformation, 168, 170,
    172
Arteritis
  cysticercosis, 98
  giant cell, 146
  granulomatous angiitis, 148
  Heubner's, 80
  luetic, 80
  polyarteritis, 148
  temporal, 146
  tuberculous, 80
Aryl sulfatase, deficiency, 268
Aspergillosis, 88
  predisposing factors, 88
  Aspergillus fumigatus, 88
Asphyxia, acute, 226
Astrocytes
  Alzheimer type I and II, 302
  in Alexander's disease, 278
  in Canavan's disease, 280
Astrocytoma
  anaplastic, 348
  cerebellar, 354
  cerebral, 352
  diencephalic, 354
  fibrillary, 352, 354
  juvenile pilocytic, 354
  pilocytic, 354
  protoplasmic, 354
  subependymal giant cell, 32
Atherosclerosis
  basilar artery, 32
  carotid artery, 120, 142
  complications, 120, 142, 188

Atherosclerosis (*cont.*)
  emboli secondary to, 142
  extracranial, 120
Atrophy
  "knife–edge," 288
  caudate in Huntington's disease, 300
  caudate in Pick's disease, 288
  cerebellar in ceroid–lipofuscinosis, 308
  cerebellar in epilepsy, 248
  cerebellar vermal, 238, 246
  in Alzheimer's disease, 284
  in ceroid–lipofuscinosis, 308
  in Creutzfeldt–Jakob disease, 292
  in Huntington's disease, 300
  in Pick's disease, 288
  lobar, 288
  neurogenic of muscle, 314
  nerve roots in amyotrophic lateral sclerosis, 314
  optic nerve, 220
  progressive sclerosing cortical, 50

B_{12} deficiency, 248
Babes nodes, 116
Balo's syndrome, 260
Basal ganglia
  in Hallervorden–Spatz disease, 302
  in Huntington's disease, 300
  in Parkinsonism, 296
  in Pick's disease, 288
  in Wilson's disease, 302
Basal nucleus of Meynert, 284, 288, 300
Blindness
  secondary to methanol intoxication, 244
  secondary to temporal arteritis, 146
Body (ies)
  Bielschowsky, 312
  Bunina, 314
  corpora amylacea, 312
  Cowdry type A inclusion, 104
  curvilinear, 308
  fingerprint, 308
  Hirano, 284
  Lafora, 312
  Lewy, 296
  Negri, 116
  Pick, 288
  polyglucosan, 312
  Verocay, 336
Border zone infarcts, 120
Brain stem necrosis, 52
Brun, pontoneocerebellar hypoplasia of, 30
"Burst lobes," 194

Canavan's disease, 280
Candida albicans, 86

Candidiasis, 86
"Candle gutterings," 32
Carbon monoxide
  acute effects, 230
  delayed effects, 232
  demyelination, 232
  pallidal necrosis, 232
Carboxyhemoglobin, 230
Carcinoma, metastatic, 324, 328
  lobar hemorrhage from, 160
Carcinomatosis, meningeal, 328
Cardiac arrest
  delayed effects, 228
  sites of injury, 228
Carotid stenosis, infarcts secondary to, 120
Carotid thrombosis, 122
Cavernous angioma, 174, 176
Cebocephaly, 22
Central pontine myelinolysis, 240, 242
Ceramide, 264
Cerebellar
  astrocytomas, 354
  atrophy, 238, 246
  hemorrhage, 38
  hypoplasia, 14, 30
  infarct, 136, 138
  sarcoma, 368
Cerebrohepatorenal syndrome, 276
Cerebrospinal fluid
  in Alzheimer's disease, 284
  in bacterial meningitis, 58, 64, 66, 68
  in candidiasis, 86
  in carcinomatous meningitis, 328
  in cryptococcal meningitis, 84
  in granulomatous angiitis, 148
  in herpes simplex encephalitis, 104, 108
  in Krabbe's disease, 264
  in leptomeningeal carcinomatosis, 328
  in multiple sclerosis, 256
  in subacute sclerosing panencephalitis, 112
  in toxoplasmosis, 94
  in tuberculosis, 80
Cerebrotendinous xanthomatosis, 276
Ceroid, 308
Ceroid–lipofuscinosis, 308
Ceruloplasmin in Wilson's disease, 302
Charcot–Bouchard aneurysm, 152
Charcot–Marie–Tooth disease, 318
Chiari I malformation, 12
Chiari II malformation, 12
Chloroma, 344
Choroid plexus papilloma, 362
Cirrhosis in Wilson's disease, 302
Colloid cysts, 364
Congophilic angiopathy, 162
Contusions, 194, 200
Copper metabolism in Wilson's disease, 302
Corpora amylacea, 312

Corpus callosum, agenesis of, 20
  and lipomas, 342
Cowdry type A inclusions, 104
Coxsackievirus infection, 102
Craniopharyngioma, 378
Creutzfeldt–Jakob disease, 292
Cryptococcal meningitis, 84
Cryptococcus neoformans, 84
Cushing's disease, 374
Cysticercosis, 98
Cyst(s)
  cerebellar, 334
  colloid, 364
  dermoid, 340
  enterogenous, 346
  epidermoid, 340
  epithelial, 346
  germinal matrix, 36
  in craniopharyngiomas, 378
  in Dandy–Walker malformation, 14
  in Zellweger's syndrome, 36, 276
  intraspinal, 346
  porencephalic, 46
  subependymal, 36
Cytomegalovirus encephalitis, 110

Dandy–Walker malformation, 14
Davidoff–Masson Syndrome. *See* Dyke–Davidoff–Masson Syndrome
Deficiency
  B_{12}, 248
  dopamine, 296
  thiamine, 236
Degeneration
  granulovacuolar, 284
  subacute combined, 248
  tract, 128
  transsynaptic of inferior olives, 38, 136
  transsynaptic of lateral geniculate, 220
  Wallerian, 128
Dejerine–Sottas disease, 318
Dementia
  Alzheimer's disease, 284
  amyotrophic lateral sclerosis, 314
  ceroid–lipofuscinosis, 308
  Creutzfeldt–Jakob disease, 292
  dysphasic, 288
  Huntington's disease, 300
  Lafora's disease, 312
  multi–infarct, 284
  neurotransmitters in, 284, 288
  Parkinson's disease, 296
  Pick's disease, 288
  senile, 284
Demyelination
  acute disseminated encephalomyelitis, 262
  acute hemorrhagic encephalomyelitis, 262

Demyelination (*cont.*)
  adrenoleukodystrophy, 272
  Alexander's disease, 278
  anoxia, 228
  B$_{12}$ deficiency, 248
  Balo's syndrome, 260
  Canavan's disease, 280
  carbon monoxide intoxication, 232
  central pontine myelinolysis, 240, 242
  Devic's syndrome, 260
  histotoxic, 232
  hyperosmolality, 242
  hyponatremia, 242
  Krabbe's disease, 264
  leukodystrophy, 264, 268, 272, 278, 280
  Lichtheim plaques, 248
  methotrexate radiation, 250
  multiple sclerosis, 256, 260
  neuromyelitis optica, 260
  Pelizaeus–Merzbacher's disease, 280
  postinfectious encephalomyelitis, 262
  progressive multifocal leukoencephalopathy, 114
  radiation, 252
  segmental in Charcot–Marie–Tooth disease, 318
  Seitelberger's disease, 280
  subacute sclerosing panencephalitis, 112
  tigeroid, 280
Dermoids, 340
Devic's syndrome, 260
Diffuse axonal injury (DAI), 206, 210
Diffuse brain injury, 206
Disease
  "adult polyglucosan body," 312
  Alexander's, 278
  Alzheimer's, 284
  Batten–Vogt, 308
  Canavan's, 280
  Charcot–Marie–Tooth, 318
  Creutzfeldt–Jakob, 292
  Cushing's, 374
  Dejerine–Sottas, 318
  familial myoclonus epilepsy, 312
  Hallervorden–Spatz, 302
  Haltia–Santavuori, 308
  Huntington's, 300
  Janksy–Bielschowsky, 308
  Krabbe's, 264
  Kufs', 308
  Lafora's, 312
  Leigh's, 306
  Parkinson's, 296
  Pelizaeus–Merzbacher, 280
  Pick's, 288
  Seitelberger's, 280
  Spielmeyer–Sjogren, 308
  von Recklinghausen's, 336
  Wilson's, 302
Dissection, vertebral artery, 212

Dolichols in ceroid–lipofuscinosis, 308
Down's syndrome
  and Alzheimer's disease, 28, 284
  trisomy 21 in, 28
Dyke–Davidoff–Masson syndrome, 50
Dysphasic dementia, 288
Dystrophy, axonal in Hallervorden–Spatz disease, 302

Edema
  intramyelinic, 280
  in brain abscesses, 72
  in cerebral infarcts, 122
  in meningitis, 64
Emboli
  atheromatous, 142
  bone marrow, 144
  cardiogenic, 138
  fat, 144
  mucin, 144
  nonthrombotic, 142, 144
  tumor, 144
Embolism. *See* Emboli
Empyema, subdural, 70
Encephalitis
  amebic, 100
  coxsackievirus, 102
  cytomegalovirus, 110
  herpes simplex, 104, 108
  progressive multifocal leukoencephalopathy, 114
  rabies, 116
  subacute sclerosing (pan–), 112
  viral, 102, 104, 108, 112, 114, 116
Encephalocele, 6
Encephalomyelitis
  acute disseminated, 262
  acute hemorrhagic, 262
  postinfectious, 262
  post–measles, 262
Encephalomyelopathy, subacute necrotizing, 306
Encephalomyocarditis, coxsackie virus, 102
Encephalopathy
  anoxic, 238
  disseminated necrotizing, 250
  methotrexate radiation, 250
  multicystic, 42
  spongiform, 292
  subacute, 250
  Wernicke's, 234, 236
Endocarditis
  and intracerebral hemorrhage, 140
  and mycotic aneurysm, 188
Enterogenous cysts, 346
Ependymoma
  cerebral, 356, 362
  myxopapillary, 358
  spinal, 358
  subependymoma, 362
Epidermoids, 340

Epidural abscess, 76
Epidural hematoma, 192
Epilepsy
  complications, 198, 246
  death from, 246
  familial myoclonus, 312
  gangliogliomas and, 370
Epithelial cysts, 346
Erdeim's rests, 378
Escherichia coli, 58
Etat crible, 150
Etat lacunaire, 150
Ethylene glycol intoxication, 244

Familial myoclonus epilepsy. *See* Lafora's disease
Fascia dentata, in Pick's disease, 288
Fibers, Rosenthal, 278, 354
Fibromas
  periungual, 32
  subungual, 32
Filum terminale, 10

Galactocerebroside, 264
Gangliogliomas, 370
Genu of Wilbrand, 220
Germinal matrix, 34
Germinoma, 372
Gerstmann–Straussler syndrome, 292
Giant cell arteritis, 146
Glioblastoma multiforme, 348
  from pontine glioma, 352
  giant cell, 348
Gliomas, pontine, 352
Gliosarcoma, 348
Globoid cells, 264
Globus pallidus
  in carbon monoxide poisoning, 232
  in Hallervorden–Spatz disease, 302
Glycogenosis, type IV, 312
Granulocytic sarcoma, 344
Granulomatosis infantiseptica, 60
Granulomatous angiitis, 148
Granulovacuolar degeneration, 284
Growth hormone, 374
Guamanian amyotrophic lateral sclerosis, 314
Guillain–Mollaret triangle, 38, 136
Gunshot wounds, 214

Hallervorden–Spatz disease, 302
Haltia–Santavuori disease, 308
Hemangioblastomas, 334
Hemangiopericytomas, meningeal, 330
Hematoidin, 154
Hematoma
  acute subdural, 194
  cerebellar, 158

Hematoma (*cont.*)
  chronic subdural, 196
  epidural, 192
  intracerebral, 152, 154, 160, 168, 170
  subdural, 194, 196
Hemiatrophy, cerebral, 50
Hemophilus influenzae, 62
Hemorrhage
  cerebellar, 38, 158
  Duret, 206
  from amyloid angiopathy, 160
  from choroid plexus, 34
  from oligodendrogliomas, 366
  from pituitary adenomas, 374
  ganglionic, 152
  germinal matrix, 34, 36
  hypertensive, 152, 154, 156, 158
  intraventricular, 34
  lobar, 160, 162
  pontine, 156
  secondary brain stem, 206
  secondary to amyloid angiopathy, 162
  secondary to arteriovenous malformation 168, 170
  secondary to cavernous angioma, 174, 176
  secondary to emboli, 140
  secondary to leukemia, 160
  secondary to metastases, 160
  secondary to ruptured aneurysm, 184
  secondary to thrombocytopenia, 160
  secondary to venous thrombosis, 164, 166
  Staemmler's marginal, 152
  subarachnoid, 34, 168, 184, 200
  subependymal, 34, 36
  thalamic, 154
  traumatic, 192, 194, 200, 206
Hemosiderin, 154
Herniation
  cingulate gyrus, 196
  tonsillar, chronic, 12
  uncal, 196
Herpes simplex encephalitis
  adult infection, 104
  neonatal infection, 108
Herpes simplex type I, 104
Herpes simplex type II, 108
Herpes zoster and granulomatous angiitis, 148
Heubner's endarteritis, 80
Hippocampal sclerosis in epilepsy, 246
Hirano bodies, 284
Hirsch–Peiffer stain, 268
Histoplasma capsulatum, 92
Histoplasmoma, 92
Histoplasmosis, 92
Holoprosencephaly, 22
Homer Wright rosettes, 368
Huntington's disease, 300

Huntington's disease, neurotransmitters in, 300
Hydranencephaly, 44
Hydrocephalus, 12, 14, 36
  secondary to aqueductal stenosis, 36
  secondary to Arnold–Chiari malformation, 12
  secondary to choroid plexus papilloma, 362
  secondary to colloid cyst, 364
  secondary to Dandy–Walker malformation, 14
  secondary to ependymoma, 356
  secondary to germinal matrix hemorrhage, 36
  secondary to subependymal hemorrhage, 36
Hydromyelia, 16, 18
Hyperosmolality, complications of, 242
Hypertension, hemorrhage from, 152, 154, 156, 158
Hyponatremia, complications, 238, 240, 242
Hypoplasia, cerebellar, 14, 30
Hypotension, border zone infarcts from, 120
Hypophysitis, lymphoid, 380
Hypoxia, 226

Inclusion body (ies)
  Cowdry type A, 104
  cytoplasmic, 110, 116, 288, 296, 312, 314
  intranuclear, 104, 108, 110, 112, 114
  Lafora, 312
  Negri, 116
Infarct(s)
  acute, 122, 124, 138
  and atrial fibrillation, 138
  and endocarditis, 140
  border zone, 120
  brain stem, 130, 132
  cardiogenic, 138, 140
  cerebellar, 134, 136
  embolic, 120, 136, 138, 140, 142, 144
  hemorrhagic, 136, 138, 140
  inferior cerebellar, 134
  lacunar, 150, 152
  lateral medullary, 132
  middle cerebral, 122, 124, 126, 128
  neonatal, 54
  perinatal white matter, 40
  pontine, 130
  remote 126, 128, 132, 134
  secondary to carotid thrombosis, 122, 124
  secondary to ruptured aneurysm, 184
  secondary to vasculitis, 80, 148
  superior cerebellar, 136

Iniencephaly, 4
Injury
  diffuse axonal, 206, 210
  diffuse brain, 206
Intoxication
  carbon monoxide, 230, 232
  ethylene glycol, 244
  methanol, 244
  methotrexate, 252
  MPTP, 296
  phenytoin, 246
  Vinca alkaloids, 250
  vincristine, 250
Iron metabolism in Hallervorden–Spatz disease, 302

Jakob–Creutzfeldt disease. *See* Creutzfeldt–Jakob disease
Janksy–Bielschowsky disease, 308
JC virus, 114

Kayser–Fleischer ring, 302
Krabbe's disease, 264
Kufs' disease, 308
Kuru plaques, 292

Laceration
  ponto–medullary, 204
  vertebral atery, 212
Lacunes, 150, 154
Lafora
  body, 312
  disease, 312
Laminar necrosis, 228
Lateral medullary infarct, 132
Leigh's disease, 306
Leukodystrophy
  adrenoleukodystrophy, 272
  Alexander's disease, 278
  Canavan's disease, 280
  definition, 264
  globoid cell, 264
  Krabbe's disease, 264
  metachromatic, 268
  Pelizaeus–Merzbacher disease, 280
  Seitelberger's disease, 280
  Zellweger's syndrome, 276
Leukoencephalopathy, progressive multifocal, 114
Leukomalacia, periventricular, 40
Lewy bodies, 296
Lhermitte's sign, 256
Lichtheim plaques, 248
Lipofuscin, 304, 308
Lipohyalinosis, 150, 152
Lipomas, 342
Lipomeningocele, 10

Lipopigments in
    ceroid–lipofuscinosis, 308
Lissencephaly, 24
Listeria monocytogenes, 60
Locus caeruleus in Parkinson's
    disease, 296
Lymphomas, 344

M–protein, 112
Malaria, 100
Malformations
    agenesis of corpus callosum, 20
    agenesis of olfactory bulbs, 22
    anencephaly, 2
    Arnold–Chiari, 12
    arteriovenous, 168, 170, 172
    cerebellar hypoplasia, 30
    Chiari I, 12
    Chiari II, 12
    Dandy–Walker, 14
    Down's syndrome, 28
    encephaloceles, 6
    holoprosencephaly, 22
    iniencephaly, 4
    lipomeningocele, 10
    meningocele, 8
    meningomyelocele, 12
    myelomeningocele, 12
    neocerebellar hypoplasia, 30
    pachygyria, 24
    polymicrogyria, 26
    schizencephaly, 46
    tuberous sclerosis, 32
    vascular, 168, 170, 172, 174, 176, 178
    vein of Galen aneurysm, 172
    Zellweger's syndrome, 36, 276
Mammillary bodies
    in Leigh's disease, 306
    in Wernicke's encephalopathy, 234,
        236
Medulloblastoma, 368
Megalencephaly, 278
Melanoma, metastatic, 324
Meningiomas, 330
Meningitis
    adult, 60, 62, 64, 66, 68, 80
    appearance of exudate, 58, 66, 68,
        80, 84
    aseptic, 102, 104, 108
    carcinomatous, 328
    childhood, 62, 64, 80
    chronic, 80, 84
    complications, 58, 62, 64, 66, 80, 166
    cryptococcal, 84
    Escherichia coli, 58
    Group B streptococcal, 58
    Hemophilus influenzae, 62
    Listeria monocytogenes, 60
    meningococcal, 68
    neonatal, 58, 60
    pneumoccal, 64, 66
    predisposing factors, 58, 64, 68, 80

Meningitis *(cont.)*
    sarcoid, 82
    Streptococcus pneumoniae, 64
    tuberculous, 78, 80
    viral, 102, 104, 106
Meningocele
    cervical, 8
    lipomeningocele, 10
    lumbosacral, 8
Meningococcemia, 68
Meningomyelocele, 12
Mesial sclerosis, 246
Metabolism
    B$_{12}$, 244
    carbohydrate in Leigh's disease, 306
    carbohydrate in Wernicke's
        encephalopathy, 236
    copper in Wilson's disease, 302
    cysteine in Hallervorden–Spatz
        disease, 304
    fatty acid in adrenoleukodystrophy,
        272, 276
    iron in Hallervorden–Spatz disease,
        302
    lipopigment in
        ceroid–lipofuscinosis, 308
    thiamine, 236, 306
Metachromatic leukodystrophy, 268
Metastases
    cerebellar, 324
    cerebral, 324
    hemorrhagic, 160
    meningeal, 328
    skull, 324
    sources of, 324
    spinal, 324
Metastases from
    choroid plexus papilloma, 362
    glioblastoma multiforme, 348
    medulloblastomas, 368
    meningiomas, 330
    pituitary adenomas, 374
Methanol intoxication, 244
Methotrexate, 250
Methotrexate radiation
    encephalopathy, 250
Meynert, basal nucleus of, 284, 288,
    296, 300
Mitochondria, in Canavan's disease, 280
MPTP, 296
Mucormycosis, 90
Multicystic encephalopathy, 42
Multiple sclerosis, 256, 260
    active plaques, 256
    asymptomatic, 260
    cerebrospinal fluid, 256
    diagnosis, 256
    inactive plaques, 256
    late onset, 260
    peripheral nerves, 260
    periventricular plaques, 256, 260
Multiple sulfatase deficiencies,
Mycobacterium tuberculosis, 78, 80
Mycotic aneurysm, 186

Myelinolysis, central pontine, 240, 242
Myelinopathy, Grinker's 232
Myeloma, 344
Myelomalacia, traumatic, 216, 218
Myelomeningocele, 12
Myelopathy
    B$_{12}$, 248
    vacuolar, 248
Myoclonus, palatal, 136
Myxopapillary ependymoma, 358
Myxoviruses, 112

Naegleria fowleri, 100
Necrosis
    basal ganglia, 228, 232, 244, 302
    cortical, 228
    from methotrexate–radiation, 250
    hippocampal, 228
    hypotensive brain stem, 52
    pallidal, 228, 232
    pontosubicular, 52
    Purkinje cell, 228
    putamenal
        in Wilson's disease, 302
        in methanol intoxication, 244
    radiation, 252
Negri bodies, 116
Neisseria meningitidis, 68
Neocerebellar hypoplasia, 30
Neonatal infarct, 54
Neoplasms
    acoustic neurinomas, 336
    ACTH–MSH adenomas, 374
    anaplastic astrocytoma, 348
    astrocytomas, 32, 352, 354
    cerebellar astrocytomas, 358
    cerebellar sarcoma, 368
    cerebellopontine angle, 336
    childhood, 354, 356, 362, 368, 370,
        372, 378
    chloroma, 344
    choroid plexus papilloma, 362
    colloid cysts, 364
    craniopharyngioma, 378
    dermoid, 340
    diencephalic astrocytoma, 354
    ependymomas, 356, 358
    epidermoid, 340
    ganglogliomas, 370
    germinomas, 372
    glioblastoma multiforme, 348
    gliosarcoma, 348
    granulocytic sarcoma, 344
    hemangioblastomas, 334
    hemangiopericytoma of meninges,
        330
    juvenile pilocytic astrocytoma, 354
    leptomeningeal carcinomatosis, 328
    lipomas, 342
    lymphomas, 344
    medulloblastomas, 368
    meningioma, 330

Neoplasms (*cont.*)
metastatic, 324, 328
myeloma, 344
myxopapillary ependymoma, 358
neurilemmomas, 336
neurofibromas, 336
null–cell adenomas, 374
oligodendrogliomas, 366
optic nerve gliomas, 354
pineal, 372
pineoblastoma, 372
pineocytoma, 372
pituitary adenomas, 374
polar spongioblastoma, 368
pontine gliomas, 352
primitive neuroectodermal, 368, 372
prolactinomas, 374
Schwann cell, 336
schwannomas, 336
skull, 340
spinal, 330, 358
spongioblastomas, 354
skull, 340
spinal, 330, 358
spongioblastomas, 354
subependymal giant cell
astrocytoma, 32
subependymoma, 360
Nerves, in leptomeningeal
carcinomatosis, 328
Neurilemmomas, 336
Neurinomas, acoustic, 336
Neurofibrillary tangle, 284
globose, 296
in Steele–Richardson–Olszewski
syndrome, 296
ultrastructure, 284, 296
Neurofibromas, 336
Neurogenic pulmonary edema, 246
Neuromyelitis optica, 260
Neuronal ceroid–lipofuscinosis. (*See*
Ceroid–lipofuscinosis)
Neuropathy (ies)
B_{12} deficiency, 248
Charcot–Marie–Tooth, 318
Dejerine–Sottas, 318
hereditary, 318
hereditary sensory, 318
hypertrophic, 318
myeloma, 344
polyarteritis, 148
Neurosarcoidosis, 82
Neurosyphilis, 80
Neurotransmitters
in Alzheimer's disease, 284
in Huntington's disease, 300
in Parkinsonism, 296
in Pick's disease, 288
Nocardia asteroides, 74
Nocardiosis, 74
Nucleus basalis. See Meynert, basal
nucleus of
Null–cell adenomas, 374

Olfactory bulbs, agenesis, 22
Oligodendrogliomas, 366
Olivary hypertrophy, 136
Olivary nuclei, malformations of, 14,
24
Olive, transsynaptic degeneration of,
38, 136
"Onion–bulb" formations, 318
Opalski cell(s), 302
Opportunistic infections
abscess, 72, 74, 96
Acanthamoeba, 100
aspergillosis, 88
candidiasis, 86
cryptococcosis, 84
cytomegalovirus, 110
histoplasmosis, 92
mucormycosis, 90
nocardiosis, 74
progressive multifocal
leukoencephalopathy, 114
toxoplasmosis, 96
Optic nerve
atrophy, 220
gliomas, 300
in anencephaly, 2
in B_{12} deficiency, 248
in Leigh's disease, 306
in methanol intoxication, 244
in multiple sclerosis, 260
in temporal arteritis, 146
Optic neuritis, 256
Oxalic acid, from ethylene glycol, 244

Pachygyria, 24
Paired helical filaments, 284
Pallidal necrosis, 230
Pallidum in Hallervorden–Spatz
disease, 302
Palsy, progressive supranuclear, 296
Panencephalitis, subacute sclerosing,
112
Papilloma, choroid plexus, 362
Papovavirus, 114
Paragonimiasis, 100
Paraphysis, 364
Parkinson's disease, 296
Parkinsonism, 296
Pelizaeus–Merzbacher's disease, 280
Perinatal injuries
brain stem necrosis, 52
cerebellar hemorrhage, 38
cerebral hemiatrophy, 50
Dyke–Davidoff–Masson, 50
germinal matrix hemorrhages, 34,
36
hydranencephaly, 44
hypotensive brain stem necrosis, 52
infarct, cerebral, 54
infarcts of white matter, 40
mesial sclerosis, 246
multicystic encephalopathy, 42

Perinatal injuries (*cont.*)
neonatal infarct, 52
periventricular leukomalacia, 40
porencephaly, 46
subependymal hemorrhages, 34, 36
ulegyria, 48
Peripheral nerve
in adrenoleukodystrophy, 272
in Charcot–Marie–Tooth disease,
318
in Dejerine–Sottas disease, 318
in hereditary sensory neuropathy,
318
in Krabbe's disease, 264
in metachromatic leukodystrophy,
268
in multiple sclerosis, 260
in Seitelberger's disease, 280
Periventricular leukomalacia, 40
Peroxisomes, disorders of, 272, 276
Pick body (ies), 288
Pick cells, 288
Pick's disease, 288
Pigment metabolism in
ceroid–lipofuscinosis, 308
Pinealomas, 372
Pineoblastoma, 372
Pineocytoma, 372
Pituitary
adenomas, 374
apoplexy, 374
craniopharyngioma, 378
lymphoid hypophysitis, 380
Plaque(s)
amyloid in Alzheimer's disease, 284
amyloid in Creutzfeldt'Jakob
disease, 292
amyloid in Gerstmann–Straussler
syndrome, 292
"kuru", 292
Lichtheim, 248
multiple sclerosis, 256, 260
senile, 284
PML. *See* Progressive multifocal
leukoencephalopathy
Pneumococcal meningitis, 64, 66
Polar spongioblastoma, 368
Poliomyelitis, 102
Polyarteritis, 148
Polyglucosan deposits, 312
Polyhydramnios, 2, 4
Polymicrogyria, 26
Pontine gliomas, 352
Ponto–medullary laceration, 204
Porencephaly, 46
Postinfectious encephalomyelitis,
262
Primitive neuroectodermal tumors,
368, 372
Prions, 292
Probst's bundle, 20
Progressive multifocal
leukoencephalopathy, 114
Progressive supranuclear palsy, 296

Prolactinomas, 374
Pseudorosettes, 354, 356, 358
Psychosine, 264
Psychosurgery, 220
Pyruvate dehydrogenase in Leigh's disease, 306

Rabies, 116
Radiation necrosis, 252
Radiation, proton beam, 170
Rathke's pouch, 378
Refsum's disease, 276
Rhabdomyomas, 32
Rhinocerebral mucormycosis, 90
Rhombencephalitis due to *Listeria monocytogenes*, 60
Riley–Day syndrome, 318
Rosenthal fibers, 278, 354
Rosettes
    Homer Wright, 368
    perivascular, 356
    pseudorosettes, 354, 356, 358

Sarcoidosis, 82
Satellitosis, neoplastic perineuronal, 366
Schizencephaly, 46
Schwannomas, 336
Sclerosis
    amyotrophic lateral, 314
    cerebellar, 238, 246
    hippocampal, 246
    mesial, 246
    multiple, 256, 260
    tuberous, 32
Secondary structuring, 366
Seitelberger's disease, 280
Selective vulnerability, 228
Senile plaques, 284
Shagreen patches, 32
Simchowicz, granulovacuolar degeneration of, 284
Sinus thrombosis, 66, 166
Spielmeyer–Sjogren's disease, 308
Spina bifida
    and dermoids, 340
    and lipomas, 342
Spinal dysraphia, 8, 12
Spongioblastomas, 354, 368
Spongiform encephalopathy, 292
Stain(s)
    alcian blue, 84
    Bodian silver, 284, 288
    Congo red, 162
    for amyloid, 162, 284
    for copper, 302
    for fat, 144
    for iron, 304
    for mucin, 144
    for mucopolysaccharides, 84

Stain(s) *(cont.)*
    for neurofibrillary tangles, 284, 288
Hirsch–Peiffer, 268
immunoperoxidase
    for factor VIII, 334
    for glial fibrillary acidic protein, 278, 332
    for neuron specific enolase, 32
    for pituitary tumors, 374
    metachromatic, 268
    methenamine silver, 84, 86, 88/
    mucicarmine, 84, 144
    oil–red–O, 144
    periodic acid–Schiff, 84, 86, 88, 266, 270, 304, 308, 312
    Prussian blue, 302
Status cribrosus, 150
Status lacunarus, 150
Status spongiosus in Creutzfeldt–Jakob disease, 292
Steele–Richardson–Olszewski syndrome, 296
Stenogyria, 12, 26
Streptococci, Group B, 58
Sturge–Weber syndrome, 178
Subacute combined degeneration, 248
Subacute necrotizing encephalomyelopathy. *See* Leigh's disease
Subacute sclerosing panencephalitis, 112
Subarachnoid hemorrhage, 168, 184, 200
Subdural effusions, 62
Subdural empyema, 70
    Causative organisms, 70
Subdural hematoma, 194, 196
Subependymal giant cell astrocytoma, 32
Subependymomas, 360
Substantia nigra
    in ceroid–lipofuscinosis, 308
    in Lafora's disease, 312
    in Leigh's disease, 306
    in Parkinson's disease, 296
    in progressive supranuclear palsy, 296
Sulfatide lipidosis, 268
Syndrome(s)
    Balo's, 260
    Batten–Vogt, 308
    cerebrohepatorenal, 276
    Davidoff–Dyke, 50
    Devic's, 260
    Down's 28
    Dyke–Davidoff–Masson, 50
    Gerstmann,–Straussler, 292
    Guamanian parkinsonism dementia, 296
    Leigh's 306
    Riley–Day, 318
    Steele–Richardson–Olszewski, 296
    Sturge–Weber, 178

Syndrome(s) *(cont.)*
    von Hippel–Lindau, 334
    Wallenberg, 132
    Waterhouse–Friderichsen, 68
    Zellweger's, 36, 276
Syphilis, meningovascular, 80
Syringomyelia, 16
    associated hydrocephalus, 16
    post–traumatic, 16, 218
    secondary to ependymoma, 358
Syrinx, 16

Taenia solium, 98
Tangle, neurofibrillary
    in Alzheimer's disease, 284, 296
    in amyotrophic lateral sclerosis, 314
    in progressive supranuclear palsy, 296
Tanycytes, 354
Tau protein, 288
Telangiectases, 168, 178
Temporal arteritis, 146
Tethered cord, 10
Thalamotomies, 220
Thiamine
    deficiency, 236
    metabolism in Leigh's disease, 306
Thrombosis
    basilar artery, 130
    carotid artery, 120, 122
    congenital heart disease, 164
    cortical vein, 164, 166
    middle cerebral artery, 122, 124
    posterior inferior cerebellar artery, 132
    sagittal sinus, 164
    venous, 66, 166
    vertebral artery, 132, 134
Toxocara canis, 100
Toxoplasma gondii, 94
Toxoplasmosis, 94, 96
Transsynaptic degeneration
    in inferior olivary nuclei, 38, 136
    in lateral geniculate bodies, 220
Trauma
    "burst lobe," 194
    contusions, 200
    coup and contrecoup lesions, 200
    diffuse axonal injury, 206, 210
    diffuse brain injury, 206
    epidural hematoma, 192
    fracture–dislocation, 216
    gunshot wound, 214
    myelomalacia, 216, 218
    ponto–medullary laceration, 204
    psychosurgery, 220
    spinal, 216, 218
    spinal birth, 216
    subdural hematoma, 194, 196
    surgical, 220
    syringomyelia, 218
    vascular injury, 212

Trauma (*cont.*)
  vertebral artery dissection, 212
Triangle, Guillain–Mollaret, 38, 136
Trisomy 13
  Dandy–Walker malformation, 14
  holoprosencephaly in, 22
Trisomy 21, 28
Tuberculomas, 80
Tuberculous meningitis, 78, 80
Tuberous sclerosis, 32
Tumor(s). *See* Neoplasms
Tumors, Koenen, 32

Ulegyria, 26, 48

Vasculitis
  granulomatous angiitis, 148
  polyarteritis, 148
  secondary to amphetamines, 148
  secondary to infections, 80, 148
  temporal arteritis, 146
  ulcerative colitis, 148
Vein of Galen, 172
Venous thrombosis, 58, 66, 164, 166
  secondary to congenital heart
    disease, 164
  secondary to meningitis, 58, 66,
    166
Visceral larva migrans, 100
von Hippel–Lindau syndrome, 334

von Recklinghausen's disease, 338

Wallenberg's syndrome, 132
Waterhouse–Friderichsen syndrome,
  68
Wernicke's encephalopathy, 234,
  236
Wilbrand, genu of, 220
Wilson's disease, 302
Wounds, gunshot, 214

Zellweger's syndrome, 36, 276